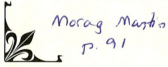

Women, Gender and Disease in Eighteenth-Century England and France

Women, Gender and Disease in Eighteenth-Century England and France

Edited by

Kathleen Hardesty Doig
and Felicia Berger Sturzer

CAMBRIDGE
SCHOLARS
PUBLISHING

Women, Gender and Disease in Eighteenth-Century England and France,
Edited by Kathleen Hardesty Doig and Felicia Berger Sturzer

This book first published 2014

Cambridge Scholars Publishing

12 Back Chapman Street, Newcastle upon Tyne, NE6 2XX, UK

British Library Cataloguing in Publication Data
A catalogue record for this book is available from the British Library

ISBN (10): 1-4438-5551-0, ISBN (13): 978-1-4438-5551-8

For our families:
Ned, Sonia and Paul
Jim, Margaret and Steve

TABLE OF CONTENTS

ACKNOWLEDGEMENTS

We are grateful to our colleagues Elaine Breslaw, Elizabeth Furdell, and Samia Spencer for their careful reading of our manuscript. Their suggestions on style and form were particularly helpful. We also wish to thank Deb Loden, Dijan Milakovic and Janelle Hamilton for technical help in producing the manuscript. Above all, we wish to thank our colleagues who contributed to this collection. Without them this book would not be possible. The patience and good humor they exhibited in response to our numerous questions are especially appreciated!

A few comments regarding editorial decisions are in order. In all cases, we respect the punctuation and spelling in quotes from original sources. The wishes of the author were also respected in cases of names or words with alternate spellings, including British conventions. Accents were added where necessary for comprehension. Capitalization in titles was changed only when necessary. Since the essay by Felicia Berger Sturzer is a reprint, no changes were made other than in style of references and in some cases, punctuation.

INTRODUCTION

FELICIA BERGER STURZER

This collection of essays focuses on the intersection of women, gender, and disease in England and France during the eighteenth and the beginning of the nineteenth centuries. The essays represent diverse critical perspectives on women's participation in the scientific and medical communities of the period, spaces that were dominated by men. Referencing encyclopedias, medical journals, historical, literary, and non-literary sources, the authors address the role of women within the medical establishment and the perception and treatment of diseases specific to women. They demonstrate that in spite of the obstacles they encountered, women made significant contributions to health care and scientific knowledge.

During the course of the eighteenth century, a philosophical shift occurred that placed greater emphasis on empirical analysis and envisioned a "science of man" informed by biomedical conjecture. During the Enlightenment, medical explanations of the female body and how it differed from that of males, the physical and emotional health of women, their medical care and contributions as caregivers within a broader socio-economic context became increasingly important as the focus of scientific, literary, and philosophical texts.[1]

When discussing sex and gender in the eighteenth century, we must do so with caution and the understanding that boundaries between disciplines and social categories were in a state of flux. While it is problematic to use the concept of "gender" and its post-modern meaning when referring to Enlightenment perspectives on sexual difference, a preoccupation with all aspects of sexuality was pervasive during the period. Sexuality and gender became significant topics of discussion within the broader context of a body of knowledge rooted in the fields of anatomy and physiology. While "there was a growing scientific literature during the eighteenth century on the nature of woman," such inquiry did not adequately account for women and sexual difference.[2] Eighteenth-century concepts of masculinity and femininity are difficult to assess, since such binary oppositions were only used by writers "to bring social differences to the fore" or "to consider a particular form of social organization" that invariably relegated women to the private sphere of domesticity.[3] Even though the majority of women were indeed denied a voice in the public sphere, as evidenced by the medical and scientific communities that excluded them, many women became well-known midwives, and some wrote self-help manuals on women's health, domestic economy, and general hygiene. They were able to make significant scientific contributions as anatomists, botanists, herbalists, and public health advocates, all without any formal university training.

What defines a woman? This seemingly simple question has been the subject of debate from antiquity into the twenty-first century. Essays by Sean Quinlan, Mary McAlpin, and Kathleen Doig provide a context to help us address the "woman question."

Quinlan's essay focuses on "the natural history of woman" as conceived in the late eighteenth and early nineteenth centuries. This topic, "unique to French sciences and letters—no exact corollary exists in English, German, or Italian," is the subject of numerous "medico-scientific" books (p. 16). Quinlan discusses writers whose works incorporated contemporary scientific discourse into an analysis of women's minds and bodies. Rather than cures for diseases, they raised issues relevant to the discussion of sex and gender. Patriarchal authority, the status of women, and their relationship to the public and private spheres were debated by physicians and intellectuals who "believed that women's status was the greatest public issue of the day, and they hoped to shape general social thought" (p. 17). Pierre Cabanis, Jean-François de Saint-Lambert, Jacques-Louis Moreau de la Sarthe, Jules-Joseph Virey, Gabriel Jouard, and Louis-Victor Bénech contributed to these exchanges. Sex and gender were important topics, attracting the interest of a general public as well as the medical and scientific communities. Influenced by theories of a "science of man," "natural history," and the philosophy of the Montpellier medical school, these

> doctors tried to explain how vital properties manifested themselves across the diverse stages and conditions of human life: age, environment, occupation, temperament, race, and sexuality (p. 21).

Quinlan notes that while women were viewed as biologically determined to be wives and mothers, roles essential to the cohesiveness of society, they were also regarded as agents of moral degeneracy among the bourgeoisie and aristocracy—thus contributing to the fall of the Ancien Régime! Although familiar, these claims were more "speculative" and philosophical in nature, relying on medical facts to support their assertions. The author argues that "these doctors and moralists likely expressed their own private agendas beyond surface politics or ideology" to gain public attention (p. 37). He concludes that

> biomedical science [...] promised that progressive change and melioration *were* possible, even if human improvement was limited by technical skill and natural realities (p. 39).

Debates on women, sex, and gender were important components of these changes.

The perfectibility of "man," the search for happiness, and the progress of civilization framed Enlightenment ideology in France. Progress, however, was also linked to the decline of French civilization. Women, "*languissantes* and *débiles*," were perceived as largely responsible for this state of affairs. How could they be "cured" to save the nation? Mary McAlpin seeks answers to this question by tracing the history of the role women played in this process (p. 45). Using literary and non-literary sources, she explores

> the *longue durée* of this history of decline from the point of view of the ideal from which eighteenth-century French women are said to have degenerated (p. 46).

Medical treatises by physicians such as Théophile de Bordeu, Joseph Raulin, Jacques Ballexserd, P. Virard and J.D.T. Bienville, maintained that women differed from men, both physically and mentally, and were therefore more easily corrupted by civilization. Such female diseases as *fleurs blanches* (leucorrhaea) and nymphomania, linked to the lifestyles of women in advanced civilizations, could be potentially controlled through better hygiene. Basing her analysis on Antoine Léonard Thomas's *Essai sur le caractère, les moeurs et l'esprit des femmes dans les différens siècles*, McAlpin traces the sources for women's moral and physical decline in advanced civilizations. While works focusing on women continued to be published throughout the eighteenth century, after the Revolution interest in women's hygiene and health issues waned as women were no longer the focus of medical discourse.

Turning to literary sources, McAlpin points to Françoise de Graffigny's *Lettres d'une Péruvienne* and Nicolas Chamfort's *La Jeune Indienne* as examples of novels in which heroines from another culture are physically and mentally strong, in contrast to aristocratic French women. She concludes that when leaders of the Revolution determined "that woman's place was in the home, raising the perfected *citoyens* of the future," it marked "a radical turn in the French cultural imagination" (p. 62). Only within the domestic sphere could women contribute to the progress of society for future generations.

Kathleen H. Doig's essay discusses certain medical articles in the *Encyclopédie méthodique* (1782-1832) that focus on women. This work, a revision and modernization of Diderot's earlier *Encyclopédie*, incorporates the influence of a new, more empirical and scientific approach to the diagnosis and treatment of disease. The volumes on *Médecine* document these advances, and include such diverse topics as "personal and public health; pathology; semiotics and nosology; therapeutic medicine; military medicine" and "veterinary medicine" (p. 68). The subjects that primarily affect women were mostly written by the physician Nicolas Chambon de Montaux. His articles provide an important historical source for medical practice and scientific thinking during the eighteenth and early nineteenth centuries.

At the intersection of the old order and modernity, Chambon was influenced by contemporary knowledge of anatomy and physiology, the older "humoralist theory" of bodily fluids, and the vitalist theories of the Montpellier school. Using observation, evaluation, physical exams, clinical data, and documentation of case histories, he could more accurately evaluate and treat illnesses that affected women, such as hysteria, chlorosis, and "fleurs blanches." As a proponent of better training for midwives and physicians, he incorporated the social dimensions of women's health care and childbirth into the medical discourses of the period. Within a broader philosophic context, he discussed such controversial issues as female sexual desire versus social and moral restraints, and the relative importance of the mother's life as opposed to that of the fetus. From our contemporary perspective, the latter anticipates underlying issues in the abortion debate. The documentation of case histories adds a human dimension to the medical discourse of his entries.

Doig concludes that medical practice at the turn of the nineteenth century had a life of its own and was "open to new methods, marked by discoveries and successes thanks to the empirical spirit that was now valued, and practiced by physicians like Chambon" who shared their knowledge with their colleagues and "readers of encyclopedias" (p. 84).

Women with scientific aspirations experienced hostility both from the medical establishment and cultural norms that relegated them to the private sphere. Nevertheless, the essays by Morag Martin, Valérie Lastinger, and Patsy S. Fowler highlight the contributions of women as healers, researchers, and teachers in the fields of anatomy, domestic economy, and hygiene.

Morag Martin's essay documents the case of Augustine Debaralle, an "unofficial healer" in the latter part of the eighteenth century and the Empire. Against a background of discrimination, complex and conflicting laws regulating the practice of medicine, the advertising and selling of medical "recipes," and the publication of scientific tracts, Debaralle demanded acceptance by scientific and medical communities monopolized by men. Marginalized and stigmatized as a crazy charlatan, her physical and mental health, along with her professional reputation, suffered. An intelligent, aggressive self-promoter, she was ultimately forced to curtail her activities, but her spirit was not destroyed.

A program for midwives at the Hospice de la Maternité in Paris opened opportunities for Debaralle in the field of women's health care, particularly for pregnant women. Exposed to lectures on complex medical topics, and supported by strong female role models, she studied independently, conducting research, and writing tracts on various medical topics that she published without authorization. Ambitious, stubborn, and persistent, Debaralle rejected acceptable standards of feminine behavior. She frequently changed her activities, promoting "herself as a healer and an inventor of patent remedies, leaving behind the respectable titles of 'midwife' and 'scientist'" (p. 98). Debaralle appealed to a rural populace who rejected the "new theories" proposed by the medical establishment. After the Revolution, laws limiting the practice of medicine were unsuccessful, resulting in lax enforcement and untrained medical practitioners who operated with little or no supervision. Yet, women were still excluded from medical schools and the health care professions.

Unable to patent her medicines, and challenging the official bureaucracy, Debaralle's activities resulted in citations, fines, labels such as "insensée, folle, charlatane" and even imprisonment (p. 104). Increasingly delusional and paranoid, she transformed herself into a human rights activist and a "femme de lettres" (p. 109). The author concludes that Debaralle was ultimately

> silenced […] not just because she challenged the official medical world's monopoly but because she insisted on speaking louder than those who opposed her (p. 110).

Valérie Lastinger introduces us to the famed anatomist Marie Marguerite Biheron, who became a master of ceroplastics, mentoring other women, and encouraging them to pursue their scientific interests. Marie Armande Gacon-Dufour wrote manuals of domestic economy, invented culinary substitutes to alleviate poverty during food shortages, and authored numerous works of fiction and non-fiction. Marie de Maupéou, mother of Nicolas Fouquet, distributed medicine to the poor while Suzanne Necker became administrator of a hospital that bears her name.

Lastinger maintains that as women moved from the "boudoir" to "the laboratory," they contributed to scientific and medical knowledge outside the universities from which they were excluded. By the end of the eighteenth and the beginning of the nineteenth centuries, however, women met with increasing resistance to their participation in scientific and medical communities. The author emphasizes, nevertheless, that

> Anatomy, botany, chemistry, physics, mathematics—no branch of science seems to have been off limits, no laboratory seems to have been able to keep women out (p. 130).

Between 1780 and 1840, women's involvement in medicine expanded to include charitable work, the compilation of formulas in recipe books, and especially the study of botany. Gacon-Dufour is a particularly interesting example of a woman knowledgeable in all aspects of domestic economy who helped develop food substitutes during times of famine. Lastinger concludes that women always found new outlets for their scientific curiosity and innovation:

> It is not to say, however, that science, medicine and women parted ways at the end of the long eighteenth century. Rather, I would propose that we look in the domestic space to find the women scientists of the nineteenth century, as kitchens, dairies, stables, and fields could easily be transformed into laboratories (p. 139).

By exploiting resources available to them within the private sphere, these women made a significant impact on the scientific discourse from which their male counterparts excluded them.

The importance of midwives within the shifting landscape of women's health care is illustrated by Patsy S. Fowler who studies representations of "copulation, contraception, conception, and childbirth," as well as the role of the midwife, in order to understand the cultural manifestations of reproduction in the eighteenth century (p. 149). Using examples from novels such as Laurence Sterne's *Tristram Shandy,* Eliza Haywood's *Anti-Pamela*, and Daniel Defoe's *Moll Flanders*, Fowler also addresses the role of female and male midwives such as William Smellie, who became popular among the "*beau monde* and the *nouveaux riches*" (p. 150). Competition from men, however, reduced the number of female midwives and decreased their income, while shifting control of women's health care to male physicians and surgeons. The latter were more concerned with money, reputation and pro-natalist policies than the needs of their female patients. Refusing to be marginalized, women used recipe books as one method to transmit their knowledge.

Basing her comments on historical sources in dialogue with literary texts set in London, Fowler takes us into the private sphere of women's lives. Their knowledge of herbs and plants, passed on from one generation to the next, provided women with control, although limited, over their reproductive lives. Such knowledge enhanced a mentoring system that empowered women.

> […] eighteenth-century women turned to midwives, prostitutes, servants, apothecaries, female relatives, and even family recipe books for information on the use of herbal remedies as birth control and abortifacients (p. 154).

Her discussion of childbirth, lying-in, confinement, the role of friends and family, the special beds and chairs invented to facilitate childbirth, and the changing social status of women provides a window into their private lives as women adopted the new role of mother. In spite of advances in health care for women, the author nevertheless concludes that:

> the medical advancements in women's reproductive health seen throughout the eighteenth century were not necessarily indicative of improvements in the overall lives of women—sexual, professional, or otherwise (p. 160).

Many diseases in the long eighteenth century were regarded as gender specific by the medical establishment. In some cases, disease functioned as a metaphor for a woman's moral deficiencies or emotional instability. Felicia Berger Sturzer, Elizabeth Kuipers, Marialana Wittman, and Ivy Dyckman present varying perspectives on specific diseases, their treatment, and their function as literary and cultural markers.

Sturzer's article on disease as metaphor focuses on the correspondence between the salonnière Julie de Lespinasse and the Comte de Guibert, as well as Nicolas de Condorcet, between 1770 and 1776. As Lespinasse creates a literary "myth" of the romantic heroine who dies of a broken heart, she also documents the symptoms and treatment of the illness that consumes her body—tuberculosis.

This lethal disease, which affected large segments of the European population, was nevertheless romanticized in many artistic and literary works well into the modern era. As a more empirical approach to the study of disease favored the observation of signs rather than the indirect, abstract classification of symptoms, "the discursive distinction between *symptom* and *sign* was at best blurred throughout the eighteenth century," with the two terms used interchangeably in the article on "Phtisie" in the *Encyclopédie* (pp. 168-169). Within this context, Julie's letters represent "the relationship between a writing subject, the patient [...] and the shifting parameters of medical discourse during the Enlightenment" (p. 165).

Merging fact and fiction, the Lespinasse letters become medical bulletins describing a body ravaged by disease, and the anguish of a mind obsessed with erotic desire and death. They document a regimen of symptoms—insomnia, lethargy, muscular stiffness—and medications, treatments, as well as the opinions of the physicians that Lespinasse consults. Nothing alleviates her suffering except Guibert's letters declaring his love, Glück's opera *Orphée* and opium. As metonym for the absent lover, the letter is both a poison and a balm that controls her existence. Letters to Condorcet also confirm the multiple physical and mental ailments that characterized her illness. Sturzer concludes that the Lespinasse correspondence is "important to our understanding of women and disease in the eighteenth century" and "the broader issue of the relationship between the female body as text and an instrument of literary inscription" (p. 180).

In her essay on breast cancer, Elizabeth Kuipers maintains that historically, the discourse on the causes and treatment of this disease has been dominated by men, and the long eighteenth century was no exception. Jean Astruc, Bernardio Ramazzini, Friedrich Hoffman of Prussia, Johannes de Gorter, and Jean Louis Petit contributed to the literature on breast cancer, and perpetuated many of the stereotypes associated with the disease. Nevertheless, as knowledge about breast cancer progressed, so did approaches to treatment and a cure, with surgery recommended only as a last resort.

Basing her analysis on personal narratives and literary texts, Kuipers provides a much-needed feminist perspective through the voices of the women victimized by breast cancer. She focuses on accounts of how three women experienced this disease—Mary Astell, Frances Burney, and Lady Delacour in Maria Edgeworth's novel *Belinda*. By daring to speak, these women not only broke the silence but challenged the negative moral connotations and shame associated with the disease. Private suffering enters the public domain through their stories, which inscribe the changing ideas regarding breast cancer toward the latter part of the eighteenth and the beginning of the nineteenth centuries.

Mary Astell underwent a mastectomy without anesthesia and died of the disease. Frances Burney's letter to her sister in 1811 constitutes "the earliest known account [of the operation] written by the patient" (p. 185). In spite of her desire to keep the correspondence private, the very act of writing marked it as a public document. Edgeworth emphasized the importance of a female support system in confronting breast cancer through the experience of the fictional Lady Delacour. In her novel, she questions the role of women as wives and mothers, and cancer as a metaphor for moral laxity.

Kuipers concludes that all three authors argued for "the need of a women's community in times of crisis" (p. 198), thus anticipating our contemporary struggle for greater emphasis on women's health issues.

Marialana Wittman's essay concentrates on the perception of venereal disease in eighteenth-century France as documented in journals, medical treatises, letters, and police reports. With few visual images, the existing information was "painted through words rather than brushes" (p. 201). She argues that contrary to earlier views of women as diseased and men as healthy, in the eighteenth century the medical discourse on venereal disease "shows clearly that culpability for" its spread "was almost exclusively assigned to men." Medical, sociological, and economic factors converged in contradictory discourses on the disease (p. 202). Shifting populations between country and urban spaces further impacted the effects of venereal disease on the development of healthy families.

Women, especially wives, were considered victims of their husband's infection, and even prostitutes were ancillary to discussions on the etiology and spread of venereal disease. The prominence of men in the medical documentation was due to many factors. The contagion theory maintained that the virus more easily penetrated the pores of the male sexual organ, while the "theory of relative female immunity" linked menstruation to the expulsion of fluids and protection from the disease. Thus,

> the gendered visions of venereal disease depicted in the theories on vulnerability gave a particular shape to the conceptualization of culpability in eighteenth-century France (p. 212).

The lack of unbiased sources regarding patients and the larger number of men than women who sought medical attention also account for the emphasis on males in the medical literature. Wittman concludes that while we cannot determine precisely why visual representations of venereal disease were rare,

> by incorporating the gendering of vulnerability and the focus on healing the male body into the history of eighteenth-century France, we can come

> closer to seeing the complex vision of venereal disease that was influential in the period (p. 221).

She demonstrates that the century's gendering of disease anticipated debates that inform the medical discourses of our own time.

In eighteenth-century France and England, literary and medical references to women who have the "vapors" are numerous, with the nature of the condition described in vague terms. Within the context of changing medical philosophies during the Enlightenment, Ivy Dyckman's essay traces references to this illness and its particular association with women. Two medical treatises in French, by Jean Astruc and by Samuel Auguste André David (S.A.D.) Tissot, and three in English, by John Ball, A. Hume, and John Leake, form the basis of her study. Confronted by rivalries between physicians, surgeons, apothecaries, licensed and unlicensed medical practitioners, women struggled to overcome their consignment to the private sphere of domesticity. Some managed to publish homemade "recipes" for cures to a variety of illnesses, the vapors among them.

Dyckman traces the etymology of vapors and notes references to it in such literary works as the letters of Mme de Sévigné, *Robinson Crusoe*, and Henry Fielding's *Amelia*. A poem by Lady Mary Wortley Montagu and Rétif de la Bretonne's novel *Les Nuits de Paris* provide a variety of contexts for eighteenth-century views on this condition. Today, it incorporates depression, "bipolar disorder, post-traumatic stress disorder" while "In the eighteenth century it was considered one of many illnesses—hypochondria, hysteria, the spleen, dyspepsia—categorized as 'nervous disorders'" (p. 238). It is noteworthy that a nervous disorder was linked to various illnesses involving the "bowels" and of course, the uterus.

The author concludes that self-help manuals, written primarily by men in the latter half of the eighteenth century, had both positive and negative results on the health care of women. On the one hand, they were

> a step forward, a written confirmation of women as individuals who were capable of taking care of their own bodies, even if men were telling them how to do it.

On the other, they promoted the place of women "as dutiful wives and mothers" who were too delicate to actively participate in the public sphere (p. 246).

The essays represented in this volume raise questions regarding the importance of women as subjects of empirical and historical discourse. Furthermore, a critical reading of the relationship between women, gender, and disease allows us to evaluate how readers reacted to medical writing, philosophical debates, and new scientific discoveries. These textual productions both challenged and reinforced traditional modes of thought in the eighteenth and early nineteenth centuries. Ultimately women, long regarded as counter-examples, as the quintessential "other" in relation to the norm of universal man, found a voice. Their contributions continue to impact our own era.

Notes

[1] Roy Porter, "Medical Science and Human Science in the Enlightenment"; Ludmilla Jordanova, "Sex and Gender" in *Inventing Human Science—Eighteenth-Century Domains*, ed. Christopher Fox, Roy Porter, and Robert Wokler (Berkeley: University of California Press, 1995).

[2] Jordanova, pp. 154, 155, 158-159.

[3] Jordanova, p. 176.

PART I:

THE NATURAL HISTORY OF WOMEN

CHAPTER ONE

WRITING THE NATURAL HISTORY OF WOMEN: MEDICINE, SOCIAL THOUGHT, AND GENRE IN POST-REVOLUTIONARY FRANCE

SEAN QUINLAN

In France, following the Reign of Terror, there appeared a steady stream of lengthy books whose authors discussed an intriguing subject-matter: "the natural history of women." The eminent physician and politician Pierre Cabanis introduced the theme in his inaugural lectures at the Institut National de France starting in 1796 and the books then started rolling off the presses: Jean-François de Saint-Lambert's *Analyse de l'homme et de la femme* (1800-1801), Jacques-Louis Moreau de la Sarthe's *Histoire naturelle de la femme* (1803), Gabriel Jouard's *Nouvel essai sur la femme* (1804), Louis-Victor Bénech's *Considérations sur les rapports du physique et du moral de la femme* (1819), and Jules-Joseph Virey's *De la femme, sous ses rapports physiologique, moral et littéraire* (1824). To this mix, one could also add the well-known text by poet and critic Antoine-Léonard Thomas (1732-1785), whose *Essai sur le caractère, les moeurs et l'esprit naturel de la femme*, a spirited apologia for female talents, appeared in a new edition in 1803.[1]

These books were written by an eclectic group of doctors, naturalists, and self-styled men of letters, all of whom claimed to explain the "physical and moral" qualities of women in their entirety. In their eyes, previous intellectual authorities—doctors, anatomists, naturalists, metaphysicians, moralists, and *philosophes*—had all failed to grasp women's true inner nature and the role they were supposed to play in society. "On a beaucoup écrit sur les femmes," regretted one doctor, "on a célébré leurs charmes, leur mérite, leur beauté; mais ces objets d'un culte universel n'ont presque jamais été pour les savants un sujet de recherches et de méditations."[2] Yet, by writing the natural history of women, these savants could penetrate the female mystique and lay bare her mind and body: an attitude later captured, for example, in Louis Ernest Barrias's sculpture "Nature Unveiling Herself Before Science," a work prominently displayed at the Paris medical faculty.[3] In so doing, scientific authorities could discover women's true vocation: the family.

This natural history of women was unique to French sciences and letters—no exact corollary exists in English, German, or Italian—and so historians might profitably approach these books as constituting a special medico-scientific genre. This genre differed from other biomedical writings on gender and healing, notably gynecology and obstetrics, because its scope was decidedly *non-therapeutic*. By this I mean that the writers focused less upon women's diseases and their cures than they asked more speculative questions about women's minds, their bodies, and their diverse ethnic varieties. In adopting this approach, these writers distilled an array of cutting-edge scientific and social thought: the Montpellier vitalists' so-called medical science of man; Charles-Louis de Secondat de Montesquieu's and Nicolas de Condorcet's sociological works; Jean-Jacques Rousseau's moral anthropology; recent ethnographic and travel literature; Félix Vicq d'Azyr's and Georges Cuvier's work on comparative anatomy; Charles Bonnet's and Lazzaro Spallanzani's embryological researches; and new clinical theories associated with the Paris hospitals.[4]

With these books, obviously, these writers wanted to disseminate medical, naturalist, and social-scientific ideas to lay readers. Nonetheless, I should emphasize that the texts also contained a personal agenda: namely, they wanted their popularizations to contribute to public discourse and thus shape general attitudes and behavior. Though these writers often hearkened back, as we shall see, to mid-Enlightenment debates about women's role in society,[5] they were also responding to experiences arising from the French Revolution itself: how leading figures such as Condorcet, Charles-Maurice de Talleyrand, and L.-M. Le Peletier de St. Fargeau had debated women's education; how ordinary women had participated in civic debate, revolutionary clubs, and collective action; and how feminist luminaries such as Marie Olympe Aubry de Gouges had challenged patriarchal authority and asserted women's rights in public life.[6] French society, it seems, was rethinking conventional gender roles—for some critics it created tremendous sexual anxiety and loathing[7]—and so now public authorities and intellectuals wanted to examine women in a new light and understand what was changing.

In what follows, I suggest that the natural history of women should be understood on three levels. First, the authors composed their books so they could influence how their readers thought about gender roles following the French Revolution. In this regard, they sought to bring their specialized knowledge to bear upon women's character and physical constitution and thus determine whether men and women were truly equal beings and what this meant for their respective social duties. Though the writers diverged in opinion and emphases, they believed that women's status was the greatest public issue of the day, and they hoped to shape general social thought.

Nonetheless, these books were not "hegemonic" in that doctors and intellectuals were imposing a coherent vision upon the lay public, as though we could speak of a "sovereign" professional consciousness when discussing women and gender relations (as Edward Said spoke of a "sovereign Western consciousness" when discussing Orientalism).[8] When these writers proffered their books to general readers, they were not just constructing political and social arguments, but they were also trying to establish themselves in the scientific and literary community and thus accrue cultural capital for themselves (to borrow Pierre Bourdieu's sociological concept).[9] Surely they hoped to sell books, but it's also likely that they wished to distinguish themselves in the medical marketplace and thus attract patrons and patients.

To achieve this goal, the authors employed a writing strategy that differed from the clinical style found in standard textbooks on women's health. They sought to delight and entertain their readers, serving them a dish of science seasoned with political ruminations and literary verve. In so doing, they offered less a shared worldview than a particular "take" on revolutionary social conditions. Sometimes the writers combined political agenda and professional ambition in ways that belied the political points they sought to establish.

Above all, doctors and intellectuals used the natural history of women to address fundamental issues regarding self and identity: they wished to determine, in the words of philosopher Charles Taylor, "where they [stood] on questions of what is good, or worthwhile, or admirable, or of value."[10] Seen in this light, the writers wanted to uncover the true and authentic self and understand what it meant to be a man or a woman in this new age and then live out these natural roles in everyday life. For these writers, the natural history of women explained what women truly were and how they should act in a rapidly changing society. It offered them an objective measure to set the world a bit straighter in a time when the path forward seemed dangerous and unclear.

***

To understand this genre, one must start with the writers themselves, for their biographies provide an important perspective. The most prominent of them was Pierre Cabanis (1757-1808), who was a leading physician and Idéologue philosopher. In the waning years of the Old Regime, he joined Madame Helvétius's salon circle and befriended the philosopher and mathematician Condorcet; from these interactions, in part, he forged his materialist philosophy and outlook on social improvement. Under the Directorial republic (1795-1799), he served as a legislative deputy and later conspired with Napoleon Bonaparte to overthrow the republic. For his support, Napoleon awarded him a senatorial post, but Cabanis later incensed the First Consul because of his liberal sympathies.[11]

The other writers lacked Cabanis's status. Jean-François de Saint-Lambert (1716-1803) was a well-known poet and man of letters. Though contemporaries praised him for his lyrical poem *Les Saisons* (1769)—a work that shows why the Enlightenment isn't known for its poetry—historians chiefly remember him today for his liaisons with mathematician Émilie du Châtelet (1706-1749), who died giving birth to his illegitimate child, and Sophie d'Houdetot (1730-1813), who inspired Rousseau's character Julie in *La Nouvelle Héloïse* (1761).[12] By the time Saint-Lambert published his work on women, he was already in his late seventies and contemporaries found him more a curiosity than a serious intellectual.

By contrast, Dr. Jacques-Louis Moreau de la Sarthe (1771-1826) belonged squarely to the revolutionary generation. He was born in Montfort and, as a young adult, moved to Paris in 1791. He trained first as a surgeon, later receiving a post as librarian at the medical faculty library in 1795. Afterwards, he earned his medical degree and taught medical history. Friend to Cabanis and Cuvier, Moreau de la Sarthe helped edit the prestigious medical series for the *Encyclopédie méthodique* (taking over for the late Vicq d'Azyr), and he directed a massive revision of Johann Kaspar Lavater's multi-volume work on physiognomy. In addition, he wrote about various medical innovations, psychiatric treatment, and vaccination.[13]

Like Moreau de la Sarthe, Julien-Joseph Virey (1775-1846) was a provincial who came to Paris during the revolution to make his career. Originally trained in pharmacy, he later took a medical degree and affiliated himself with the prestigious Société des Observateurs de l'Homme. He wrote prolifically on natural history, physiology, *and materia medica*, and he also helped edit the *Nouveau dictionnaire d'histoire naturelle* and Georges-Louis Leclerc de Buffon's monumental *Histoire naturelle*. Later he was elected a national deputy from his native Haute-Marne and distinguished himself with his liberal sympathies and political engagement—an outlook that, under the Restoration, might have cost him a faculty appointment.[14]

The remaining writers are more obscure. Doctor Gabriel Jouard (17[??]-18[??]) published some literary criticism and submitted a medical thesis on the natural history of women. He wrote two other short books—one on contagion and the other on Montpellier medical doctrine—but beyond this, we know little about his life. Finally, Louis-Victor Bénech (1787-1855[?]) was born in Saint-Cirq in Lot and trained in Paris. Of these writers, he alone experienced the French Revolution as a child. Beyond his ruminations on women, Bénech wrote several short works on disease, environment, and cancer, and he seems to have incited public controversy in his native province with his unorthodox treatments for chronic disease.

Several points emerge from these short biographies. All these writers—excepting Bénech—formed powerful firsthand impressions of the French Revolution, and, in the case of the medical men, benefitted from its institutional reforms, participating in the innovative and exciting environment of the Paris hospitals. Though they possessed some intellectual status, none of them—save Cabanis—was a major player in the scientific and literary establishment. For example, Moreau de la Sarthe benefitted from Cabanis's patronage and published widely, but he never received a prestigious university position; Virey's sentimental attachment to Rousseauian philosophy and his liberal politics annoyed his medical colleagues and public authorities alike. In other contexts, figures such as François-René de Chateaubriand dismissed Saint-Lambert as a relic from a bygone Rococo era,[15] whereas Jouard and Bénech remain complete unknowns. Surely, then, all these figures craved greater status in the republic of letters, and so they picked up the subject of women and sexuality, hoping to advance their careers.

Ultimately, then, these male writers—excepting Cabanis—were not major luminaries within the Parisian *monde*; they are perhaps best characterized as average or even mediocre thinkers. Like many other thinkers of their caliber, they became fixated on one hot-button issue—in this case, sexuality and gender relations—and elevated it to a causal factor, one that explained everything in French society. In this sense, they engaged in special interest pleading, appearing as what today we'd call single-issue voters. And like many single-issue voters, they wanted to find like-minded souls and convert them to their cause.

***

These writers functioned in a larger biomedical context. One important impetus came from a growing medical literature on what contemporaries called "les maladies des femmes": not just obstetrics and gynecology, but the range of diseases that afflicted women.[16] Strikingly, the medical authors expanded upon the old Aristotelian-Galenic tradition—seen in books such as Jean Liébault's *Trois livres des maladies des femmes* (1649) and Jean Varandée's *Traité des maladies des femmes* (1666)—and treated women as a distinct group, in pathological terms, "à raison de la constitution qui leur est propre."[17] Following Jean Astruc's pioneering works, these practitioners argued that women suffered from special diseases "dépendant des parties particulières aux sexes": menstruation, procreation, gestation, childbirth, and nursing.[18] This understanding informed most notably Nicolas Chambon de Montaux's lengthy trilogy on female pathology: *Des Maladies des femmes* (1784), *Des Maladies de la grossesse* (1785), and *Des Maladies des filles* (1785). In 1794, when revolutionaries transformed the medical faculties and hospitals, reformers placed these ideas in the new medical curriculum, and they were reflected in major textbooks such as François Vigarous's *Cours élémentaire des maladies des femmes* (1801) and Joseph Capuren's *Traité des maladies des femmes* (1812).[19]

At the same time, the natural history of women drew upon two other traditions in learned medicine: the so-called "science of man" and "natural history," both of whose content and conventions shaped the genre's content and style.

The science of man meant complex things for contemporaries. Following David Hume, they believed that the science of man constituted the science of human nature itself, the means by which they applied "experience and observation" to understand the moral realm of the mind.[20] Through this experimental philosophy, they could explain human consciousness and activity, both on the individual and collective level. Strikingly, the science of man boasted a clear Enlightenment agenda. For these philosophers, this study was the first step towards comprehending the human condition so that they could change that condition, making people more happy and useful, if not perfecting them outright.[21]

Natural history also had its own formal conventions, practices, and philosophic agenda.[22] Whilst empirical in scope, natural history featured an observational and taxonomic dimension—"la description fidèle des singularités de la nature"—that distinguished it from the more analytical science of man.[23] Given these qualities, natural history appealed to the erudite and leisured public, as seen by the proliferation of naturalist books and curiosity cabinets. However, some critics found that this fashionable quality rendered the tradition scientifically suspect, its methods and practices "mal conçus."[24] So, by the early 1800s, its practitioners tried to elevate natural history to a more rigorous experimental science, analyzing its subjects from "le point de vue de leur utilité réelle, de leur application aux arts, au commerce, et à l'agriculture."[25] This was particularly true for those savants who wished to apply natural history techniques to study human diversity—what we now call physical anthropology—and these interests were expressed in the new courses on the "histoire naturelle de l'homme," taught first at the Muséum d'Histoire Naturelle by Bernard-Germain Lacépède (who had collaborated with the great naturalist Buffon) and later at the École Normale with his colleague Jean-Louis-Marie Daubenton (who was editing Buffon's posthumous works).[26]

Both factors, the science of man and natural history, coalesced in a medical tradition that Elizabeth A. Williams has called "anthropological" or "physiological" medicine, a tradition which was famously associated with the doctors of the Montpellier medical school: François Boissier de Sauvages, Théophile de Bordeu, and Paul-Joseph Barthez.[27] These medical writings strongly influenced post-revolutionary writings on women and healing. In them, doctors wanted to explain mind-body relations by identifying the discreet physical property that animated the human frame. This knowledge would allow them in principle to explain human nature, that is, what made individuals feel, think, and act, and thus they would make medicine integral to philosophic and scientific thought. In this process, doctors tried to explain how vital properties manifested themselves across the diverse stages and conditions of human life: age, environment, occupation, temperament, race, and sexuality.[28]

When doctors analyzed these different stages, they thought that women presented a special case study: a pathological state of exception. "Hors de-là," wrote Dr. Victor de Sèze, "la femme est un être à part, qui a ses passions, ses mœurs, son tempérament, sa santé, et ses maladies."[29] The most important work, in this regard, was Pierre Roussel's *Système de la femme*, which he first published in 1775 to wide acclaim.[30] In this book, Roussel argued that doctors and *philosophes* must consider women in their physical totality, not just as reproductive machines. For him, women possessed "une différence radicale, innée, qui a lieu dans tous les pays et chez tous les peuples," and their study thus required a holistic approach typical of the Montpellier school.[31] In this regard, he considered his work as complementing the pedagogical and moral ideas that Rousseau advanced in his *Émile* (1762), as well as the strong anxieties about luxury, fashionable refinement, and nervous disease advanced by medical reformer Samuel Tissot, amongst others. Roussel thus wanted to naturalize women and regenerate them by recalling them to their domestic destiny. Like other Enlightenment critics, he believed that something had gone horribly wrong with women during the eighteenth century, and it was up to doctors and moralists to cure these pathological relations.[32] The health and vitality of the body politic depended upon it. Following the revolutionary upheaval, with all its questions about women and gender, legislative and intellectual authorities returned to this theme with new energy and determination.

***

Pierre Cabanis picked up this theme about women in his lectures at the Institut National, the crown jewel of the Directory's new educational system, and he later compiled them in his *Rapports du physique et du moral de l'homme* in 1802. In this text, so important for philosophic and scientific thought in the nineteenth century, Cabanis promised that the medical science of man could heal a country torn apart by revolution and war. In essence, he built upon Claude-Adrien Helvétius's materialist monism, in which physical sensibility and environment shaped human experience, and superimposed upon it Condorcet's vision of perfectibility that he had outlined in his posthumous work, *Des progrès de l'esprit humain* (1795).[33] Here Cabanis promised that he would treat three qualities as interdependent: the physiological, the moral, and the world of ideas. Throughout, he insisted that intellectuals should never separate mind and body, as the sensory organs determined all feeling and thought.[34]

To understand human nature, then, physicians must study how this physical sensibility functioned in the body and then determine how it affected mental and moral functions. To do so, Cabanis identified what he considered to be the most important facets of sensibility: the basic sensations; the influence of age, sex, temperament, disease, regimen, and climate or geography; the formation of ideas and "affections morales"; the qualities of "animal" life such as instinct, sympathy, sleep, and deliria; mind-body relations; and education and temperament.

When Cabanis expounded upon this physical sensibility, he argued that sexuality utterly shaped humanity's physical and mental experiences, marking men and women as radically different beings (p. 338). He began with the reproductive organs. Here the uterine system seemed to provide a centripetal force that governed the female organism and this force extended throughout the whole body: the bones, the muscles, the fibers, and, especially, the brain and nervous tissue, which Cabanis characterized as soft and pulpy when contrasted to a man's. These constitutional weaknesses subjugated women to powerful internal and external stimuli, so they couldn't dominate their desires and emotions (pp. 334-335).

Moreover, these physical factors determined women's character, behavior, and moral and intellectual aptitude. From the start of a woman's life, he asserted, sickness and death haunted her:

> Pour une nécessité sévère, attachée au rôle que la nature lui assigne, la femme se trouve assujettie à beaucoup d'accidents et d'incommodités; sa vie est presque toujours une suite d'alternatives de bien-être et de souffrance; et trop souvent la souffrance domine (p. 350).

Nonetheless, nature's "severe necessity" illustrated the part that women ought to play in society, because biological determinants destined them for procreation, nursing, and primary education.

To fulfill this domestic vocation, then, nature had given women one set of skills, namely sentiment and devotion, but had denied them a strong and fertile mind. Like Roussel, Cabanis drew upon Rousseau and claimed that women were attracted to objects and sentiments that underscored their innate maternal instincts and skills: qualities, he lamented, that men themselves often lacked. Yet women's affective qualities meant that they couldn't concentrate their minds, particularly when they tried to grasp abstract ideas associated with science and math. Even "les femmes savantes," said Cabanis, "ne savent rien au fond" (p. 362).

When Cabanis compiled his examples, he rebuked recent philosophers and legislators who claimed that men and women were equal in their intellectual and moral aptitudes and so society should grant women the same opportunities (this group included Cabanis's late friend, Condorcet). No belief, he said, could be more pernicious to the commonwealth: for him, women were only happy when they made men happy, and he dismissed those radicals who claimed to represent women's best interests. In rhetorical style, Cabanis wondered whether feminists truly believed that women should pick up arms to defend their country or mount the public tribunal to debate "les intérêts d'une nation" (pp. 364-365). It was clear that Cabanis himself didn't think so, and he asserted that his opinions were grounded in biomedical fact. To believe otherwise, he concluded, would do violence to women, who should rather live in mutual dependency with men. As he saw it, "Il faut que l'homme soit fort, audacieux, entreprenant; que la femme soit faible, timide, rusée. Telle est la loi de la nature" (p. 348).

Two points should be made about Cabanis's attitudes towards women. First, Cabanis truly thought that biomedicine offered insights into the moral nature of both men and women. It provided not just a vision of social and natural reality, but also a means to ground moral-ethical behavior and to turn individuals into responsible and dutiful moral agents. Biomedicine thus allowed people to understand their inner selves and personal identity and thus become authentic and useful individuals. Through this science, his contemporaries could reconcile personal liberties and social duties to the natural order.

At the same time, Cabanis saw himself as moderate, if not liberally minded, in how he understood women and sexuality. At no point would he have characterized himself as reactionary, obscurantist, or simply old-fashioned. Throughout his work, he believed that his ideas steered a middle ground between two extremes: on the one hand, reactionary or traditionalist attitudes towards womanhood (that is, the Christian view of woman as either saint or harlot); and, on the other, more revolutionary and subversive views about women's emancipation and autonomy (which he found equally unnatural and untenable). In the face of extremes, Cabanis believed that the medical science of man provided physicians, moralists, and legislators the means to discover the just balance and put it into practice. Other doctors and *philosophes* shared his faith and developed it further in their own works.

***

The first writer to expand upon Cabanis's agenda was Saint-Lambert in his *Analyse de l'homme et de la femme*, a work he published as part of his two-volume *Oeuvres philosophiques* (1800-1801). In this grand analysis, the former poet purported to study human nature and then apply his insights to control and contain the passions: an essential task, he thought, given the violent emotions unleashed by the French Revolution. Like the urbane *philosophes* whose company he had kept during the Old Regime, Saint-Lambert identified with Epicurean principles, and he called upon legislators and moralists to take people as they "really were" and not as rational abstractions that leaders needed to change through legislative force or violence.[35]

Saint-Lambert divided his philosophic works into four sections. In the first, he treated men and women separately, describing the inner nature of each. Then, he outlined explicit pedagogical approaches that he hoped would change parental attitudes and give them good skills for molding their children's beliefs and behavior. Next, Saint-Lambert commented on how readers could learn to control their emotional passions and appetites, thereby sustaining the social peace. Last, he sketched historical progress in law, institutions, and philosophy (especially science), providing a summary that evoked Jean Le Rond d'Alembert's celebrated "Discours préliminaire" to Diderot's and d'Alembert's *Encyclopédie* (1751).

Throughout, Saint-Lambert drew upon different genres and expository techniques, all which gave his book a digressive feel, a series of Lockean associations, as seen in Laurence Sterne's and Denis Diderot's literary experiments. Originally, when Saint-Lambert analyzed the male character, he used an analytic framework derived from Descartes and Hume, focusing upon human nature, the passions, and moral ideas. However, when he turned to women, he changed his style, declaring that this "doux emploi" required a more imaginative form. He tried to achieve this effect by casting this section as a dialogue between two noted figures from the age of Louis XIV: François Bernier (1620-1688), the Montpellier physician, voyager, and Epicurean disciple of Pierre Gassendi; and Anne "Ninon" de l'Enclos (1620-1705), a famous courtesan and freethinker, who was one of the great salonnières of the period and mistress to François de La Rouchefoucauld and Christian Huygens, amongst others. Throughout the dialogues, however, it's the male philosopher who does the heavy intellectual lifting. It's this persona, and not the *femme d'esprit*, who gets in the last word about women.

Saint-Lambert's dialogues take place in the Tuileries palace and Ninon's home and garden (he included one as an epistolary exchange), and the subject-matter ranged from women's character to her passions and virtues. Bernier begins by asking Ninon why women seemed in "un état moins heureux que le nôtre," despite their physical, intellectual, and moral qualities, which liken them to a beautiful work of art. When responding to his gallant statement, Ninon rebukes him. She declares that the more she thinks about women the more their condition revolts her. It's as though she refuses the existential fate that nature and society have prepared for her. More pointedly, she doubts whether men could ever divest themselves of their prejudices when they assessed women, acknowledging that they too possessed reason and "esprit." In her eyes, men had failed to study women in a fair and systematic fashion.[36]

In some ways, Bernier invokes Rousseau's claim in *Émile*—"en tout ce qui ne tient pas au sexe, la femme est homme"—and he declares that men and women possessed on the surface the same intellectual aptitude: "des principes de la morale conviennent également à l'un et l'autre sexe."[37] Nonetheless, when observers studied women, they must begin with physical and not moral qualities, for the former determined women's experiences. One must acknowledge these biological realities before contemplating inequalities between the sexes.

In this regard, Saint-Lambert echoed Cabanis. For him, women were simply weaker than men. They possessed great beauty but lacked physical force, and this lack undermined their mental faculties. Consequently, women "n'ont pas la force d'examiner, de méditer, de raisonner."[38] Of course, men could be weak-minded as well, but this condition was more common in women. In response, Ninon complains that "vous ne nous donnez pas ... un caractère fort noble," but Bernier doesn't respond to her.[39]

As Bernier describes it, women's sensible nature denied them "un esprit supérieur."[40] They lived only in the present moment and their feelings were only reactive. They resembled more a mirror than a living being, reflecting passively rather than actively representing anything on their own. As a result, women lived in a world of illusion, surrendering themselves to imaginative desires. Indeed, Bernier asserts that women often abandon everything to satiate their passions, above all that of love, and in the process they become capricious, unjust, and cruel. Love seasons life, he declares, but deep down people needed friendship. Unfortunately, women cannot endure this true sincerity and instead employed tactics of flattery and coquetry—tactics, Bernier found, which were both the pride and shame of Gallic culture.

Consequently, when Bernier asks Ninon whether women could ever unite against men, she responds that such a movement would be impossible: women lack solidarity because they see each other as rivals for male love and attention. Like Mary Wollstonecraft—who complained that women acquired "manners before morals"—Saint-Lambert suggested that women relied too much upon other people's opinions when they formed their self-worth and this slavish attention to personal taste and fashion hampered their authentic inner nature: that interior realm where they could fortify their moral nature and then emancipate themselves.[41] Instead, as in Montesquieu's *Lettres persanes*, women engage in seraglio politics, pleasing despotic men for their private gain and aggrandizement.[42] Male tyranny had stripped women of their true moral nature and ultimate destiny.

Nonetheless, morals and customs degraded women even more than any intrinsic "natural" weaknesses. Initially, Ninon declared that women learn from an early age that they are at men's mercy, subject to force and violence: first from their fathers, then later from their husbands. This reality governed their whole outlook and behavior. Women learned to alleviate their "slavery" by using sentiments against their "tyrants." They acted passively and indirectly so they could endure their daily subjugation, and they treat men seductively and with charm because their oppressors never tolerated women being direct and assertive with them. Above all, women cultivate pity in men by their tears and emotional displays. In Ninon's words: "c'est en l'excitant en vous que nous échappons à une partie de vos injustices."[43]

Still, Saint-Lambert said that women possessed virtues. Though women seemed weaker than men in their minds and bodies, they possessed canny qualities. Bernier wryly notes that women grasped the male character and they knew more about men than men knew about themselves: a quality, he adds, that all slaves developed with their masters. Not surprisingly, he underscores that women loved children more than men did and without this maternal instinct the family unit could not exist. This virtue pointed to a deeper morality. Since women pitied more than men, they considered not just children but all people who were weaker and dispossessed, such as the sick and the poor, and thus demonstrated a higher ethical calling.[44] With their love and pity, women moderated male avarice and violence and taught them empathy. They became the carriers of a secularized agape: love for one's neighbor.

Saint-Lambert's conventionality notwithstanding, he concluded his work with a degree of self-criticism. In the final dialogue, Bernier composed a long letter to Ninon in which he summarizes what he's learned about the female condition. He confesses freely: he's long blamed women's weaknesses on their physical nature, but now he recognizes that men and men alone had created their "sad" state. Playthings of male desire and bigotry, women couldn't unite with each other to overcome their servitude. Yet it isn't Ninon's reasoning that convinces Bernier, but rather her desultory attitude, so pessimistic about women's fate. Social convention and hypocrisy had covered up a deeper natural reality between men and women. In the end, Saint-Lambert cannot share Cabanis's certainties about women's destiny.

Gabriel Jouard presented a different understanding of women in his *Nouvel essai sur la femme* (1804). Apparently Jouard made women's conditions into a personal crusade. The year before, in 1803, he had submitted a thesis to the Paris medical faculty entitled, *Essai sur quelques points de l'histoire naturelle de la femme*,[45] and, even earlier, he had published a literary critique of the poet and academician named Gabriel Legouvé (1764-1812), whose elegiac *Mérite des femmes* (1801) had been received warmly and was translated into Italian and Catalan. In this analysis, Jouard developed a point to which he returned in his medical writings: namely, that men subjugated their weaker counterparts to a "déspotisme virile" and themselves caused all the faults they blamed on women.[46]

According to Jouard, society misunderstood women for two reasons: men scorned and slandered women and then judged them in a biased way. For this reason, he hoped his book would change public discourse and raise male awareness. Despite his protestations to the contrary, he followed his colleagues and believed that women had become utterly pathological during the Old Regime and French Revolution. However, by studying women in a scientific and objective manner, learned authorities could discover their true nature and make them more happy and useful. Yet this task, he felt, was for men alone.

To study women scientifically, then, observers must first confront sexual difference, as it determined women's experience. Throughout the living world, vast differences existed between males and females and these differences extended into the human world, as well. In biological terms, these markings appeared at the earliest stages of fetal development: sexuality, for Jouard, was an impulsive force that shaped human experience. In his words: "Ainsi dans châque âge, depuis la naissance jusqu'à l'extrême vieillesse, on retrouve dans la femme des caractères généraux qui la distinguent de l'homme du même âge."[47] Consequently sexual dimorphism clarified one's biological destiny as well as social duties: "pour le complément et pour la reproduction de l'espèce."[48]

Given the universal nature of women, Jouard dismissed travel writers who suggested that women in different cultures could assume dominant social roles. For him, nothing could be farther from the truth. Physical factors always limited what women could think and what they could do. They had smaller brains and inconstant nerves, and the uterine system influenced the entire animal *economy.* Even their skeletons reflected their procreative destiny. Accordingly, he said that men and women seemed so different it was best to consider them separate species.[49] For these reasons, Jouard dismissed an "auteur très moderne et encore plus célèbre"—likely Helvétius or Condorcet—who had "refusé à ces organes tout espèce d'influence, tant au moral qu'au physique, sur l'organisation et la manière d'être de l'individu qui en est pourvu."[50]

That said, society had abused these biological differences. According to Jouard, men had exploited women's physical dependencies, abusing their dominion over women and turning them into slaves. Men thus annihilated women's status as moral beings. He wrote:

> de l'infériorité de la structure de la femme et de l'infériorité de ses organes [...] résulte la plus grande et la plus importante des différences physiques qui existent entre les deux individus de l'espèce humaine; je veux parler de l'inégalité extrême de leurs forces, inégalité sur l'effet de laquelle sont fondés tous les rapports respectifs, dans lesquels se trouvent les deux

> sexes; soit dans l'état naturel, soit dans l'état social, inégalité si fort à l'avantage de l'homme qui en a tant usé et abusé.[51]

"Inequality" and "difference": strange words to invoke repeatedly in a democratic age. Nonetheless, Jouard believed that he was rejecting traditional prejudices against women. He dismissed doctors such as Pierre Roussel who had characterized women as children or castrated males. They weren't, he said, "imperfect men": anatomical lack didn't define them, and it was morally wrong to approach women in these terms. Rather, Jouard struggled with how revolutionary transformations, both in political and scientific cosmology, had transformed understanding of men and women and what roles they were supposed to play in this new world. For by knowing what one is one can become what one should be. Like others, he wondered if biomedical science could help contemporaries imagine a more natural society, one stripped of the Old Regime's decadent artifices. At the same time, he still worried about what biological determinism meant for moral liberty and individual responsibility. He didn't think that he was substituting Christian servitude with a new biological ideal. Rather, he thought he was liberating women and letting them be what they truly were. He wanted to discover for women an authentic self.

***

The longest and most influential of these books were written by Jacques-Louis Moreau de la Sarthe and Jules-Joseph Virey. Both doctors were avid naturalists and consummate popularizers. Though neither was a major player in the scientific establishment, on par with the cutting-edge clinicians at the Paris hospitals or the naturalists at the Muséum National d'Histoire Naturelle, both men moved in these intellectual circles and published enough that they did achieve status in the Paris intellectual scene. For these reasons, their books weighed significantly in the world of ideas—indeed, Moreau de la Sarthe's book found its way into the university curriculum[52]—even if one senses that top figures found their writings too facile, geared more towards fashionable readers.

Moreau de la Sarthe's *Histoire naturelle de la femme* was a two-volume opus filled with striking engravings, scientific tables and figures, and literary digressions. In all this, he addressed a broader reading audience, making his book "agréable" in style and "utile" in content, so that men of letters, fashionable elites, and, above all, women might be drawn to his work and instruct themselves "à leur bonheur et à leur conservation."[53] In this regard, as Sergio Moravia observed, Moreau de la

Sarthe's work achieved a "notable echo."[54] Following the example that Voltaire had established when he popularized the Newtonian system, Moreau de la Sarthe said that the writer must soften the "thorns" of science with the humanistic "flowers" of style.[55] Therefore, he engaged readers by juxtaposing the informative and the fantastic, the technical and the pleasing.

Moreau de la Sarthe organized his book around four primary topics. Foremost, he wanted to explain fully women's physiological nature by drawing upon the gamut of post-revolutionary science and medicine, whether new work on respiration and digestion, Volta's electrical experiments, new embryological data on development and regeneration, comparative anatomy and taxonomy, and clinical advances in pathology and hygiene. From here, he looked to analyze female form and beauty and he distilled the aesthetic writings of Hogarth, Winckelmann, and Burke. Next, he applied Buffon's model established in his "Discours sur la nature des oiseaux" so he might distinguish "la somme et la quantité totale des différences, des qualités et des attributs qui distinguent le sexe."[56] Finally, he provided lengthy passages expounding anthropological and ethnographic data on women—particularly with racial classification—and treated "des principales variétés que présentent le physique et le moral de la femme considérée dans les différentes circonstances d'âge, de climat et de civilisation."[57]

In all this, Moreau de la Sarthe followed Cabanis's pattern of elaborating on women's biology, how it influenced character and behavior, and what roles and duties society should establish for them. Indeed, his expansive scope suggests how deeply social and political elites had begun worrying about women's status following the French Revolution. In this regard, Moreau de la Sarthe believed that the medical community had liberated itself from old religious and scholastic prejudices and moved beyond the Aristotelian model of women as an imperfect male. Rather, readers must take women for what they were: "la partie essentielle de l'espèce, puisqu'elle concourt davantage à la reproduction."[58]

Like Roussel and Jouard, Moreau de la Sarthe wanted to prove that sexuality transcended procreation. Reproduction alone, he declared, did not a woman make. By contrast, sexuality saturated the whole body, concentrating itself in women's nature. In his words: "la femme n'est pas seulement femme par un appareil d'organes, ou par ses formes extérieures qui nous séduisent." Rather, "elle est femme [...] dans toutes ses manières d'exister, dans ses affectations morales comme dans son système physique, dans ses jouissances comme dans ses douleurs." He concluded:

> toutes les parties, tous les points de son être relèvent son sexe, et présentent avec tous les points et toutes les parties correspondantes de l'homme, une série d'oppositions et de contrastes.[59]

For these reasons, woman was woman and no one could do anything to change this biological fact. Surely Moreau de la Sarthe was responding, as his colleagues had done, to Helvétius and Condorcet. He wanted to demonstrate the unique but integrated nature of a woman's body, which he said the scientific practitioners could not reduce to a single physical part.

When making this point, Moreau de la Sarthe multiplied his examples. He drew upon recent works in which anatomical practitioners created either exact or idealized models of the female skeleton. In particular, he referenced the famous texts by Albinus and Thomas von Soemmering, among others, whose works seemed to establish that the female pelvis predominated and thus demonstrated a woman's natural childbearing role.[60] Next, Moreau de la Sarthe turned to embryological research and expounded upon Spallanzani's work on animal generation, which built upon Albrecht von Haller's and Charles Bonnet's preformation theories, and which seemed to confirm ovist pre-existence: the idea that the embryo pre-existed in the female ovaries and subsequent generation was the unfolding of this original germ structure. From this evidence, Moreau de la Sarthe speculated that sexual difference existed in embryonic form—if not a priori—in the uterine system, perhaps even before fertilization.[61]

In other passages, Moreau de la Sarthe argued that women suffered from hypersensitive nerves and a weak muscular apparatus, both which meant that they easily succumbed to exaggerated feeling. These determinants extended even to physiological processes such as absorption and nutrition and apparently predisposed women to plethora and discharge (as seen with menstruation). Given these collected observations, Moreau de la Sarthe arrived at a similar conclusion as Jouard: women were less imperfect men than a different species.

Moreover, these physical determinants shaped moral qualities: mind, character, and behavior. Indeed, Moreau de la Sarthe claimed that women underwent no less than twelve distinct life stages, ranging from birth to post-menopause, each which altered basic female experiences. Her corporeality thus determined her entire personal experience. This muscular weakness and excessive sensibility made them mentally inconsistent, unable to reason properly, though their nervous energy gave them powerful motor skills and social graces. However, this hyper-sensibility also rendered women prone to emotional outbursts and deadly nervous diseases, notably the vapors and syncope (as seen with coma or trancelike states).

Moreau de la Sarthe linked physicality and character most strongly when he discussed female beauty. In this discussion, he drew upon Burke's aesthetic theory of the beautiful and the sublime—a political contradiction, given Moreau de la Sarthe's republican sympathies—and argued that female beauty inspired neither fear nor respect but rather weaker feelings associated with "tendre prédilection, le désir, l'amour."[62] Unlike the male sublime, which evoked for the spectator images of power and horror, femininity inspired images of delicacy, refinement, and gentle beauty. For Moreau de la Sarthe, these aesthetic qualities reflected what he believed were a woman's inferior creative and rational qualities.

These characteristics suggested women's proper roles and duties. In his mind, the uterine temperament predominated in the female body and thus marked her reproductive destiny. Further, ovist pre-existence suggested that women possessed all possible embryos in their ovaries, which meant that the fetus constituted a part of the female body, like a nose or an ear, an appendage for which she alone was responsible. At the same time, women's sensible and sentimental nature prepared her for domestic duties, making her respond lovingly to these duties, particularly her children's needs. That said, Moreau de la Sarthe railed against what he considered to be reactionary and bigoted Christian attitudes towards sex, above all celibacy and ascetic denial. Both he felt were inherently unhealthy and incited sexual pathologies such as nymphomania, "habitudes lesbiennes," and "l'onanisme anglais."[63] Rather, he promoted a more moderate but natural sexual ethic as seen in Diderot's "Supplément au voyage de Bougainville" and his *La Religieuse* (which was published posthumously in 1796).

To behave properly, women must always practice moral and physical hygiene. Following the claims set out in Thomas's *Essai sur la femme*, Moreau de la Sarthe said that women shared the same health dangers as men, but then nature inflicted upon them even more deadly disorders. In this regard, medical science could help women by teaching them hygienic precepts and giving them the peace of mind that only good health provides. Hygiene, he promised,

> peut au moins en affaiblir les effets par d'heureuses applications; signaler des écueils; donner des avis utiles; prévenir des abus; éclairer, améliorer l'emploi de la vie, dont les femmes sont si portées à abuser; enfin, conduire, surveiller ces êtres si faibles, si intéressants; les guider au milieu des périls; les soutenir au moment des crises les plus redoutables, dans les transitions les plus orageuses, dans l'exercice des fonctions les plus délicats; et assurant ainsi leur existence au milieu des dangers qui la menacent, conserver leur santé ainsi que leurs charmes, et leur préparer une vieillesse sans infirmités et une mort sans agonie.[64]

***

In his *De la femme*, Virey recapitulated many themes established by Cabanis, Jouard, and Moreau de la Sarthe, but he added the literary flair characteristic of Saint-Lambert's dialogic text. In this work, Virey concerned himself strongly with perceived moral degeneracy and sexual perversion amongst women. In many ways, he moved beyond the monist materialism associated with Cabanis's Idéologue circle, and he instead promoted a more sentimental and pastoral worldview, one that evoked Rousseau's and Bernardin de St. Pierre's "natural man" and primitive moral virtue. In this regard, he mimicked the great Enlightenment health crusader Doctor Samuel Tissot. Tissot, as is well known, had styled himself as the "friend" of the people's health and had launched endless jeremiads about the perceived debauchery of Enlightenment society.[65] Like Tissot, Virey felt a special animus against upper-class elites and fashionable society, particularly well-heeled women. Throughout, one personal issue determined Virey's thought: class and sexual resentment.

Like Moreau de la Sarthe, Virey wrote his natural history of women in an accessible and engaging style. Despite his generalist tone, however, he didn't wish to curry favor amongst women; following Cabanis, he assumed that his readers were all male. In this spirit, he divided his book into three main parts. In the first section, he surveyed physiological considerations, making general remarks about corporeal function and racial varieties of women across the globe. Then Virey discussed the female life course, ranging from youthful virginity to marriage, before turning to moral questions: women's intellectual qualities, their feelings and passions, and lastly their proper social roles. In the final section, entitled "De la femme considérée sous le rapport littéraire," he discussed women luminaries and what role they played in politics, letters, arts, and sciences. To close, he appended a short "dissertation" on the sexual dangers of libertinism in which he fully indulged his sexual anxieties and fixations.

According to Virey, the learned observer must combine natural history, comparative anatomy, and physiological science when discussing women. Only through this means, he insisted, could one grasp the physical and oral functions that shaped human experience. In so doing, he returned to Rousseau by distinguishing between nature and artifice, arguing that civilization utterly altered humanity's natural body and mind. Consequently, humanity's

> divers états de civilisations et d'éducation, ses genres de vie si variés dans toutes les situations et les conditions politiques, parmi toutes les contrées du globe, exaltent ou dépriment, altèrent ou déforment son type originel.

Here, however, he put women at the center of this evolutionary drama, making them the primary motor behind generation, degeneration, and regeneration. Unfortunately, woman—"cet être si délicat, cette fleur de la nature vivante"—underwent these physical alterations more profoundly than their male counterparts, marking them for disease and disorder.[66]

To make this point, Virey drew upon a wide range of anthropological and travel literature, much as he had done in his two-volume *Histoire naturelle du genre humain* (1800-1801). He filled these chapters with prurient ethnographic details about women across the globe and divided them between what he called whites, blacks, Mongolians, Malaysians, and Amerindians. He focused heavily upon sexual custom and practice—surely the only other contemporary to fixate so much upon the sex habits of other societies was the Marquis de Sade—and he characterized non-Western sexuality as alien and barbarous. In particular, he believed that menstruation marked civilized over-refinement, in which early onset of the menses revealed a deep-seated moral pathology; and he claimed that matriarchy (or any other form of female authority) suggested either capricious barbarism or anarchy—that is, any society in which people failed to achieve a balance between nature and civilization.

Unsurprisingly, all this detail coalesced in angry critique of contemporary gender relations and sexual emancipation. From the onset of his book, Virey railed against those thinkers he saw to be the deluded "partisans de l'égalité des deux sexes."[67] In other writings, he had described human beings as split, in almost Manichean fashion, between two "poles" of existence—the intellectual and the genital—and he said that individuals must struggle throughout their lives to balance these powerful internal impulses.[68] Given these conditions, he characterized a woman as "an extreme being," one consumed by powerful biological drives and appetites. In addition, sensibility overcharged her brain and nervous system, which overwhelmed her muscular apparatus and drove her spongy tissue to states of hysterical display. In this hapless state, women thus "presque toujours" resembled dependent children.[69]

While extreme and volatile, women had also been marked by nature as the source of all life. Like Moreau de la Sarthe, Virey followed Bonnet and Spallanzani and posited that women were the depositories of all possible embryonic germs, rendering them "la tige essentielle de notre espèce" and the "âme de la reproduction."[70] But if she possessed the embryonic germs, making procreation the principle of her life, she lacked one key ingredient: the seminal fluid whose spirituous qualities animated the germ and caused it to develop. In Virey's view, this animating substance gave men their powerful minds and bodies, and its spirituous qualities infused all levels of male activity. However, since women lacked semen, they felt aimless and despondent; and Virey even speculated that women's inability to ejaculate during orgasm left them emotionally unfulfilled and sexually insatiable. Hence they could never moderate their desires and live responsibly.

From here, Virey inveighed on broader social problems and currents. In his mind, women's physical and moral degradation signaled a deeper rot in French society; indeed, it was this deep strain of moral vice that had caused the Old Regime to collapse in revolution. Yet, Virey said, upper class and bourgeois women had started it all. He complained how they lived frivolous lives to please corrupt men and ambitious mothers. These factors rendered young women spiteful and embittered. Meanwhile at home domestic servants waited upon them hand and foot, instilling in them a taste for sadistic caprice. Then it was off to enjoy the nightlife, attending parties and dances, where endless pleasures battered their fragile nerves. When they combined these activities with other ruinous conventions—coffees, teas, sweets, spirits, suffocating dresses, crass novels—young women found themselves in a deadly physical state and easily fell victim to nervous diseases such as the vapors.[71]

This inappropriate lifestyle spread throughout society and infected even the male ruling order. And as these men succumbed, women readily usurped their power and inverted the natural order. Indeed, this process had occurred under the Old Regime. According to Virey, women had always exercised more influence in French society than any other place and they dominated courtly life and letters (despite Salic law). However, the situation exploded when Louis XIV died and high society abandoned the old king's Baroque piety. In Virey's estimation, under the Regency and Louis XV, the upper classes abandoned themselves to scandalous debauchery—above all women, who profited from this dissipated state and abandoned their sacred duty to be good wives and mothers. Here, under Louis XV's mistress, Madame de Pompadour, fashionable women got their hands into every shady deed, ranging from Jansenist controversies to fiscal bankruptcy. The nation enervated itself, abandoned its patriotic sentiment, and became "indifférent à tout."[72]

To cure this unnatural state, Virey claimed that male authorities must re-establish marital authority by imposing the male order upon women. Apparently he was satisfied that revolutionaries had taken initial steps, especially with the Civil Code (which denied women active citizenship), but he felt that legislators needed to do more.[73] In his words, "La femme ne pouvant pas subsister seule, devient, par sa faiblesse, ses grâces et les fonctions auxquelles son sexe la destine, le premier lien de la vie civile"—

and so civil law and custom must do all it could to guarantee that women anchored the social order.[74]

Here Virey returned to his greatest theme: love. Indeed, this theme preoccupied social thinkers and literary men in the post-revolutionary age—notably Antoine-Louis-Charles Destutt de Tracy, Étienne Pivert de Senancour, Stendhal, Henri de Saint-Simon, Charles Fourier, Honoré de Balzac, and Jules Michelet—each of whom wrote extensively and even lyrically upon this subject, wondering how men and women could be reconciled with each other and how their mutual love and understanding could transform the family and regenerate society.[75]

Not surprisingly, love also concerned medical practitioners. As Doctor Louis-Victor Bénech observed in his *Considérations sur la femme*, published in 1819, love bonded the two sexes together, calmed their mutual anxieties, fulfilled their existence, and helped create the human community. In a highly eroticized passage, Bénech insisted that the sentiment was always strongest amongst women, whose bodies—"l'économie entière"—seemed constructed around it, as their charm and beauty enticed men to reproduce the species. At the same time, however, female modesty counterbalanced male sexual desire and forced them to control and domesticate their passions, almost sublimating love: first in the family unit and later in society itself.[76]

Virey echoed Bénech's sentiments, though he seemed less gallant. Through the power of love, he said, God had breathed boundless invention into his creation and given men and women the affective bond that held society together. In his words, love made life and perpetuated it: "c'est la force, le principe de notre existence, comme il est la source de toute reproduction."[77] Love makes and preserves humankind, because "[a]imer, c'est vivre pour son espèce."[78] He went on to say that women bore a central role in this process, because they alone carried all the embryonic germs that make the human species: past, present, future. In a biological sense, humanity had evolved to such a degree that people felt more deeply than any other being in nature. This biological progress marked women more strongly than men and made them experience love to the depth of their being.

Despite these evolutionary adaptations, love tormented women and this torment made them emotionally extreme. Hence they desperately needed to marry men, an arrangement that somehow could alleviate their emotional agony. At the same time, Virey also expounded a "free love" argument and claimed that men and women should marry whom the pleased. When they could choose their "douce sujétion" for themselves, they loved their partners more constantly and happily. Women could then embrace the "modest servitude" that anchored their health and well-being. Above all, he said, men and women loved best when men were manly and women more feminine, all of which gave each other a "certaine harmonie d'inégalités correspondantes." In this state,

> Nous voyons que chaque sexe déployant ses vertus et ses vices, mais d'une qualité différente, il n'y a point de comparaison exacte à faire à cet égard entre l'homme et la femme.[79]

In such passages, Virey outlined what he believed was a more "natural" sexuality between men and women. Like the republican and Idéologue Moreau de la Sarthe, he denounced as archaic traditional Christian morality, above all celibacy and abstinence, which, in his view, debased natural instincts and desires. Rather than unrealistic self-control, individuals needed modesty, a sentiment that developed only in the tender love experienced between a man and a woman. Only this quality could mend the social fabric and thus transcend political violence and confusion—particularly in a revolutionary age, when individuals and families lurched from one political extreme to the other.

***

The natural history of women, thus, addressed personal, professional, and broader cultural concerns in post-revolutionary France. Foremost, the authors intended their works to contribute to the general thought of the period, particularly the more materialist and liberal attitudes associated with the Idéologues and their circles. In this sense, the natural history of women lacked the therapeutic or practical elements normally associated with technical books on women's disease and cures. Rather, these books engaged in a more philosophic and speculative analysis, one purportedly anchored in biomedical fact, which aimed at uncovering women's so-called true nature and what society should do with it. With these books, these doctors and moralists intervened in public discourses about changing gender roles: the social and public role of women, especially their rights and duties, as well as questions of public education. These writers had personal stakes in each of these questions, and so they wrote to influence readers on what were, for them, pressing social and political concerns.

At the same time, as I've tried to suggest, these doctors and moralists likely expressed their own private agendas beyond surface politics or ideology. They used gender concerns to insert themselves into public consciousness and thus situate themselves in the broader medical and intellectual community. In their eyes, their books could potentially accrue cultural capital and thus give them intellectual status by establishing their bona fides as both doctors and men of letters. The medical practitioners likely hoped to distinguish themselves in the medical marketplace proper, selling their theories of domestic bliss and sexual relations, and thus attract patrons and patients in Paris fashionable society: either by appealing to women directly (as with the case of Moreau de la Sarthe), or by appealing to husbands and fathers, who may have been looking to find a good doctor for their wives and daughters. This private agenda is not unusual. In the early 1800s, for example, a similar trend appears with doctors who wrote on sexual hygiene and reproductive strategies: they sought to establish their names in the intellectual scene and increase their professional recognition.[80]

With the natural history of women, authors sought to attain this recognition by entertaining their audiences with a good read. Consequently the books themselves were often fragmentary, digressive, and filled with literary pretention—collections that mixed medicine, physiology, embryology, natural history, and history proper—and they were narrated in imaginative and non-linear ways (unlike the objective clinical style that characterized works on pathology and comparative anatomy). In short, the writers wanted to entertain and delight their readers, perhaps evoking "wonder" in the old naturalist tradition, especially when associated with curiosity cabinets.[81] In this regard, the book served as a substitution, a simulacra, for the naturalist collection, replacing the direct visual or tactile experience with the textual medium.

Most importantly, the natural history of women offered a way for readers to explore ideas of self and society. Through this self-knowledge, they might discover their true inner nature, one that allowed them to live more authentic and meaningful lives as men and women. And medicine, they believed, was fundamental for this self-discovery. Nonetheless, in the post-revolutionary period, this biomedical discourse about self and society was but one of many competing visions about the social order: human rights, nationalism, sentimental pastoralism, neo-Christian sensibility, ultra-montanism, romanticism, and so on.[82] This rich ideological and cultural mosaic should not surprise. As Karl Manheim originally observed, modern democratic societies, by virtue of their participatory nature, produce more and more cultural perspective as increasing numbers of people participate in public life and debate.[83] It is a precondition of modern pluralism that no single framework governs the collective imagination.

Biomedical science, then, fits into this general pattern. Yet, it was different in an important way. These new biomedical ideas generated enormous excitement and even hope within the literate public, as they provided new secular ways to think about human nature, the body, and society. They allowed people to make sense of momentous sociopolitical changes and made them think that they could control and master these events. More importantly, biomedical science also promised that progressive change and melioration *were* possible, even if human improvement was limited by technical skill and natural realities. Here, as these writers suggested, a little medical perspective could open an enormous vista on the human condition.

Notes

[1] See Yvonne Knibiehler, "Les médecins et la 'nature féminine' au temps du code civil," *Annales E.S.C.* 31 (1976): 824-845; Paul Hoffman, *La femme dans la pensée des Lumières*, 2nd ed. (Geneva: Slatkine, 1995), pp. 157-171; Sean M. Quinlan, *The Great Nation in Decline: Sex, Modernity and Health Crises in Revolutionary France, ca. 1750-1850* (Aldershot, UK: Ashgate, 2007), pp. 128-134.

[2] Jacques-Louis Moreau de la Sarthe, *Histoire naturelle de la femme*, 2 vols. (Paris: I. Duprat, Letellier, 1803), vol. 1, p. 1.

[3] On this image, see Ludmilla Jordanova, *Sexual Visions: Images of Gender in Science and Medicine between the Eighteenth and Twentieth Centuries* (Madison, WI: University of Wisconsin Press, 1989), pp. 87-88.

[4] On science in the French Revolution, see especially Michel Serres, "Paris 1800," in Serres, ed., *A History of Scientific Thought: Elements of a History of Science* (Oxford: Blackwell, 1995); Charles C. Gillispie, "Science in the French Revolution," *Behavioral Science* 4 (1959): 67-73; Gillispie, "The *Encyclopédie* and the Jacobin Philosophy of Science: A Study in Ideas and Consequences," in *Critical Problems in the History of Science*, ed. M. Clagett (Madison, WI: University of Wisconsin Press, 1969), pp. 255-289; and Gillispie, *Science and Polity in France: The Revolutionary and Napoleonic Years* (Princeton, NJ: Princeton University Press, 2004).

[5] Madelyn Gutwirth, *The Twilight of the Goddesses: Women and Representation in the French Revolutionary Era* (New Brunswick, NJ: Rutgers University Press, 1992); and Dena Goodman, *The Republic of Letters: A Cultural History of the French Enlightenment* (Ithaca: Cornell University Press, 1994).

[6] Lynn Hunt, *The Family Romance of the French Revolution* (Berkeley: University of California Press, 1992); Joan Landes, *Women and the Public Sphere in the Age of the French Revolution* (Ithaca, NY: Cornell University Press, 1988); Dorinda Outram, *The Body and the French Revolution: Sex, Class, and Political Culture* (New Haven, CT: Yale University Press, 1989).

[7] On the sexual panic thesis, see especially K. Binhammer, "The Sex Panic of the 1790s," *Journal of the History of Sexuality* 6 (1996): 409-435; and Dror Wahrman,

"*Percy*'s Prologue: From Gender Play to Gender Panic in Eighteenth-Century England," *Past and Present*, 159 (1998): 113-160.

[8] Edward Said, *Orientalism* (New York: Vintage, 1979), p. 95.

[9] Pierre Bourdieu, *La distinction: critique sociale du jugement* (Paris: Éditions de Minuit, 1979), pp. 22-23.

[10] Charles Taylor, *Sources of the Self: The Making of Modern Identity* (Cambridge, MA: Harvard University Press, 1989), p. 27.

[11] On Cabanis, see Sergio Moravia, *Il tramonto dell'illuminismo: filosofia e politica nella società francese (1770-1810)* (Bari: Laterza, 1968), and *Il pensiero degli Idéologues: scienza e filosofia in Francia (1780-1815)* (Florence: La Nuova Italia, 1974), pp. 13-288, esp. pp. 13-23 (for basic data). The best biographical study remains Martin S. Staum, *Cabanis: Enlightenment and Medical Philosophy in the French Revolution* (Princeton, NJ: Princeton University Press, 1980).

[12] Roger Poirier, *Jean-François de Saint Lambert, 1786-1803: sa vie, son oeuvre* (Sarreguemines: Pierron, 2001).

[13] Véronique Signoret, "La féminité vue par deux médecins des Lumières: Roussel et Moreau de la Sarthe" (MA thesis, Université de Paris XII [Val-de-Marne], 1992), pp. 33-44.

[14] Claude Bénichou and Claude Blanckaert, eds., *Julien-Joseph Virey, naturaliste et anthropologue* (Paris: Vrin, 1988).

[15] Poirier, *Saint-Lambert*, p. 304.

[16] See especially Jacques Gélis, *L'arbre et le fruit: la naissance dans l'Occident moderne (XVIe–XIXe siècle)* (Paris: Fayard, 1984); Lindsay Wilson, *Women and Medicine in the French Enlightenment: The Debate over Maladies des Femmes* (Baltimore, MD: Johns Hopkins University Press, 1993); and Nina Rattner Gelbart, *The King's Midwife: A History and Mystery of Madame du Coudray* (Berkeley: University of California Press, 1998).

[17] Bibliothèque de l'Académie Nationale de Médecine (henceforth ANM), ms. 1025, fol. 1: Coutouly, "Des maladies des femmes en général" (1786), p. 1a. On this point, see François Azouvi, "Woman as a Model of Pathology in the Eighteenth Century," *Diogenes*, 115 (1981): 22-36.

[18] Bibliothèque de la Faculté de Médecine de Paris (henceforth FMP), ms. 5192, fol. 572: Astruc, "Traité des maladies des femmes en général" (n.d.), 3ff. See also FMP, ms. 5087: "Extrait des leçons de Mr. Astruc (manuscrit provenant du Dr. Andry)" (1737); as well as Archives de la Société Royale de Médecine, carton 201, dos. 14: Gautier (maître-ès-arts et en chirurgie à Saint-Hilaire), "Mémoire sur les règles des femmes" (1788).

[19] ANM, ms. 1062, vol. XI: Dr. Desormaux, "Cours de maladies des femmes et des enfants" (11 Apr. 1820). This source constitutes the classroom notes of a medical student named Jules Cloquet, in which direct references are made to Pierre Roussel, Pierre Cabanis, J.-L. Moreau de la Sarthe, and François Vigarous.

[20] David Hume, *A Treatise of Human Nature*, ed. Ernest C. Mossner (London: Penguin, 1969), p. 43.

[21] Peter Gay, *The Science of Freedom*, vol. 2, *The Enlightenment: An Interpretation* (New York: Knopf, 1969), chap. 4, "The Science of Man"; Sergio

Moravia, *La scienza dell'uomo nel settecento* (Bari: Laterza, 1978), esp. pp. 15-47; idem, *Filosofia e scienze umane nell'età dei Lumi* (Florence: Sansoni, 1982), especially chap. 1, "L'origine teorica delle scienze umane nel Settecento"; and Elizabeth A. Williams, "The Science of Man: Anthropological Thought and Institutions in Nineteenth-Century France" (PhD thesis, Indiana University, 1983), pp. 1-28.

22 See especially Emma C. Spary, *Utopia's Garden: French Natural History from Old Regime to Revolution* (Chicago, IL: University of Chicago Press, 2000).

23 Antoine Furetière et al., ed., *Dictionnaire universel: contenant généralement tous les mots François tant vieux que modernes, et les termes des sciences et des arts*, 2nd ed., 3 vols. (La Haye and Rotterdam, 1701), s.v. "Histoire."

24 *Encyclopédie, ou dictionnaire raisonné des sciences, des arts, et des métiers*, Denis Diderot and Jean Le Rond d'Alembert, eds., (28 vols., Paris, 1751-1772), s.v. "Histoire naturelle" (quote in vol. 8, p. 229).

25 *Nouveau dictionnaire d'histoire naturelle, appliquée aux arts, à l'agriculture, à l'économie rurale et domestique, à la médecine, etc.*, 36 vols. (Paris, 1816-1819), s.v. "Avis."

26 Moravia, *La scienza dell'uomo*, pp. 70-85, especially pp. 73-74.

27 On Montpellier medical thought, see Elizabeth A. Williams, *The Physical and the Moral: Anthropology, Physiology, and Philosophical Medicine in France, 1750-1850* (Cambridge: Cambridge University Press, 1994), and *A Cultural History of Medical Vitalism in Enlightenment Montpellier* (Aldershot, UK: Ashgate, 2003); as well as Roselyne Rey, *Naissance et développement du vitalisme en France de la deuxième moitié du 18e siècle à la fin du Premier Empire* (Oxford: Voltaire Foundation, 2000).

28 Paul-Joseph Barthez, *Nouveaux élémens de la science de l'homme*, 2nd ed., 2 vols. (Paris, 1806).

29 Victor de Sèze, *Recherches physiologiques et philosophiques sur la sensibilité ou la vie animale* (Paris, 1786), pp. 217-218.

30 See Anne C. Vila, "Sex and Sensibility: Pierre Roussel's *Système physique et moral de la femme*," *Representations*, 52 (1995): 76-93.

31 Pierre Roussel, *Système physique et moral de la femme* (Paris, 1775), pp. 16-17.

32 Quinlan, *Great Nation in Decline*, pp. 19-51; Michael E. Winston, *From Perfectibility to Perversion: Meliorism in Eighteenth-Century France* (New York: Peter Lang, 2005).

33 On Cabanis's sensationist philosophy and his understanding of social improvement, see Moravia, *Il pensiero degli Idéologues*, 165-79; Staum, *Cabanis*, pp. 207-243.

34 Pierre Cabanis, *Rapports du physique et du moral de l'homme*, 2 vols. (Paris, Year X [1802]), vol. 1, p. xiii. Future references will be given in the text.

35 See especially Catherine Wilson, *Epicureanism at the Origins of Modernity* (Oxford: Oxford University Press, 2008); as well as Thomas Kavanagh, *Enlightened Pleasures: Eighteenth-Century France and the New Epicureanism* (New Haven, CT: Yale University Press, 2010); and John Robertson, *The Case for the Enlightenment: Scotland and Naples, 1680-1760* (Cambridge: Cambridge

University Press, 2005).

[36] Saint-Lambert, *Analyse de l'homme et de la femme*, in *Oeuvres philosophiques* (Paris, Year IX [1800-1801]), vol. 1, p. 45.

[37] Saint-Lambert, *Analyse*, vol. 1, p. 169. Cf. Rousseau's dense comments in *Émile, ou de l'éducation*, ed. Michel Launay (Paris: Garnier-Flammarion, 1966), 465-470 (quote on p. 465).

[38] Saint-Lambert, *Analyse*, vol. 1, p. 227.

[39] Saint-Lambert, *Analyse,* vol. 1, p. 230.

[40] Saint-Lambert, *Analyse,* vol. 1, pp. 184-185.

[41] Mary Wollstonecraft, *A Vindication of the Rights of Woman*, edited and with an introduction by Miriam Brody (London: Penguin, 1975), p. 106. On this question of moral autonomy in eighteenth-century thought, see especially Taylor, *Sources of the Self*, pp. 355-390.

[42] On this point, see Hoffmann, *La femme dans la pensée des Lumières*, pp. 338-339.

[43] Saint-Lambert, *Analyse*, vol. 1, pp. 193-194.

[44] Saint-Lambert, *Analyse*, vol 1, p. 235.

[45] Gabriel Jouard, *Essai sur quelques points de l'histoire naturelle médicale de la femme* (Paris, 16 fructidor an XI [16 September 1803]).

[46] [Gabriel Jouard], *Un mot sur le mérite des femmes* (Paris, Year IX [1800-1801]), p. 17.

[47] Gabriel Jouard, *Nouvel essai sur la femme* (Paris, Year XII [1804]), p. 11.

[48] Jouard, *Nouvel essai*, pp. 2-3.

[49] Jouard, *Nouvel essai*, p. 69.

[50] Jouard, *Nouvel essai*, p. 4.

[51] Jouard, *Nouvel essai*, p. 12.

[52] Desormaux, "Cours des maladies," n.p.

[53] Jacques-Louis Moreau de la Sarthe, *Histoire naturelle de la femme*, vol. 1, p. 5.

[54] Moravia, *Il pensiero degli Idéologues*, p. 173 n. 146.

[55] On Newtonian popularizations in France, see J. B. Shank, *The Newton Wars and the Beginning of the French Enlightenment* (Chicago: University of Chicago Press, 2008).

[56] Moreau de la Sarthe, *Histoire naturelle de la femme*, vol. 1, p. 17.

[57] Moreau de la Sarthe, *Histoire naturelle de la femme*, vol. 1, pp. 4-5.

[58] Moreau de la Sarthe, *Histoire naturelle de la femme*, vol. 1, p. 69.

[59] Moreau de la Sarthe, *Histoire naturelle de la femme*, vol. 1, pp. 69-70.

[60] On this discussion, see Londa Schiebinger's classic essay, "Skeletons in the Closet: The First Illustrations of the Female Skeleton in Eighteenth-Century Anatomy," in *The Making of the Modern Body: Sexuality and Society in the Nineteenth Century*, eds. Catherine Gallagher and Thomas Laqueur (Berkeley: University of California Press, 1987), pp. 42-82.

[61] On Spallanzani's theories, see Walter Bernardi, *Le metafisiche dell'embrione: scienze della vita e filosofia da Malpighi a Spallanzani (1672-1793)* (Florence: Olschki, 1986); and on reception of generation theories in the Paris medical community, see Sean M. Quinlan, "Heredity, Reproduction, Perfectibility: Early

Ideas about Eugenics during the French Revolution," *Endeavour* 34.4 (December 2010): 142-150.

[62] Moreau de la Sarthe, *Histoire naturelle de la femme*, vol. 1, pp. 334-335.

[63] Moreau de la Sarthe, *Histoire naturelle de la femme*, vol. 2, pp. 269-270.

[64] Moreau de la Sarthe, *Histoire naturelle de la femme*, vol. 2, pp. 223-225.

[65] See Antoinette Emch-Dériaz, *Tissot: Physician of the Enlightenment* (New York: Peter Lang, 1992).

[66] Jules-Joseph Virey, *De la femme, sous ses rapports physiologique, moral et littéraire*, 2nd ed. (1824; Paris, 1825), pp. 1-2.

[67] Virey, *De la femme*, pp. 3-4.

[68] For helpful discussion, see Robert A. Nye, *Masculinity and Male Codes of Honor in Modern France* (Oxford: Oxford University Press, 1993), pp. 59-62; and Anne C. Vila, "Sex, Procreation, and the Scholarly Life from Tissot to Balzac," *Eighteenth-Century Studies*, 35 (2002): 239-246.

[69] Virey, *De la femme*, pp. 182-183 & p. 215.

[70] Virey, *De la femme*, pp. 2-3.

[71] Virey, *De la femme*, pp. 96-97.

[72] Virey, *De la femme*, p. 312.

[73] On family law, see Marcel Garaud and Romuald Szramkiewicz, *La Révolution française et la famille: histoire générale du droit privé française (de 1789 à 1804)* (Paris: Presses universitaires de France, 1978); and especially Suzanne Desan, "Reconstituting the Social After the Terror: Family, Property, and the Law in Popular Politics," *Past and Present,* 164 (August 1999): 81-121.

[74] Virey, *De la femme*, pp. 266-267.

[75] On this subject, see Sergio Moravia, "Stendahl, l'amore e la scienza dell'uomo," in *Filosofia e scienze umane*, pp. 392-405.

[76] Louis-Victor Bénech, *Considérations sur les rapports du physique et du moral de la femme* (Paris, 1819), pp. 31-35.

[77] Virey, *De la femme*, p. 189.

[78] Virey, *De la femme*, pp. 193-194.

[79] Virey, *De la femme*, p. 214.

[80] See Sean M. Quinlan, "Sex and the Citizen: Reproductive Manuals and Fashionable Elites under the Napoleonic Consulate, 1799-1804," in *Views from the Margin: Creating Identities in Modern France*, eds. Kevin J. Callahan and Sarah A. Curtis (Lincoln: University of Nebraska Press, 2008), pp. 189-217.

[81] Lorraine Daston and Katharine Park, *Wonders and the Order of Nature, 1150-1750* (New York: Zone, 1998).

[82] On this intellectual landscape, see Martin S. Staum, *Minerva's Message: Stabilizing the French Revolution* (Montreal: McGill-Queen's University Press, 1996); as well as George Boas, *French Philosophies of the Romantic Period* (New York: Russell & Russell, 1964).

[83] Karl Manheim, *Ideology and Utopia: An Introduction to the Sociology of Knowledge,* trans. Louis Wirth and Edward Shils (San Diego: Harvest/Harcourt Brace Jovanovich, 1936).

CHAPTER TWO

HEALTH AND THE EIGHTEENTH-CENTURY FRENCH WOMAN: A HISTORY OF DECLINE

MARY MCALPIN

> C'est que vos femmes sont languissantes, débiles;
> J'en ai déjà vu deux tout à fait immobiles;
> Mais pour moi le travail eut toujours des appats;
> Dans nos champs, dès l'enfance, il exerça mes bras.
> —Nicolas Chamfort, *La Jeune Indienne* (1764)

Although critics tend to focus on the controversy generated by Rousseau's denunciation of progress in the *Discours sur l'origine de l'inégalité* (1755), this view of human affairs met with considerable agreement among the era's cultural commentators. The belief that the French populace had reached a state of crisis caused by an overly "civilized" lifestyle was something of a commonplace among the intellectuals of the French Enlightenment.[1] While both sexes were said to display the moral and physical results of this decline, women, given their supposedly "softer" (more malleable) tissues and organs (brains included), were cast as affected both earlier and more dramatically than their male counterparts. The host of illnesses diagnosed as ravaging the female population of France includes a roll call of extremes: excessive languidness, or to the contrary, hyper-excitability; overly abundant, or absent menstrual flow; and, most disturbingly, an excessive—unless entirely absent, of course—sexual appetite. For the physiologists who wrote on these issues, the state of French womanhood put the future of French civilization in serious danger. With increasing intensity as the century progressed, these medical theorists warned that creatures so *languissantes* and *débiles*, to quote Chamfort's young American Indian woman, were able to produce only equally weak and unimpressive offspring, if any. Given that such characteristics were believed to become inheritable over time, the need to "cure" the female population of France was presented as a major public health issue.

The conviction that one's culture is undergoing a moral and physical collapse of unparalleled intensity is of course by no means unique to eighteenth-century France. This belief is most often intimately connected, as was the case in the France of the Enlightenment, to the assumption that one's society has reached a *nec plus ultra* of technological development, sedentariness, licentiousness, and moral decay. What sets the French eighteenth century apart from a more general rhetoric of decline is the central role assigned to women's physiology. Women had of course long been associated with moral corruption; the novelty was the belief that women's moral failings were not a manifestation of some inherently feminine sinfulness, but rather the result of insidious cultural forces at work upon the minds and bodies of the "weaker" sex. The cure in question was equally physiological, and involved, as I have explored elsewhere, a rigorous course of hygiene aimed at prepubescent young women (and men) in particular.[2]

Eighteenth-century meliorism has attracted a number of critics in recent years, but most have ignored the supposition behind this rhetoric of a dramatic and tragic decline: the assumption that at one point in the not-too-distant past, the French "race" embodied a universal ideal. In this article, I explore the *longue durée* of this history of decline from the point of view of the ideal from which eighteenth-century French women are said to have degenerated. The questions I ask include: What characterized the lost paragon of French womanhood, in comparison to whom contemporary women are found so very lacking? What confluence of causes is said to have resulted in the robust health and strong moral sensibilities of this avatar—and what caused the subsequent degradation of her progeny? At what historical moment is the degradation in question supposed to have begun? In exploring these questions, I look for common threads in works by representative eighteenth-century authors, without attempting to conflate these different narratives of decline into one coherent narrative. What interests me is rather the multifariousness of this deep history of feminine decadence as recounted in eighteenth-century France, in both the physical and the moral realms, and in a variety of genres. I follow this circuitous path up to the beginning years of the Revolution, when this particular manifestation of the "problem" of the second sex is solved by reassigning women to the protected environment of hearth and home.

The most systematically developed eighteenth-century theory of woman's physical-moral failings is found in the numerous medical treatises on female hygiene published around mid-century. These treatises, authored primarily by doctors, were imbued with the vitalist philosophy associated with Montpellier School of Medicine. These works, aimed at a lay readership comprised for the most part of concerned parents, assume a profound (post-Cartesian) interconnectedness between mind and body.[3] Relying on theories originally put forward by the Montpellier-trained Théophile de Bordeu and other specialists in *les maladies des femmes*, the authors of these works diagnosed French women living in an urban environment as the most severely affected by their society's advancement. The urban woman in question is to be understood as a member of the elite upper class of French society, be she noble or bourgeois (although generally the former); she is most certainly not a member of the urban poor. The paradox at the heart of this assumption of decline, in other words, is that the endangered and/or debased eighteenth-century woman in question is to be found at the epicenter of her culture's economic and artistic brilliance, with that culture understood to represent the acme of world cultural achievements. Her access to her society's technological and cultural achievements means she experiences all of the nefarious consequences of their influence.[4]

Before turning to a brief survey of these medical treatises, I first outline the proto-anthropological writings of Georges-Louis Leclerc, Comte de Buffon, insofar as this eminent natural historian's writings on racially-inflected climate theory both reflected and influenced the rhetoric of degradation underlying the other works of interest to me. The underlying logic of the history I am tracing holds that only that singular racial group—understood as French—capable of creating a culture in which humankind's artistic, social, intellectual, and technological potential was fully realized, could suffer the debilitating effects of these same accomplishments. I then consider several representative treatises on female hygiene from the 1760s and 1770s, before turning to the history of this supposed decline as recounted in an essay by Antoine Léonard Thomas. The *Essai sur le caractère, les moeurs et l'esprit des femmes dans les différens siècles* (1772) by this member of the Académie Française, renowned for his style, traces the history of the devolution of French women's morals over the centuries. I end my essay as this fascination with women's physiology ended: with a shift in focus to the "new man" of the Revolutionary period. By relegating women to the home, at least symbolically, the republicans made the moral and physical health of this half of all citizens a non-issue, for this claustration served as an efficient manner of "protecting" women from the culture at large.

Buffon's contribution to eighteenth-century racial theory is found primarily in the *Histoire naturelle de l'homme* (1749), the third volume of his enormous, and enormously influential, *Histoire naturelle, générale et particulière* (36 volumes, 1749-1788). Andrew Curran has recently emphasized that Buffon's theory of racial difference was profoundly monogenetic, in that it was based on a relativity-inflected discourse of *cousinage*.[5] Buffon, that is, postulates an original model—white, of course, and based in the temperate zone that includes France. All other "races" are then given to be the result of a "regression" from this ideal caused by harsh climatic conditions.[6] The issue of how many generations it might have taken to achieve these various "degradations" from the originary population, as human beings migrated to Africa or the Americas, is held by Buffon to be merely a matter of scientific observation, albeit on a multi-generational scale that allows him to gloss over the need for any hard evidence of his theory's veracity. That these changes might be "reversed," should Africans be brought "back" to Europe, is the most important aspect of Buffon's theory for my purposes. If the French are to be "saved" from moral and physical decline, the process of racial "degradation" that they are undergoing as a result of their high level of civilization must be reversible, through the science of hygiene.

It is important to note that Buffon did not share the belief that his own culture was in a state of degeneration; he belonged to an earlier, and far more self-satisfied, intellectual mindset, as did that other influential climate theorist from the first half of the century, the Baron de Montesquieu. The belief in humankind's inherent perfectibility—the Enlightenment thesis that has, in critical writing on this period, for so long eclipsed the related belief that over-civilization was leading to a cultural implosion—was a central component of the thought of both Buffon and Montesquieu.[7] Buffon's humans tend to return to their originary state, in accordance with the famous Buffonian concept of the *moule intérieur* that fixes the form to which each species must remain faithful, even as it is modified by the forces of climate and multiplication.[8] In the case of human beings, part of this fixed nature is the "instinct" to reach as high a degree of civilization as possible, and the rewards for this effort, when climatic conditions are right, are considerable, for Buffon:

> un peuple policé qui vit dans une certaine aisance, qui est accoûtumé à une vie réglée, douce et tranquille, qui par les soins d'un bon gouvernement [...] sera par cette seule raison composé d'hommes plus forts, plus beaux et mieux faits qu'une nation sauvage et indépendante.[9]

Better looking and better made women as well, one might add. Although Buffon's references to women in his *Histoire naturelle de l'homme* are sparse, the women of other countries are generally presented as at a disadvantage, and are at times given to be truly hideous.[10] As for differences within the French population, Buffon elevates the educated city woman over her ignorant peasant cousin, with the latter described as "robotic":

> Dans l'espèce humaine, que d'automates! combien l'éducation, la communication respective des idées n'augmentent-elles pas la quantité, la vivacité du sentiment! quelle différence à cet égard entre l'homme sauvage et l'homme policé, la paysanne et la femme du monde.

He even elevates domesticated animals above their wild counterparts:

> Et de même parmi les animaux, ceux qui vivent avec nous deviennent plus sensibles par cette communication, tandis que ceux qui demeurent sauvages n'ont que la sensibilité naturelle, souvent plus sûre, mais toûjours moindre que l'acquise.[11]

What changes in the realm of scientific discourse with the rise of the Montpellier School is, first, an insistence on the decline ineluctably associated with so-called advanced cultures. The writers of the hygiene treatises of interest to me, which appeared in force beginning around 1760, focus their attacks on degeneracy within their own society, rather than listing the deleterious effect of environment on such far-flung peoples as Buffon's Laps, Greenlanders, Africans, and Americans.[12] The principal argument of these theorists is that moral laxity leads to physical degradation when the effects of lascivious living pervert the development of pubescent children. This disturbance of the "natural" process of puberty—with "natural" corresponding to puberty as it manifests itself in simpler peoples, including country-dwelling French girls—is said to produce the languid, potentially infertile creatures described above.

The focus on women's health that is so marked in proponents of Montpellier-style vitalism has been ascribed to a paradigm shift, christened "the invention of sex" by Thomas Laqueur.[13] This new, "two-sex model" of sexual differentiation meant that women were no longer viewed as merely inverted variants on the male model, but were rather endowed with a fascinating physiological "otherness." As the moral was inseparably tied to the physical in vitalist doctrine, women's moral failings were said to be the result of their experiencing to a greater degree the deleterious effects of life in an "advanced" civilization: the consumption of exotic foodstuffs and of immoral entertainment such as plays and—above all—novels, coupled with a striking lack of physical exertion. Women were also, by this theoretical model, excluded from contributing directly to the advancement of their race; as Michael Winston notes of the work of Pierre Roussel, the most famous proponent of the Montpellier vitalists' view of women: "Unlike Helvétian or Buffonian views of progress, whereby all humans are theoretically capable of improvement, only the man possesses the physiological attributes necessary to advance in Roussel's system."[14]

But while viewed as constitutionally incapable of advancing civilization, they nevertheless served an important role as the proverbial canaries in the coalmine, so to speak: charming, decorative warning mechanisms in a male-dominated environment. The physician Joseph Raulin, for example, who worked as a specialist in women's diseases in Paris, was educated in Bordeaux, but his *Traité des fleurs blanches* (1766) is one of the most virulent mid-century attacks on French womanhood, and his approach reflects many of the key assumptions of the Montpellier theorists. Raulin's treatise is, predictably, climate based, for he insists that the passage of air through the pores of the body is a determining factor in establishing temperament and thus, according to the theory of the humors, of establishing a healthy constitution or of bringing on an illness. The following quote from the *Traité* is useful to understanding how national character, understood as racial characteristics, was commonly believed to be established at this time:

> L'air est imbibé d'ingrédients différents, selon la nature des différents pays & des différents terrains: car tout transpire, jusqu'à la glace des hivers. Les eaux, les mines, les volcans, les mouffettes, la terre, les substances animales, les végétales, les minérales, fournissent des vapeurs, des exhalaisons qui causent à l'air des changements selon leur nature; & aux hommes, si elles sont altérées, autant de causes de maladies différentes.[15]

Sickness is endemic to any climate, we are to understand, although some geographical locales are more nefarious than others, but the healthy body, after "inhaling" both the good and the bad (through its pores, principally) is able to expel the harmful "exhalations" of its particular geographical location. Should "unnatural" living pervert one's body, however, this process is blocked. All too often, Raulin ominously declares, when Nature tries to rid a woman's body of harmful liquids,

> les voies des évacuations naturelles se refusent à ses vues; elle [la Nature] est forcée de se faire de fausses routes; elles suivent les pentes les moins

difficiles; elle les trouve vers l'utérus; l'écoulement se forme: ce sont des fleurs blanches.

These "white flowers" (leucorrhaea, understood as any whitish vaginal discharge)—all but unknown in fourteenth-century France, Raulin tells us—are become endemic in French women of all ages and estates. The result is disaster on a species-wide scale: "C'est principalement cette maladie qui fait dégénérer l'espèce humaine, & qui allarme la Nature."[16] Raulin's diagnosis is the usual condemnation of soft living, racial mixing, and exotic foodstuffs.[17] The list of causes and symptoms attributed to women in these treatises does vary somewhat, and the proposed solution for these *maladies des femmes* varies as well, in accordance with each author's physiological obsession. Raulin is interested in immediate cures (cold baths, bleeding), while the Genevan physician Jacques Ballexserd emphasizes diet. In his *Dissertation sur l'éducation physique des enfants, depuis leur naissance jusqu'à l'âge de puberté* (Paris: Vallat-La-Chappelle, 1762), Ballexserd offers parents a disquisition on the proper diet for children raised in the European climate, the diet best suited, that is, to prepare them for the "revolution" of puberty. P. Virard, in his *Essai sur la santé des filles nubiles* (1767), focuses more on the role of physical exercise in determining the frequency and quantity of menstrual flow.

While menstrual flow in all its aspects (quantity, age of onset, color, etc.) is presented in these treatises as a highly important element in judging a woman's overall health, the rules for making such a judgment are somewhat vague. Most physiologists did agree that excessive flow was the sign of a serious problem, and that premature onset was a disaster, as it warped the developing mind and body. The timing of the onset of puberty was of course given to be a factor of climate, understood primarily as temperature in this case, with hot climates predictably said to cause early puberty. But even in colder countries, unnatural (premature) puberty can be brought on by, in Virard's words,

une atmosphère échauffante, par l'oisiveté, la mollesse, l'usage des aliments incendiaires, par la lecture de certains livres, la contemplation de certaines estampes, par la fréquentation de certaines compagnies, ce qui forme autant de causes qui réveillent de bonne heure l'imagination.[18]

Virard excepts the hard-working peasant girl, who sweats during physical labor and thus dispenses a caloric count already reduced by her healthier diet. We are to pity the rich, sedentary city girls, "chargées de graisse," those "filles oisives, qui nagent comme je l'ai dit, dans une atmosphère échauffante," and bleed earlier and far more abundantly, both in terms of flow and frequency (up to three times a month) than do their active country counterparts, who "vivent moins incendiairement."[19]

The most damning condemnation of the effects of over-civilization on women comes from one J.D.T. Bienville, whose *De la nymphomanie ou traité de la fureur utérine*, inspired by Samuel August David Tissot's *Onanisme* (1760), was published in 1771.[20] Bienville's list of the potential causes of nymphomania (a "hidden" malady defined as "un mouvement déréglé des fibres dans la Partie Organique de la femme") demonstrates how closely this illness is linked, in Bienville's system, to the accoutrements of the civilized life. He begins with the influence of that strongest of emotions, love, understood as sexual desire:

> Cette maladie [nymphomania] surprend quelquefois les jeunes filles nubiles dont le coeur prématuré pour l'amour a parlé en faveur d'un jeune homme dont elles sont devenues éperdument amoureuses, & pour la jouissance duquel elles trouvent des obstacles insurmontables (p. 12).

This disease can also be brought on, we are told, by lascivious novels, music, conversation, or by masturbation (inspired by the former causes, one understands), but also by incessant drinking of strong wine or liqueurs, or even the abuse of coffee and chocolate, the excessive use of which is said to be "prodigious" among women. The result is the corruption of "l'harmonie naturelle" of the female body, and an accompanying inflammation of the passions (pp. 14-15). In a poetic, nightmarish scenario, Bienville warns that the "tourbillon de flammes" that makes up the corrupted "atmosphère" of these young women creates "traits de feu" that, sparking from their eyes, may transform a Vulcan into an Adonis (p. 17).

Translated into more common terms, the process is the following: sexual desire born of an over-heated body affects the young girl's brain so dramatically that the most unattractive of young men—a "Vulcan"—may appear to be a veritable Adonis. The young girl is soon whispering the most shocking proposals into this young man's (no doubt astonished) ear, and even physically attacking those individuals who refuse her requests (pp. 17-19). Why, Bienville then asks, have previous authors not written about this problem? Because it was assumed, he answers, that this malady was absent in women of colder climates; yet it is clearly the result of forces stronger than climate, he concludes (p. 20).

These (admittedly extreme) theories of female sexual development and desire are in the service of convincing parents of the need to "protect" their daughters from the harmful effects of their perverse cultural situation. But while these authors do propose pragmatic solutions to the Armageddon-like cultural situation they describe, they rarely enter into the historical arc of the decline they are intent on curing. For a chronology of this supposed feminine decline, I turn to Antoine Léonard Thomas's *Essai sur le caractère, les moeurs et l'esprit des femmes dans les différens siècles* (1772). This sweeping historical survey was first given as a speech at the Académie Française, and is best known today for Diderot's review, or rather response essay, *Sur les Femmes* (1772). Liselotte Steinbrügge observes that the *Essai* constitutes something of a summary of the debates on the nature of woman at this time, and is thus "just the place to learn which aspects of the mid-century *querelle* had gained intellectual influence."[21]

I am of course interested above all in what this piece tells us about the Golden Age of French womanhood, and about what led, in Thomas's opinion, to its disappearance. Our author does not disappoint on this topic, for his stated goal in the *Essai* is to explore women's (shifting) virtues in relation to the particular cultural situations in which one finds them. By examining

> les qualités et les diverses sortes de mérite dont les femmes sont susceptibles, jusqu'où le gouvernement, les circonstances et les lois peuvent les élever, et le rapport secret de la politique avec leurs moeurs,

he will show us "ce que les femmes ont été, ce qu'elles sont, et ce qu'elles pourraient être."[22]

The one thing that women are not, have never been, and, we are left to assume, will never be, is a force pushing humankind to its full potential. This point is crucial, for Thomas is best known as a panegyrist, and won, on a remarkable four occasions, the "prix de l'éloquence" of the Académie Française. But while Thomas's subjects include Marie-Thérèse Geoffrin (whose salon he frequented), and while he repeatedly stresses the reasoning ability of women in his *Essai*, as well as the ability of superior women to write on profound topics, he reserves his greatest admiration for those young married beauties of his era—few in number, we are told—who spend their time at home caring for their children rather than out in the world seeking lovers. In a telling moment near the end of his essay, Thomas exclaims: "Oh! si ces exemples pouvaient ramener parmi nous la nature et les moeurs!" (p. 85).

In setting up this exclamation, that is while describing the lost era of French womanhood in which Nature-inspired mores ruled supreme, Thomas follows Montesquieu, Buffon, and many other commentators in placing climate and its myriad influences first among the determining causes of any culture's specific make-up. His historical account of the fate of French women is also clearly based on the firm belief that there is a fixed ladder of civilization that cultures climb, when they are capable of doing so—and the vast majority are not, or are at least not able to reach the most desirable top rungs. The result for women is said to be devastating, for the most part, for Thomas argues that although Nature made the fair sex charming, "She" neglected to provide for women's happiness. Society, in its earliest stages of development, is said to add to women's sufferings, because savage men possess no moral notions: "Plus de la moitié du globe est couverte de sauvages; & chez tous ces peuples les femmes sont très-malheureuses" (p. 1).

Thomas may well be echoing Buffon, although the assumption that Native American women, in particular, were treated as "beasts of burden" by their "savage" husbands was a commonplace. In such a "cold" climate, it was declared, men's level of sexual desire never rises to that degree required to constitute love, rather than mere enjoyment in the possession of what other men cannot have. As for hot climates, heat is presented, unsurprisingly, as inimical to both advanced culture and to women's happiness. As Thomas would have known, Montesquieu presented the early puberty and intense lasciviousness of "Eastern" women as necessitating their sequestration.[23] Thomas follows suit in declaring that only in temperate countries do women enjoy the liberties associated with man's increased confidence in their virtue—a confidence born of women's supposedly more tepid capacity for physical lust in cooler locations ("le climat, donnant moins d'ardeur aux désirs, laisse plus de confiance dans les vertus," p. 2).

That Thomas is also familiar with the conclusions of the later, Montpellier-inspired physiological texts on women is clear when he refers to how the natural "weakness" of women's organs (a category that includes, as mentioned above, the brain) causes them to be highly nervous and to receive a multitude of (distracting) sensations. He also echoes the physiologists in remarking that while this organic "fluidity" gives rise to French women's soft beauty and attractive gaiety, it prevents "cette attention forte et soutenue qui peut combiner de suite une longue chaîne d'idées; attention qui anéantit tous les objets pour ne voir qu'un et le voir tout entier" (p. 42). Women, however well educated, however capable of producing creative works (novels and poetry, in particular), serve as the charming accoutrements of an advanced society, not as its engines. An educated woman is a sign of her society's moral health, for Thomas, and of its placement on the top rung of the ladder of civilization. While she does not help to ascend a single rung of this ladder, she embodies the pleasures inherent in the attainment of this goal, a goal programmed into the instincts of the male of the human species, we are to understand. Women may thus be viewed as "mirrors" of their culture, and this mirroring includes their educational levels and their production of literary and other texts.

Thomas's historical overview presents the women of ancient Greece, unsurprisingly, as among the first to enjoy the pleasures of a developed culture, although he postulates that courtesans were a necessary outlet for a masculine population that enjoyed the arts as much as did Greek men. These "public" women, that is, allowed the virtuous wives to spend their days in a soul-fortifying "retreat" (p. 7). Roman women are said to have enjoyed a similar austere virtue,

> Renfermées dans leurs maisons; là, dans leur vertu simple & grossière, donnant tout à la nature, & rien à ce qu'on appelle amusements, assez barbares pour ne savoir être qu'épouses & mères, chastes sans se douter qu'on pût ne pas l'être, sensibles sans jamais avoir appris à définir ce mot, occupées de devoirs, & ignorant qu'il y eût d'autres plaisirs (p. 19).

Their ignorance protected them, that is, from the burgeoning decadence that would eventually destroy their culture. Six hundred years of such development is said to have led, however, to such a steep decline in morals that even these virtuous matrons would be affected:

> Cette dernière révolution se fit sous les Empereurs, & mille causes y contribuèrent. La grande inégalité des rangs, l'excès des fortunes, le ridicule attaché dans ces cours aux idées morales, & à Rome l'excès des âmes fortes, impétueuses dans le mal comme dans le bien, tout précipita la corruption (pp. 14-15).

The entrance of Christianity onto the European scene around the third century is, of course, presented as a force for good where women were concerned, primarily in that it strengthened the bonds of marriage (p. 21). But the "surprise" that follows—a surprise only for those not familiar with the commonplaces of this version of the history of French civilization, that is—comes when the "barbarians" invade, following the fall of Rome. "Jamais peut-être il n'y eut de révolution plus singulière," we are told, for it was these

> sauvages qui portèrent avec les embrasements & les ruines, l'esprit de galanterie qui règne encore aujourd'hui en Europe: & le système qui nous a fait un principe d'honneur de regarder les femmes comme souveraines, système qui a eu tant d'influence, nous est venu des bords de la mer Baltique & des forêts du nord (p. 24).

One should not be "astonished" by this apparent paradox, Thomas insists, adding, in yet another nod to the primacy of climate, that northern peoples always demonstrate greater respect for women (lower male sex drive, in this case, leading to better treatment; climate theory being, if nothing else, extremely malleable). Thomas also notes that once men have advanced from the first level of savagery to a point where large groups gather and begin to govern themselves,

> les femmes ont naturellement & doivent avoir le plus grand empire. Déjà la société est assez établie pour qu'il y ait en amour des idées de préférence: elle ne l'est point assez pour que les sens soient affaiblis, & l'imagination usée par l'habitude (p. 24).

In France, this stage of development is seen by eighteenth-century commentators as having taken place when the Franks invaded during the senescence of the Roman empire. The influence of the Franks is a key component of the standard narrative on the development of civilization in France, and of particular importance to theorists of nobility. The (unlikely) claim that the blood of the Franks still runs in the veins of the eighteenth-century French *noblesse d'épée* is central to the argument of Henri de Boulainvilliers, the most often cited theorist of nobility in the eighteenth century. In his *Essais sur la noblesse de France, contenant une dissertation sur son origine & abaissement* (Amsterdam: [s.n.], 1732), Boulainvilliers evoked the Franks in order to argue for the overthrow of the absolute monarchy and the return to collective leadership by an elite. For Thomas the "barbarian invasions" mark the point when, no longer under the yoke of Roman rule, the French finally reached a state of cultural adulthood (albeit young adulthood). So strongly do men at this state of societal development begin to feel for women, Thomas declares (foreshadowing the Age of Chivalry as he does so) that for tribes such as the Franks, love for a woman is mixed with "quelque chose de religieux" (p. 25).

Another result of reduced sex drive in the barbarian "hordes" is said to be that less "reserve" is required in communication between the two sexes. As a result, "Pendant des invasions qui durèrent trois ou quatre cents ans, on s'accoutuma à voir les femmes mêlées aux guerriers" (p. 25). In imitation of this practice, the original inhabitants of the area that would one day include France are said to have relaxed their rules concerning the sequestration of women, a change in mores that resulted in the *mixité* considered by such commentators as Buffon and Montesquieu to be the principal delight of French culture.[24] The melding of the superior mores of the "simpler," virtuous, northern Franks with the advancements of Gallo-

Roman culture resulted in a unique, superior cultural configuration, we are to understand. After a period of strife and conflict (Christianity needing to triumph, among other issues), the descendants of the Frankish invaders—the ancestors of the eighteenth-century French nobility—acted to establish a regulated society, in the absence of a public will to do so on the part of the mass of (one assumes) Gaulish folk ("pour faire ensemble ce que la force publique ne faisait pas, ou faisit mal," p. 26). Along with instigating principles of hospitality inspired by the Romans ("comme faisaient autrefois les Hercule & les Thésée"), these proto-Frenchmen established rules concerning the role of women in society inspired by their Frankish ancestors, and designed above all to "défendre l'honneur & les droits du sexe le plus faible, contre le sexe impérieux, qui souvent opprime & outrage l'autre" (p. 27).

On to the Renaissance, and page after page of examples and edifying notes in which Thomas stresses the intellectual production of European women during this period and the corresponding outpouring of books by men recognizing the accomplishments of such women. He then proceeds to undermine women's accomplishments during this time, not only by declaring that the rare, true genius—he who transforms knowledge—is indeed always a "he," but also by making a sharp turn toward the physiological:

> Il semble que pour terminer cette grande question d'amour-propre & de rivalité entre les sexes, il faudrait examiner la force ou la faiblesse des organes; le genre d'éducation dont les deux sexes sont susceptibles; le but de la nature en les formant (p. 42).

Woman's role—designated by nature, and confirmed by Thomas's historical overview—is not to move society forward, as do men of true, globalizing genius (however rare), but rather to soften men's virile edge and to add charm to their lives.

Following a lengthy digression on whether women are capable of love and friendship, Thomas returns to his historical overview. We see Chivalry, the ultimate byproduct of the Frankish invasion, die out in Europe. Its death throes come last in France, with the blame assigned to François I, who during his reign (1515-1547) is said to have given "le signal de la corruption" that would lead even the French to abandon gallantry, albeit centuries later (p. 63). A different sort of *mixité*, that of the classes, will cause the French to begin treating their women badly, for as Thomas follows the downfall of "la galanterie," he insists above all on the invisible moral barriers that had previously kept the estates separate.

The vices of the court stayed at the court, while the "grossièreté" of the lower ranks served to keep the nobles safe from their debasing influence. "Mais sous Louis XIV tout changea […] tout se rapprocha" (p. 69). By the Regency, and after six centuries of triumph, French "galanterie" is said to have degenerated quite entirely, replaced by "un sentiment vil, qui supposa toutes les faiblesses, ou les fit naître" (p. 78). With fewer barriers holding them apart, men and women spend far too much time together, and as a result, "les deux sexes se dénaturent"—lose, that is, their complementary specificity. More and more drawn into society, women stopped spending time at home ("dans la retraite") and as a result become "moins épouses et mères" (p.79). Little wonder, Thomas observes, that there are few panegyrics written to the fair sex today by men in whom "une habitude froide et factice, ne réveille plus nulle part ni l'imagination ni l'esprit" (p. 83).

It is at this concluding point that Thomas evokes the young Beauty who chooses to stay at home rather than chase lovers in high society, "tour-à-tour pressant dans ses bras ou sur son sein le fils qu'elle nourrit de son lait, tandis que l'époux en silence partage ses regards attendris entre le fils & la mère" (p. 84). This young paragon is, significantly, also a reader, perhaps even a writer, but engages in these activities for their own value, "non pour une réputation vaine et frivole" (p. 86). How preferable is this life of quiet retreat, Thomas concludes, to "cette vie inquiète & turbulente, où l'on court sans cesse après un sentiment qu'on ne trouve point! Ah!," we are told, on a brief note of meliorism, "c'est alors que les femmes recouvreraient leur empire" (p. 85).

Thomas does acknowledge the existence of one contemporary French woman writer, Françoise de Graffigny, referring to her as "une femme de beaucoup d'esprit" (p. 96). He refers specifically to Graffigny's *Lettres d'une Péruvienne* (1747), one of the century's best-selling novels, and a work in which the sad state of eighteenth-century French womanhood is put into relief by a comparison to a princess of the Golden Age of the Incas (the anachronism was deliberate, if a bit unsettling).[25] The first-person narrative covers the travels and travails of Zilia, and opens with her dramatic kidnapping by Spanish soldiers (conquistadors) intent on plundering the gold-filled Temple of the Sun in which she has spent her life. Torn from her homeland and her fiancé, Aza, by these marauding thugs, on her wedding day no less, Zilia is placed on a ship bound for Spain that is in its turn attacked by a French warship. In a letter to Aza, she describes these kidnappers as far more benevolent and attractive, indeed as a race that seemingly escaped from Nature's hand "lorsqu'il n'était encore entré dans leur composition que l'air et le feu" (water and earth, those heavier elements, being left out of their makeup).[26] Thomas quips that this description applies to French women only, but that Graffigny has attributed it to French men as well in an attempt to keep the "secret" of her sex. Rather than a gendered observation, however, Zilia's impression of the French is very much a contrast between nations (understood as racial types), for the Spanish are said to be "composés de la matière des plus durs métaux" (p. 34).

Zilia's initially flattering portrayal of the French is quickly replaced by a more tempered judgment, based on the common criticism that the French are all about appearances and neglect the reality of their moral and intellectual states. Installed in the Parisian home of her savior (and suitor), the noble Déterville, Zilia encounters declining European mores on a grand scale. Among the "discoveries" that Zilia makes once she is established in France and able to speak and read French is that this alien culture's men have abandoned the type of gallantry that Thomas characterizes as central to the heyday of the French aristocracy. Not that French women are worthy of much respect, for Zilia (presented as having received a superior education in Peru) laments the weak intellectual development of the women who surround her.

The true cause of the decline in French morals is given in Letter XXIX, one of the two harshly critical letters added to the 1752 edition of the novel. Giving us a fictionalized rendition of Boulainvilliers's ode to the virtues of the original French nobility, and painting, as will Thomas and so many other writers, an appealing portrait of the Golden Age of French (elite) morals, Graffigny has Zilia recount a typical conversation, in the course of which her companions

> [...] insultent gaiment à la mémoire de leurs ancêtres, dont la sage économie se contentait de vêtements commodes, de parures et d'ameublements proportionnés à leurs revenus plus qu'à leur naissance. Leur famille, dit-on, et leurs domestiques jouissaient d'une abondance frugale et honnête. Ils dotaient leurs filles et ils établissaient sur des fondements solides la fortune du successeur de leur nom, et tenaient en réserve de quoi réparer l'infortune d'un ami, ou d'un malheureux (pp. 121-122).

Zilia writes that this description of French ancestral practices left her feeling as if she were again among the virtuous Peruvians; she is rudely awakened from her reverie when her spoken admiration for this frugal lifestyle is met with peals of laughter.

Graffigny's Zilia can be seen as a precursor of such characters as the heroine of Chamfort's *Jeune Indienne* (1764), quoted in the epigraph above as to her astonishment at the physical weakness of the European women she observes during her first visit to the Anglo-American colony of "Charles Town." She is with the hero of the play, one Belton, a young man of British descent who has just returned after having been stranded in the wilderness for five years. Belton owes his survival during this ordeal to the young Indian woman, whom he calls "Betti." He is nevertheless about to break with her, in order to set himself up in a style that will permit him to count for something in white society. Betti is quite confused when the man she considers to be her husband attempts to explain to her why they need money. He tells her that it is impossible for her to work the land as she has been doing, for in his world, "On épargne à ton sexe un travail odieux."[27] Ah, that clarifies something, says Betti, for I have already noticed how languid and debilitated your women are; why, I've seen two who are positively immobile. To Betti's suggestion that Belton now repay her by doing the fieldwork necessary to keep them alive in white society, he explains that doing so would shame him. He must marry another. "O ciel!" Betti cries, have I not risked shipwreck for you, have I not saved you from (highly unlikely) tigers, and from starvation, on a daily basis? To the spectator's relief, in something of a *deus ex machina*, Belton's Quaker (and therefore simple and virtuous) uncle overhears this conversation and saves the day by handing over 50,000 *écus* (money he just happens to owe to Belton's father).

That the couple is mixed race is a moot point, because "Betti" is no less French than Zilia. The true difference between Belton and his bride is chronological, for she is of a different, better "age of man." The pre-Romantic nature of this rather overwrought play does not overshadow the very eighteenth-century concerns it reveals—Betti is no sentimental Atala, in other words. There are several revealing similarities between these two *jeunes indiennes*, but the most important aspect of Betti's character, indeed, the one point that brings her alive as an interesting individual, is the least "romantic" of her qualities: her ability, indeed her eagerness, to engage in hard, physical labor. Just as Zilia's exceptional and anachronistic "health" is indicated by the state of her fine mind and her unshakeable moral virtue, Betti, imagined later in the century, possesses a physical energy that is a reproach to the supposedly sedentary lives of eighteenth-century French women. Like Belton, these women are presented as the debilitated products of an over-civilized society obsessed with appearance and legalisms, and blind to what really matters.

Chamfort's emphasis on the physically debilitating nature of the lifestyle of contemporary French women (displaced as English in his play) is indicative of the increasingly medical nature of the causes diagnosed as driving the degeneration of the French women during the 1760s and 1770s. The assumption that these symptoms might be reversed by proper hygiene—that is, sufficient exercise and a proper diet, alongside the avoidance of lascivious cultural productions—reveals a simultaneous shift from a concern with the morality of the French nobility (as epitomized by Graffigny) to the health of the French population as a whole.

In the following decades, women's health will be pushed to the background, alongside their importance to the history of their culture. Works on the "natural history of women" do not disappear any time soon, and indeed continue well into the nineteenth century. Jacques Moreau de la Sarthe's *Histoire naturelle de la femme, suivie d'un traité d'hygiène*, 3 volumes (Paris: Duprat, Letellier, 1803) is one example, in addition to a work by Julien-Joseph Virey some twenty years later, *De la femme sous ses rapports physiologique, moral, et littéraire* (Paris: Crochard, 1823). Overall however, women are of less interest to social commentators as the Revolution nears.

One example of this disappearance of what had been something of a cultural obsession is Jean-Nicolas Démeunier's *L'Esprit des usages et des coutumes des différents peuples, ou Observations tirées des Voyageurs & des Historiens* (Paris: Pissot, 1776). Démeunier was of a later generation than the authors considered above—he was only twenty-four when this work was published—and thus better represents the values of the coming Revolution, in which he would play an important role.[28] The basic tenet of *L'Esprit* is that the "progress" of civilization is accompanied by an increase in folly, caprice, and corruption. Démeunier's goal is to trace how this process has led, over time and with increasing intensity, to the development of perverse cultural practices that run counter to "nature's" logic. Women are important to Démeunier's argument, but only to the extent that they become increasingly necessary to men as civilization develops. They are not even given primacy of place as a need, however, for Book Two, "Des Femmes," follows on the heels of the topic treated in Book One: food ("Aliments, Repas").

The diminution of the role of women is also evident in the far more hopeful vision of mankind's "progress" presented in Condorcet's *Esquisse d'un tableau historique des progrès de l'esprit humain* (1793-1794). Condorcet wrote this work in hiding, and would soon die in somewhat mysterious circumstances in a prison cell, but in his *Esquisse* he remains positive about the long-term future of the human race. He asks three preliminary questions: Are some countries doomed to remain uncivilized? Is class inequality a necessary result of the civilizing process? Will the human race as a whole continue to progress? His answer:

> En répondant à ces trois questions, nous trouverons, dans l'expérience du passé, dans l'observation des progrès que les sciences, que la civilisation ont faits jusqu'ici, dans l'analyse de la marche de l'esprit humain et du développement de ses facultés, les motifs les plus forts de croire que la nature n'a mis aucun terme à nos espérances.[29]

Condorcet was of course one of the few Revolutionary figures to argue that women should be educated to the same degree as men, but he mentions women only infrequently in his study, as when he remarks that the servitude to which women are everywhere subject is attenuated as societies develop.[30] Women no longer serve as cultural barometers, and even the medical theoreticians of this time focus rather on the maladies (and thus the potential rejuvenation) of French men. In an essay on what would become better known as hysteria (*Recherches sur les vapeurs*, 1789), the Montpellier doctor Joseph Bressy speaks almost exclusively of how this illness manifests itself in men, mentioning women only briefly at the end of his study (women, said to be possessed of "extra" organs—those of generation and lactation—necessarily, we are told, exhibit more symptoms).[31] Such "causes" of hysteria cannot be removed, but Bressy's focus is after all not on "curing" women but rather on inspiring his male readers to emulate their ancestors, who had vanquished the Romans:

> [...] rappelle ce caractère qui te donnait, & par tes formes & par ton âme, la supériorité sur les maîtres du monde; bientôt le nom de vapeurs te sera étranger comme à eux. La mollesse, le luxe, l'énervation, le défaut d'âme, ont fait de ton cerveau, triste Sardanapale, un organe débile qui, usé dès ton enfance par les jouissances, ne peut plus être sensible qu'aux douleurs; redonne lui cette vigueur qui doit chasser cette cause physique qui, l'abreuvant, t'occasionne tant de maux.[32]

The role of contemporary French women, in this exhortation, is that of consorts to the Persian King Sardanapalus: so many accessories to his sloth and self-indulgence, rather than the center of attention in themselves.

The insistence by the leaders of the Revolutionary movement that woman's place was in the home, raising the perfected *citoyens* of the future, marks a radical turn in the French cultural imagination. The idea that the sequestration of women was a cure for what ailed society was of course present in the vitalist hygiene treatises, as well as in Rousseau's *Emile* and even, to a lesser degree, in Thomas's *Essai*. Of the examples given above, only Graffigny's Zilia—created, we note, by a woman author of noble birth, if limited means, writing in the 1740s—escapes the domestic maternal scenes celebrated in the other examples I have considered. Zilia does of course sequester herself in a home in the country.

A severe yet clairvoyant judge of French society, she deliberately chooses to withdraw from contact with a culture she finds so lacking in moral purity and intellectual interest. But the conditions of her retreat, in terms of both her material comfort and, more importantly, her independence (she refuses to marry Déterville), are important to note: Zilia will live out her life as the unattached, very wealthy lady of a considerable estate, attended to by devoted peasants who are as "simple" and virtuous as any imaginary Peruvian serfs. Most importantly, for this product of a French woman's imagination, isolation from cultural influences is not the precondition for Zilia's virtue—it is the consequence of her virtue.

Notes

[1] On the topic of European degeneracy, see Sean M. Quinlan, *The Great Nation in Decline: Sex, Modernity and Health Crises in Revolutionary France c. 1750-1850* (Aldershot, UK: Ashgate, 2007) and Michael Winston, *From Perfectibility to Perversion: Meliorism in Eighteenth-Century France* (New York: Peter Lang, 2005).

[2] See my recent study of the supposed relationship between premature puberty (brought on by lascivious encounters) and the perception of the physical and moral decline in the young women of eighteenth-century France: *Female Sexuality and Cultural Degradation in Enlightenment France: Medicine and Literature* (Burlington, VT: Ashgate, 2012).

[3] On the centrality of vitalism to eighteenth-century medical theory, see especially Roselyne Rey, *Naissance et développement du vitalisme en France de la deuxième moitié du XVIIIe siècle à la fin du Premier Empire* (Oxford: Voltaire Foundation, 2000), and Elizabeth A. Williams, *The Physical and the Moral: Anthropology, Physiology, and Philosophical Medicine in France, 1750-1850* (Cambridge: Cambridge University Press, 1994).

[4] Novelists who portrayed the results of this cultural degradation found a ready audience, although their heroines, not unexpectedly, tended to represent the exception to the rule. Rousseau's Julie of *La Nouvelle Héloïse* (1761), whom he placed in the relatively protected setting of the "foothills of the Swiss Alps," was the most popular eighteenth-century example of the exceptional woman struggling to live well in a corrupt world, while the infamous Marquise de Merteuil of the *Liaisons dangereuses* (1782) represented the full embodiment of cultural degradation, in contrast to her virtuous and (therefore) doomed rival, Mme de Tourvel.

[5] Andrew Curran, *The Anatomy of Blackness: Science and Slavery in an Age of Enlightenment* (Baltimore: The Johns Hopkins University Press, 2011).

[6] "Le climat le plus tempéré est depuis le 40me degré jusqu'au 50me, c'est aussi sous cette zone que se trouvent les hommes les plus beaux" (George-Louis Leclerc, Comte de Buffon, *Histoire naturelle, générale et particulière, avec la description*

du cabinet du roi, 36 vols. [Paris: Imprimerie Royale, 1749-1788], vol. 3, p. 528). Future references will be given in the text.

[7] Michael Winston emphasizes both the malleability and the perfectibility of race in Buffon: "Buffon contends the human organism is a malleable entity subject to virtually unlimited 'perfectibility.' Realizing this potential, however, depends on the ability to isolate and subsequently manipulate the factors (climate, diet, etc.) that influence human development." See *From Perfectibility to Perversion*, p. 4.

[8] For an analysis of the philosophical basis for the Buffonian *moule intérieur*, see Peter Hanns Reill, *Vitalizing Nature in the Enlightenment* (Berkeley: University of California Press, 2005), p. 47.

[9] Buffon, *Histoire naturelle*, vol. 3, pp. 446-447.

[10] The Jalofe women of Senegal are a rare exception. Said to live between two rivers (such details are key), they are described as "bien proportionnez, et d'une taille assez avantageuse, les traits de leur visage sont moins durs que ceux des autres Nègres [...] il y a parmi eux d'aussi belles femmes, à la couleur près" (Buffon, *Histoire naturelle*, vol. 3, p. 457).

[11] Buffon, *Histoire naturelle*, vol. 6, pp. 8-9.

[12] On Buffon's complex relationship to the philosophy of the Montpellier School, see Roselyne Rey, "Buffon et le vitalisme," in *Buffon 88: Actes du Colloque international pour le bicentenaire de la mort de Buffon* (Paris: J. Vrin, 1992), pp. 399-413.

[13] "Sometime in the eighteenth century, sex as we know it was invented" (Thomas W. Laqueur, *Making Sex: Body and Gender from the Greeks to Freud* [Cambridge: Harvard University Press, 1990], p. 149).

[14] *From Perfectibility to Perversion*, p. 104. The work in question is Pierre Roussel's *Système physique et moral de la femme, ou tableau philosophique de la constitution, de l'état organique, du tempérament, des moeurs, & des fonctions propres au sexe* (Paris: Vincent, 1775).

[15] Joseph Raulin, *Traité des fleurs blanches* (Paris: Herissant, 1766), p. 145. I have modernized the spelling of this and other quotes given in the text of this article.

[16] Raulin, *Traité*, p. 146; p. v.

[17] "C'est de la faiblesse des organes qu'est provenue la plus grande partie des maladies. L'oisiveté est une des principales causes: le mêlange de différens peuples les a multipliées; les richesses, surtout celles des grandes Indes, en ont rendu plusieurs héréditaires, plus fréquentes & plus dangereuses par les drogues incendiaires qu'on en retire, & dont on abuse" (Raulin, *Traité*, p. v).

[18] P. Virard, *Essai sur la santé des filles nubiles* (Londres et se trouve à Paris chez Monory, 1776), p. 11.

[19] Virard, *Essai*, p. 12.

[20] J.D.T. Bienville, *De la nymphomanie ou Traité de la fureur utérine* (Amsteram, Marc-Michel Rey, 1771). Future references will be given in the text. Other influential works of this type include Pierre Roussel, *Système physique et moral de la femme, ou Tableau philosophique de la Constitution, de l'Etat organique, du Tempérament, des Moeurs, & des Fonctions propres au Sexe* (Paris: Vincent, 1775); Guillaume Daignan, *Tableau des variétés de la vie humaine*, 2 vols. (Paris:

chez l'Auteur, 1786); and M. Desessartz, *Traité de l'éducation corporelle des enfans en bas âge, ou Réflexions-pratiques sur les moyens de procurer une meilleure constituion aux Citoyens* (Paris: Herissant, 1760).

[21] Liselotte Steinbrügge, *The Moral Sex: Woman's Nature in the French Enlightenment*, trans. Patricia Selwyn (New York: Oxford University Press, 1995), p. 35.

[22] Antoine-Léonard Thomas, *Essai sur le caractère, les moeurs, et l'esprit des femmes dans les différens siècles* (Paris: Champion, 1987), p. 4. Future references will be given in the text.

[23] Montesquieu, *De l'esprit des lois*, in *Oeuvres complètes*, 2 vols., ed. Roger Caillois (Paris: Gallimard, 1949), pp. 509-510.

[24] "Il est heureux de vivre dans ces climats qui permettent qu'on se communique; où le sexe qui a le plus d'agréments semble parer la société; et où les femmes, se réservant aux plaisirs d'un seul, servent encore à l'amusement de tous" (Montesquieu, *De l'esprit des lois*, vol. 2, p. 517).

[25] The popularity of Graffigny's novel was rivaled, Janet Altman has observed, only by that of *La Nouvelle Héloïse* and *Candide* ("A Woman's Place in the Enlightenment Sun: The Case of F. de Graffigny," *Romance Quarterly* 38.3 [August 1991]: 261-272, 261).

[26] Françoise de Graffigny, *Lettres d'une Péruvienne* (New York: Modern Language Association, 1993), p. 61. Future references will be in the text.

[27] Nicolas Chamfort, *La Jeune Indienne*, in *Oeuvres complètes*, 2 vols. (Paris: Sandre, 2009), vol. 1, p. 283.

[28] A Mason and strong supporter of the American Revolution, Démeunier served as a deputy of the Third Estate during the Estates General of 1789 and was later President of the National Constituant Assembly, before fleeing to the United States during the Terror. He returned to serve Napoleon, and is now entombed in the Pantheon.

[29] Jean-Antoine-Nicolas de Caritat, marquis de Condorcet, *Esquisse d'un tableau historique des progrès de l'esprit humain* (Paris: J. Vrin, 1970), p. 195.

[30] The moment arrives in the "Deuxième époque: Les peuples pasteurs," at least for richer women: "Les moeurs durent s'adoucir; l'esclavage des femmes eut moins de dureté; les femmes des riches cessèrent d'être condamnées à des travaux pénibles" (Condorcet, *Esquisse*, p. 54).

[31] Joseph Bressy, *Recherches sur les vapeurs* (Paris: Planche, 1789), pp. 134-135.

[32] Bressy, *Recherches sur les vapeurs*, pp. 84-85.

CHAPTER THREE

TOWARDS THE NEW MEDICINE: NICOLAS CHAMBON DE MONTAUX'S CONTRIBUTIONS TO THE *ENCYCLOPÉDIE MÉTHODIQUE*

KATHLEEN HARDESTY DOIG

We know very little about how eighteenth-century encyclopedias were actually read. Surviving subscriber lists identify some of the owners but not the articles they read or their reactions to them, except in rare instances.[1] References made in correspondences and publications are of course the best proof that purchasers actually read these texts, but specific mentions are relatively few in number. Other indications of reading are somewhat nebulous but convincing in the aggregate. The fact that thousands of sets of encyclopedias continued to be purchased throughout Europe suggests that there was a genuine reading public for them, since subscribers of the time were perhaps less prone than some of their modern descendants to make these enormously expensive investments mainly for show. Subscribers of the eighteenth century also continued to favor the alphabetical organization for encyclopedias, which greatly facilitated locating specific points of interest; they generally won out over scientific critics of this format, who lamented its destruction of a unified presentation of knowledge on a given subject.

The parts of an encyclopedia that were read in each household no doubt depended on the interests of its particular members. To speak for the moment only of the *Encyclopédie*,[2] an analysis of its technical information in areas such as military strategy, mathematics and industrial processes suggests that the work could serve as a resource for many professionals. Amateur collectors could find useful classificatory information about their plants, shells or coins. Readers with intellectual interests could find background on philosophy, literary rules, or any of dozens of other topics.

All of these offerings were magnified in the *Encyclopédie méthodique*, the huge revision and reconceptualization of the *Encyclopédie* that began to appear in 1782 under the direction of the publishing magnate Charles Joseph Panckoucke. The methodical format of this new encyclopedia consisted of individual subject dictionaries.[3] Specialist editors were in charge of each dictionary, assisted by collaborators as necessary. Panckoucke claimed that the *Méthodique* would have approximately 100,000 more articles than the *Encyclopédie*.[4] In reality the number is far more, since the originally projected forty-six volumes of text expanded to approximately 177, accompanied by twenty-six volumes of plates.[5] The publishing timeline was extended in equally stunning proportions, from the anticipated five years to exactly fifty, with the last installments delivered on 29 September 1832.

The dictionary of medicine is responsible for a considerable percentage of the expansion both in number of volumes and in the number of years required for completion of the entire encyclopedia. Originally projected to be two to three volumes and slated to be completed, along with the rest of the encyclopedia, by 1787, *Médecine* did not even begin to appear until that year. By the time of its completion in 1832, *Médecine* filled not two to three volumes but thirteen.[6] As recent scholarship has demonstrated, the decades around the turn of the nineteenth century were a pivotal moment in medical thought, as a clinical, empirical approach replaced the systematizing of earlier times. The training of physicians evolved to correspond, the pharmacopoeia became less fanciful, and new fields such as mental illness were delineated.[7] *Médecine*, written and published during this seminal period, reflects the changes that were underway, fulfilling its promise to be an up-to-date work composed by a team of specialists. The six editors who successively edited *Médecine* were all prominent, from the first, Félix Vicq d'Azyr, an important anatomist and physician, to the last, Auguste Thillaye, author of several medical texts. The team of collaborators numbered at least seventy over time and included many names that figure prominently in the history of medicine.[8]

The size of the team is explained by the range of sub-areas delineated by Vicq d'Azyr and maintained by all the editors: personal and public health; pathology; semiotics and nosology; therapeutic medicine; military medicine; veterinary medicine; forensics; regulations concerning medicine; mental illness (added as of volume 10); and biographies of important physicians. As in the *Méthodique* project as a whole, where many subjects resisted compartmentalization in a single dictionary, so also articles in *Médecine* often did not fit neatly under one of these ten headings, two of which in fact—military and veterinary medicine—were actually sub-groups of pathology.[9] Nor did each of the ten areas receive the same proportion of coverage. The biographies and the articles on regulations constitute relatively minor wings of the dictionary, for example, while pathology, often with the article designation "Médecine pratique," is dominant, used with perhaps two-thirds of the entries.

The prospectus elaborated on pathology by featuring a list, printed in italics for emphasis, of various illnesses that would be covered in this area by experienced specialists in *Médecine*: "*Les maladies des prisons & des armées, les maladies vénériennes, celles des gens de mer, celles des femmes & des enfans, celles des artisans, celles des animaux, celles des yeux, celles qui sont propres aux différens climats & aux saisons, les lésions que produisent les maladies des blés*" (*Beaux-arts*, vol. 1, p. xii). We note, wedged here between sailors and artisans, the category of women and children. That it represented a vast swathe of the population as compared with the other categories listed, and that women and children represent quite disparate groups whose alliance in a single phrase suggests that the author conflated them to some extent, are observations that a modern reader makes. An original subscriber was probably more likely to be impressed by the very existence of the category, with its implication that this was a modern work presenting medical advances which were improving the chances that children would survive the first several years of their lives,[10] and that their mothers would survive the process of bringing them into the world as well as the other diseases that threatened women of the time.

The verso of the title page of *Médecine* lists major contributors in various areas. Among them is "Chambon, Les maladies des femmes." Nicolas Chambon de Montaux was not the only contributor in this area—others include Augustin Olivier Mahon and Louis Charles Henri Macquart—but Chambon's prominent billing here and the number of articles he contributed, approximately forty,[11] several of which are more than ten pages, make him the major contributor on women's illnesses and health care. His articles are of interest from several perspectives. They reveal the limits of medical care available to the late eighteenth-century woman because of the limits of medical knowledge at the time, and to some extent they reveal the gender biases of the age and the theorizing approach characteristic of virtually all French physicians in the preceding centuries. But the corpus of Chambon's articles also shows very clearly how medicine was evolving towards a modern form that stresses clinical observation and evaluation of multiple types of data. As Joseph Génévrier notes of Chambon's medical writings,

> En somme nous nous trouvons en présence de deux tendances bien différentes; ce contraste se retrouve à chaque instant dans les ouvrages de Chambon; tantôt il obéit à la tradition, tantôt il s'abandonne aux nouveaux courants d'idées; il appartenait à une époque de transition, son œuvre est également *une œuvre de transition.*[12]

Because Chambon writes in the first person and recounts many case histories from his own practice, and because he expresses firmly held views, a sense of the personality of this physician also emerges from his contributions to *Médecine*. The full biography, especially of his later years, adds dimensions to this portrait that are surprising at first glance, less so when the historical context is considered. Chambon was born in Champagne on 21 September 1748, to a surgeon and a mother descended from an ancestor who had been ennobled under Louis XIV for battlefield heroism—hence the "de Montaux" often attached to Chambon's name. The son's medical studies consisted first of lessons learned by observing his father and later of a formal course of study in Paris. He returned to Langres for a short while and then opened a practice in Paris that became increasingly successful. Chambon also devoted considerable time to the hospitals and was named an official physician of Salpêtrière in 1786. From his earliest days, Chambon had been an indefatigable collector of clinical data, which led to the publication of a series of works in the 1780s on the illnesses of women and girls.[13] There is overlap between these books and his contributions to the *Méthodique*, which began during this same decade. But the *Méthodique* contributions are not a mere regurgitation of the earlier publications; he edits the material and, as we shall see, adds references to cases encountered after the books were published.[14] In 1790 Chambon lost the Salpêtrière post, perhaps because of his *Notice sur les Moyens de rendre les hôpitaux utiles à la Nation* (Paris, 1787), in which he criticized the organization and management of the hospital as well as the disproportionate preponderance of surgeons over medical doctors in an establishment where illnesses far outnumbered surgical cases.[15] In 1791, at the age of forty-two, he married Augustine-Épiphanie Barbe Bateste, age nineteen, a union apparently of both heart and mind and which survived the many trials that they were to endure.

Chambon, who frequented liberal circles, supported many of the reforms proposed during the early phase of the Revolution and by late 1792 was playing a public role in events, as the administrator of Paris taxes and finances. Two additional posts were offered to Chambon, those of hospital inspector and of chief inspector of the army. But the physician declined both, although he was apparently proud of the nominations because he signed documents with these titles for the rest of his life. The title which has made his name appear in histories of the Revolution was acquired on 8 December 1792: the moderate Gironde elected Chambon mayor of Paris. He struggled to keep order in the city and to save the king as the radical Montagne became more powerful. He failed, of course, and took the dangerous step of resigning on 4 February 1793, a few weeks after the execution of the king.[16] Chambon and his wife managed to escape to Blois but were eventually arrested and imprisoned. They were released after Robespierre's fall and remained in Blois, where Chambon resumed practicing medicine and doing research. He published a second edition of *Maladies des femmes* and a treatise on vaccination, the latter interest occasioned by his wife's nearly fatal case of smallpox. His health, never robust, steadily worsened, so he tried to obtain a government post that would provide better income with less stress than a demanding provincial practice. But Chambon was not successful, even after the couple returned to Paris in 1803.[17] They appear to have welcomed the Restoration. Mme Chambon had come into possession of a lock of Marie-Antoinette's hair and returned it in 1814 to the late queen's daughter, the Duchesse d'Angoulême, who seems to have rewarded the donor for her good deed. Mme Chambon further indicated her political allegiance by publishing a book-length defense of the divine right of kings, *Réflexions morales et politiques sur les avantages de la monarchie* (Paris: P. Didot l'Aîné, 1819). Chambon continued to produce medical manuscripts, none of which he managed to publish. He died on 2 November 1826, in straitened circumstances. His widow was saved from penury by a small pension provided by the Duchesse d'Angoulême.

In the following pages, we shall examine articles by Chambon on the physical constitution of women and the various illnesses to which they are subject. In a second section, we shall concentrate on key concepts in articles related to pregnancy and childbirth. As we shall see, Chambon's approach to medicine is based on several theoretical constructs. There is first a physiological underpinning. He attempts to describe the exact site in the body of the medical problem under discussion. The extensive knowledge of anatomy demonstrated here was acquired in part through performing autopsies, which he mentions frequently. Secondly, like many contemporaries, he continued to adhere to a humoralist theory going back to Antiquity.[18] According to this interpretation of phenomena, the movement, quantity and type of fluids in the body explain its functions and malfunctions. Another major influence reflected in Chambon's work was the vitalist theory propounded at the Montpellier École de Médecine. Elizabeth A. Williams summarizes the scientific ideas of these physicians as follows:

> the Montpellier vitalists posited an absolute distinction between living, 'organized' being and brute, inert matter. They attributed this life to the action of a force, principle, or power whose origin and ontological status were unknowable. They saw life as enabled by the interrelated and harmonious activities of the 'body economy' and as engaged in a constant struggle against processes of disharmony, destruction, and disintegration commonly conceived of as illness. They perceived ceaseless interactions of internal disposition and external milieu that eventuated in distinctive human types formed by age, sex, temperament, region, and other powerful influences on the vital economy.[19]

These influences are much in evidence in "Constitution des femmes" (*Médecine*, vol. 4, p. 88). Chambon begins with a physiological description of the internal differences between the female and the male, such as less voluminous muscles and more supple veins in the female, as well as of the more obvious external differences. Humoralism comes into play at several points, for example, women's greater serosity is said to make them more subject to colds and related ailments; it also rounds out their bone structure in pleasing ways, and it is responsible for their hair lasting longer than men's. Having established that physical differences between the sexes exist and having attempted to explain their causes, Chambon places the female in a social context and analyzes the role of nurture (what he calls "des institutions humaines," *Médecine*, vol. 4, p. 91). Well-versed in ancient authors, who are referred to in nearly every article, he turns to them for observations that contradicted contemporary views of the inferiority of women—the views that would become the established norm for decades to come. According to Chambon, the Greeks knew that women required exercise as much as men in order to promote both physical health and mental acuity, and were thus able to produce not just eminent women poets, who developed the natural feminine proclivities for imagination, but also eminent women scientists and intellectuals who excelled in the pursuits "qui exigent plus d'application & de savoir réel" (*Médecine*, vol. 4, p. 92). The Romans took a different view, however, and promoted mental improvement through physical training only for men; their great women are distinguished for their virtue, not their learning. Chambon does not make an explicit connection at this point with the physical degradation of modern woman and the concomitant wasted potential of this half of the species, but the implication is obvious.

The modern female's physical life is then summarized in a narrative characterized by the affective terms and physiological personifications that enliven many of Chambon's texts. Nature makes the woman walk, he says, "à côté d'un précipice prêt à l'engloutir"; the power "qui a voulu que son cœur se livrât aux charmes de l'amour" hides from her "les cruels & périlleux travaux de l'enfantement"; old age brings circulatory perturbations, "ces affections terribles," that are quite simply incurable (*Médecine*, vol. 4, p. 93). These dangers are compounded by modern customs, at least those practiced among the better-off. Chambon's recurring criticism of the unhealthy lifestyle imposed on the urban and/or wealthy female is now forcefully stated. In "Constitution des femmes," the harmful practices include subjecting girls to hours of sedentary needlework and lessons. The boned corsets worn by most of them are especially dangerous, in that they compress the viscera and prevent proper digestion, blood flow to the liver, and breathing. Most girls, says Chambon, "respirent à la manière des agonisants" (*Médecine*, vol. 4, p. 94). Unable to eat properly during meals, they also experience terrible hunger pangs when decorseted at night. These instruments of torture are further blamed in "Gonflement douloureux des seins, sans tumeur contre nature," along with other kinds of metal or wooden plates and tight clothing, for impeding breast development. Chambon notes that the problem is prevalent in religious houses. The constrictions are particularly dangerous if a cancer develops, because the tumor is flattened and spread through a larger area.[20]

A companion text to "Constitution des femmes" is "Filles (Maladies des)." The article repeats Chambon's contentious view that the female body contains a plethora of fluids, especially in the gastric area; that the female's nerves are more sensitive; and that modern lifestyles in certain classes weaken her by blocking various kinds of secretions. Chambon's accounts of where these secretions go are ingenious and theoretical rather than based on empirical data. He believes, for example, that blocked menstrual blood can seep into the lungs and cause pulmonary diseases. A new element that we shall note in other articles appears here: a conflict between natural sexual impulses and moral restrictions on them. In extreme and rare cases, the latter lose, and the girl throws herself "sans ménagement comme sans honte" at the first male she encounters (*Médecine*, vol. 6, p. 401). In less severe cases, the girl suffers from hystericism, which we shall discuss below; even in the mildest attacks, she risks suffering such serious melancholy that she may ultimately lose her mind completely. Lest readers think that masturbation might be a cure for the unmarried young woman, Chambon warns that this "libertinage secret" causes its own devastation (*Médecine*, vol. 6, p. 401).[21]

The ailment of hystericism is covered in the nine-page "Hystéricisme." The article is an excellent example of Chambon's efforts to establish a more exact nosology for diseases, even when the conditions are ill-defined and diffuse. He quotes at length from Aretaeus of Cappodocia, a Greek physician on the numerous possible symptoms of hystericism, including paleness, insensibility and gastric problems among many others. But Chambon is careful to also note Aretaeus's errors, the chief one of which was to regard the uterus as an independent animal capable of moving about in the abdomen, not a muscle. Chambon also distinguishes hystericism from other nervous maladies such as epilepsy and hypocondriacism. Fluid imbalance, in the uterus in this case, is again cited as the cause of an illness, but Chambon adds a new element, the influence of the imagination. It is said to be so strong in some women that hystericism can be exacerbated in them by licentious gatherings and plays or books that remind the woman of sexual pleasure.[22] As for cures, Chambon observes that debauched women are never afflicted with hystericism, but, as a careful observer, he also notes various situations where "marriage" is helpful. More prosaically, irritating odors and various medicines can be used to counteract the disease. Certain mysterious "moyens cruels & indécens" used by the lower classes are alluded to but not explained; Chambon finds them less reliable than other treatments (*Médecine*, vol. 7, p. 459, misprint for p. 457).

A related uterine disorder is described with many rhetorical flourishes in "Fureur uterine." This illness is defined as

> cette fureur avec laquelle une jeune personne, sage et modeste jusqu'à ce moment, se trouve agitée d'un trouble qui anéantit sa raison et qui la précipite dans les désordres d'une luxure effrénée (*Médecine*, vol. 6, p. 536).

Uterine fury differs from hystericism in some ways, for example, the sufferer tends to lose consciousness, but the cause, a plethora of uterine fluids, is similar. The signs of an onset seem to be more the stuff of a novel than a medical article: the young women make constant reference to the men they fancy, their eyes sparkle, they blush and engage in bold behavior, and so forth.[23] These signs and actions can lead to dramatic situations where the young woman commits suicide to avoid dishonor or else abandons all constraints and throws herself at the object of her affections. The conditions that can promote the development of the illness are quite varied. They include a warm climate, the bilious-sanguine temperament (an echo of Chambon's humoralist approach to medicine), rich food, a sedentary life, and warm baths, among others. If attacks are frequent, the woman will likely develop epilepsy or dementia. For Chambon, the essential goal of a cure is to empty uterine fluids as quickly as possible. In convoluted language, he hints that sexual activity is the best cure but notes that it poses other dangers:

> Mais d'un autre côté (sans parler ici des obstacles qui s'y opposent, en suivant les loix qu'une morale austere nous prescrit) quel danger ne resulteroit-il pas de l'usage des moyens qui rempliroient efficacement cette indication? (*Médecine*, vol. 6, p. 538)

Treatments that are more socially acceptable include various pharmaceutical concoctions, opium, and blood-lettings to the point that the woman is weakened.

Better that, perhaps, than "cette multitude de maladies terribles" enumerated again in "Continence (suites de la),"[24] a remarkable article from the pen of a physician ready to overthrow, in the name of nature, an old and deeply held moral code. No more convoluted language here. According to Chambon, the preservation of virginity is perhaps the most difficult virtue to achieve. If you maintain it, he declares to the young women for whose benefit he is writing, "vous éprouverez des maux infinis par la perte de la santé" (*Médecine*, vol. 3, p. 100). He gives a graphic accounting of what may follow:

> Mais que devient une femme qui résiste à tant d'orages? Souvent une épilepsie symptomatique crée une maladie habituelle; le dérangement du cerveau conduit à la folie. L'embarras des viscères du bas-ventre rend une autre mélancolique; de la mélancolie naissent les obstructions, les squirres, le scorbut, l'hydropisie, &c. Voilà donc les fruits de la continence! (*Médecine*, vol. 5, p. 102)

Chambon is skeptical about whether any young woman is able to avoid these effects permanently, for he deems that "la source qui accumule ce feu concentré, lui fournit sans cesse un aliment trop combustible" (*Médecine*, vol. 3, p. 102), and it is certain to erupt eventually in the explosion of the above-mentioned illness, uterine fury. His concluding statement in "Continence (suites de la)" is the challenge of a scientist, made not just to the lower classes named in it and who scorn loose women, but to anyone setting the demands of a harsh moral code against the equally imperious claims of nature:

> Le peuple stupide en son jugement, voit avec mépris celle qui en [uterine fury] est attaquée, tandis que le physicien instruit ne considère en elle que la victime de la vertu (*Médecine*, vol. 5, p. 102).

On a related matter, a section in "Matrice" on genital itching becomes an impassioned discussion about the dangers of masturbation. Causes of this habit include the example of parents expressing affection, since girls want to experience the same feelings they observe in their mothers. So must you edit every action? he asks these mothers. The answer is a resounding affirmative. Also dangerous are concentrated groups of young women, often located near "altars," apparently a reference to convent schools, "ces écoles de débauche," where the adept tutor initiates her charges into debauchery (*Médecine*, vol. 8, p. 635). He sermonizes young women about the increasing degradation into which they will fall, destroying their sense of family and their capacity to feel, leading them ultimately to "traîner dans l'humiliation une vie languissante, jusqu'à ce qu'une mort lente termine vos tribulations," a death that will not even elicit pity from others because of its ignoble cause (*Médecine*, vol. 8, p. 636).

The connection between chastity and the risk of illness is also drawn in other articles.[25] It is probably the most controversial of Chambon's stances against certain cultural practices and taboos, but it is not the only one. We have already mentioned his condemnation of the boned corsets girls were often forced to wear. A more delicate matter is covered in "Gonflement du bas ventre avant la menstruation," the prohibition against invasive vaginal treatments and exams for unmarried women. Chambon makes his case as a man of science interested in improving the health care of women, but also as a practitioner who is fully aware of certain disconnections between improved medicine and deeply held cultural beliefs:

> Cependant, quelque respectable que soit l'usage qui ne tolère l'introduction d'aucun corps étranger dans le vagin avant le mariage, il me semble que la circonstance dont je parle est une exception à cette règle, qu'il seroit dangereux de suivre à la rigueur, puisqu'en s'y soumettant sans réserve on s'exposeroit à des maladies difficiles à détruire et qu'en les prévenant par les moyens que j'ai indiqués, on ne porte aucune atteinte à la pureté des mœurs. Je conclus de cette réflexion que les préjugés doivent ici être subordonnés à la nécessité physique (*Médecine*, vol. 6, p. 663).

Chambon's analyses of two other illnesses that often afflicted younger women also show evidence of a highly theoretical approach that is coupled with a modern emphasis on clinical observations, the latter gathered from his own and other physicians' case histories. Chlorosis, a condition marked by paleness, weakness and lethargy, appears to a modern reader to involve anemia (and cures mentioned by Chambon include iron-rich mineral waters and hearty diets). For Chambon in the eleven-page "Chlorose," the illness occurs when weakness slows circulation and fluids stagnate in both the blood and tissues; the ensuing "fermentation" (a frequent metaphor in these articles) can result in a long list of complaints. The first goal in treatment is to reduce the mass of blood, but Chambon is too experienced and well-read to resort to the most obvious solution for such a problem, bloodlettings. Indeed, he cautions against them in some circumstances and offers various other options. They include vaginal fumigations if the hymen does not need to be preserved, horseback riding in the male style, marriage to bring on blocked menstruation, singing and dancing if the girl belongs to a social class with access to these activities, and a new electrical cure in which electrified tips are placed on affected parts of the body. Chambon ends the article by telling of a case from his own practice, a patient identified as "Mlle Val...," who developed a "trouble moral occasionné par une sédition qui menaçoit la tranquillité des citoyens de son quartier" (*Médecine*, vol. 4, p. 827). Chambon managed to cure her over a period of months by using various treatments and medicines to force blood into her uterus and improve her circulation.[26]

The second malady, covered in "Fleurs blanches," is also explained according to Chambon's theory of fluids: this discharge is a superfluous fluid that needs to be expelled; the physician's job is to facilitate the expulsion. The humoralist theory is also at play here in the recommended treatments, which vary according to whether the temperament of the woman is moist, acrimonious or sanguine. A separate article, "Injections astringents," deals with a specific side issue connected with these discharges, the astringent injections used by some women to stop the flow. Chambon rails against the practice, listing in a frightening catalogue the possible consequences and wondering how "ces vinaigres astringens, de Vénus, de Cythère, &c" are allowed on the market (*Médecine*, vol. 7, p. 597).[27]

For Chambon such treatments hold the same essential dangers as the institutions that command lively young women to preserve their virginity: these treatments and institutions thwart nature's goals for the woman, which he sees as primarily geared to reproduction of the species. Articles on obstetrics and related subjects, not surprisingly, constitute the majority of Chambon's contributions to *Médecine*, and indeed also of the other contributors who wrote on women's health. Cooperating with nature by bearing children does not, however, guarantee nature's unqualified blessing on the process. There remains an important role for nature's assistant, the physician. This is especially true because the unhealthy lifestyle of the modern urban mother is out of harmony with natural processes and tends to promote pathological conditions that require medical attention during pregnancy and childbirth. In the following discussion, we shall outline major themes surrounding child-bearing in Chambon's articles.

Chambon's humoralism and his reliance on a theory of fluids continue to inform these articles. It suffices to mention a few of many such references. On the humors, he believes, for example, that phlegmatic women are more likely to suffer from a prolapsed uterus ("Descente de matrice") and that the dry temperament is less subject to a displacement of the pubic bones ("Ecartement des os pubiques"). On fluids, the gravitational pull of blood rushing to fill the uterine cavity after birth and the subsequent need to expel it are frequently noted explicative principles ("Accouchées" for example, *Médecine*, vol. 1, p. 69). In addition, irruptions of "l'humeur laiteuse," both interior and exterior, are blamed for many complications ("Femmes en couches," *Médecine*, vol. 6, p. 276). Other irruptions that result from the suppression of the postnatal discharge are described graphically but with scientific objectivity. The following passage can illustrate many such in *Médecine*, including the distressingly large number of fatal outcomes:

> Le bas-ventre se tend dans l'espace de quelques heures; il devient douloureux; il s'enflamme; la fièvre s'allume; le délire ne tarde pas à se manifester; quelquefois même il est violent, & subsiste plusieurs jours de suite. Le hoquet survient; il est bientôt accompagné de vomissement de matières verdâtres: chez quelques sujets il y a des convulsions. Le feu que les malades ressentent dans les viscères du bas-ventre ne peut pas être modéré par les boissons. La bouche se dessèche, les lèvres deviennent arides, le teint pale & plombé [...] il n'y a sur le visage que des taches rouges, sur un fond pale & livide; la peau est sèche, mais elle conserve de la mollesse.
>
> Cependant le pouls se concentre, les extrémités deviennent froides, les yeux s'éteignent, le son de la voix s'affoiblit; une foiblesse générale s'empare des malades et les fait mourir ("Lochies," *Médecine*, vol. 8, 296).

As we have seen, Chambon holds to a humoralist interpretation of certain phenomena at the same time that he adopts principles of the "new" medicine, with clinical observation the most basic characteristic of this approach to medicine. Most articles on obstetrics therefore include case histories, and, all too frequently, reports of what he and others have learned from autopsies. Before that unhappy point, clinical observation required complete physical exams, which, as we saw, involved cultural as well as medical considerations. The scientific physician also had to carefully weigh evidence and to take a critical stance towards inherited wisdom when clinical data contradicted it.

A first example of Chambon's scientific approach is the introduction of the thirty-page article "Grossesse, Accidens qui l'accompagnent." This section of the treatise discusses the various ways suggested in the professional literature to determine early on if the woman is truly pregnant. Chambon rejects certain of these suggestions and then proposes his own most reliable method, the detection of a cervical mucus a few weeks after conception. He has even invented a small instrument for collecting the mucus.[28] A second example is in "Descente de matrice," where Chambon gives an exact description of this condition, mentions variations he has observed, and stresses the need for a thorough physical examination.[29]

In that same article, Chambon also follows a new approach in attempting to separate psychological (his term is "moral") from physical causes. The need for the distinction arises often in discussions of the painful and frequently dangerous process of giving birth. In "Délivrer," for example, he claims that excitable women have greater difficulty expelling the placenta and recommends ready use of forceps to help them through this stage of childbirth. Chambon often attempts to show the physical basis of such psychological causes, sometimes with an imaginative recreation of what has happened. In "Faux germe," he explains how a miscarriage may happen as a result of a frightening experience:

> c'est encore aux effets physiques qu'il faut rapporter le mechanisme de ces accidens, et voici, ce me semble, comment on peut expliquer cette question. Dans une frayeur, toute la machine est ébranlée; les fluides lancés par le cœur, sans régularité, dans leurs canaux, y portent des commotions violentes [...]; c'est moins l'empire de l'ame qu'on doit considérer dans ces circonstances comme l'agent immédiat de la destruction, que l'ébranlement occasionné par le trouble des nerfs et l'agitation des esprits animaux, qui rendent plus permanente les secousses dont je parle (*Médecine*, vol. 6, p. 274).

The many articles where Chambon's theory of fluids is in play also demonstrate that he was ultimately seeking physical, material causes of illnesses or complications. The concept is basic in most of the articles where he is combating a prevailing notion. "Expulsion du fœtus" provides a good illustration of this point. Against prevailing thought, Chambon maintains that it is the uterus as a muscle that forces the fetus to emerge, not the fetus itself. One of his arguments: if it were the fetus, birth would happen more easily in dead mothers, whose emotions would no longer impede the process; but such is not the case.

As in the articles on the non-obstetrical illnesses of women, Chambon occasionally alludes to or states his views about broader social dimensions of pregnancy and birth. The shame of the unwed mother is evoked in "Expulsion du fœtus." Obviously describing a pregnant woman with little material support, Chambon describes her as delaying her departure for the midwife's home until the last moment; she arrives barefoot no matter how terrible the weather; she leaves a few hours after the birth, to the great detriment of her health. "Femmes en couches" extends the discussion to three different levels of society, describing impediments to women's health in each group. The rich woman, often a city-dweller, is enervated by her sedentary life (Chambon refers to "Constitution des femmes," which, as we saw, discusses this problem). In the country, there is a tradition of over-feeding the new mother, causing fermentations that develop into fevers: "J'en ai vu un grand nombre qui ont péri des suites de cette imprudence," notes Chambon, who, as we recall, had spent several years practicing medicine in Langres and Blois (*Médecine*, vol. 6, p. 285).[30] And in the lowest ranks of society, the situation of the destitute women who give birth in the hospitals is evoked in the section on postpartum fevers. At the Hôtel-Dieu, where Chambon assisted for a period during the 1780s,

> […] les *Femmes en couches*, toujours environnées du spectacle de la mort des nouvelles accouchées, continuellement tourmentées par les cris de la douleur, n'appercevant rien autour d'elles qui ne leur annonçat une fin prochaine, tomboient dans une stupeur et un accablement qui sont les symptomes d'une grande malignité. Joignez à ces circonstances une diète mal observée, souvent des maladies anciennes qui se compliquoient avec la fièvre de lait, l'appauvrissement du sang, suite nécessaire de la misère et la désolation de la plupart d'elles, vous aurez connu les causes des morts fréquentes qu'on y observoit (*Médecine*, vol. 6, p. 296).

Abortion was not the controversial issue it is today, since no one was demanding legalization. But one aspect of the question had to be faced by physicians, the difficult cases where they could probably save the mother by aborting the fetus. The articles on the subject in *Médecine* do not call on religious or moral authorities for guidance in making this decision. Chambon employs, rather, a social calculus about which of the two lives is more valuable to the community. He disagrees on this point with his fellow contributor Mahon.[31] For Chambon, the life of the mother is to be valorized because she has a demonstrated history of survival and fertility, whereas the newborn has a statistically high chance of dying during the first few years. In the medically fraught case of a tubal pregnancy, Chambon points out that delaying an abortion in hopes of preserving both lives merely puts both in danger. "D'après ces principes," Chambon states firmly, "je conseille de pratiquer l'opération cæsarienne, aussitôt que la *grossesse* abdominale sera constatée" ("Grossesse ventrale ou abdominale," *Médecine*, vol. 6, p. 770), effectively an abortion, even if the term is avoided.

Another important element in the new medicine was better training for medical practitioners. The push was for more clinical practice for physicians and a more professional status for surgeons in order to differentiate between their medical and non-medical tasks. As pertained to obstetrics, another goal was to give midwives at least some basic training. Chambon, a well-trained and experienced physician himself, makes several statements on the subject. In "Accoucheur," he claims that women and infants are lost every day because the rules permit surgeons who have no specialized knowledge of obstetrics to deliver babies; and he develops at length his conviction that only persons with "un moral doux et patient" should be permitted to care for women during childbirth, "pour éloigner d'elles tout sujet d'inquiétude" (*Médecine*, vol. 1, pp. 84-85). The companion entry "Accoucheuse" does not mention that midwives often possessed these qualities; Chambon dwells instead on the dangers that women incur by preferring midwives to doctors. (The obvious compromise, women doctors, is not proposed.) His strong preference for physician-guided births likely explains in part why he does not express any enthusiasm for recent reforms. He recounts without any affective terms the more advanced training that midwives must now undergo and the recommendations they must obtain ("attestations de bonnes vie, mœurs & religion," *Médecine*, vol. 1, p. 86). Chambon adds that these rules are largely ignored in the countryside and that he has seen little improvement from other government efforts to give very basic training to village midwives. His conclusion: many reforms need to be effected in this area, and they will be difficult to execute.

The call for better training is implied in other articles where Chambon discusses problems aggravated or even caused by less skilled practitioners. Ordinary obstetricians are blamed, for example, for causing tears and other complications by ripping out the placenta too quickly ("Délivrer," *Médecine*, vol. 5, p. 358; "Femmes en couches," *Médecine*, vol. 6, p. 275), a criticism also voiced in "Dépression de matrice," where he attributes the haste to doctors who want to speed things along so as to treat more patients and therefore earn more fees.

Chambon criticizes fellow practitioners on other counts as well—*Médecine* in many areas is heir to the *Encyclopédie* tradition of calling for reforms within the context of an informational encyclopedia entry. In "Nymphotomie," Chambon condemns the "faste des apprêts chirurgicaux," in this case unnecessary packing and bandaging of a wound (*Médecine*, vol. 11, p. 48), and he is not averse to judging contemporaries harshly, referring scornfully, for example, to the "praticiens modernes, qu'on ne compte point parmi les hommes d'un mérite eminent" (on the subject of distinguishing among various kinds of fevers, "Femmes en couches," *Médecine*, vol. 6, p. 275), or to certain Parisian anatomists who claim that the pubic bones cannot separate because they have never seen this phenomenon, "comme s'il fallut s'en rapporter à eux pour savoir ce que l'on doit croire & penser!" ("Écartement des os pubiques," *Médecine*, vol. 5, p. 672).

Many of Chambon's recommendations for care and treatment could appear with few changes in a modern medical manual. The expectant mother should get moderate exercise (for example, "Grossesse," *Médecine*, vol. 6, pp. 752-753), and nursing the child is recommended (because it will help to draw excess abdominal fluid to the breasts, "Femmes en couches," *Médecine*, vol. 6, p. 287), although Chambon is not a crusader on this subject.[32] The new mother needs tranquility to recover from labor and delivery. On this point, Chambon twice repeats what is done in the Dutch Republic to promote the new mother's recovery: a notice on her front door warns passersby to avoid excessive noise ("Accouchées," *Médecine*, vol. 1, p. 71; "Lochies [Écoulemen excessif des]," *Médecine*, vol. 9, pp. 292-293). But many other entries remind us that we are still in the eighteenth century. Complex herbal and medical concoctions are frequently recommended. A single example is the tea of infused violets to which a few drops of spirit of stag's horn are added, administered to control milk-fever ("Femmes en couches," *Médecine*, vol. 6, p. 283). Age-old treatments are offered apparently with Chambon's approbation. The treatment for the malady called uterine fever, for example, that dated back to physicians in Antiquity was to shave the head and swathe it in bandages soaked in vinegar. Certain procedures also remind modern readers that, even if cleanliness of bandages and linen is often recommended, *Médecine* was compiled well before sterile conditions were shown to be paramount. To remove the placenta, for example, Chambon follows André Levret's recommendation to coat the hand with oil, or better yet with pork fat, and then to gradually widen the opening from two to three fingers' width before scraping off the placenta with the fingernails.

As we have seen, Chambon collects case histories as scientific support for his recommendations and conclusions. These cases are also stories that bridge the chasm between objective empirical data and the humans who gave rise to it.[33] Very subtly, these stories about mostly anonymous women serve as a counterpoint to all the biographical entries on named persons of some distinction who are covered in the various series of the

Méthodique, including *Médecine*. We would like to conclude by summarizing several of Chambon's stories, each of which enlarges his article beyond the purely medical.

In "Grossesse avec hydropisie" we read about two mothers in labor, wives of a thresher and an unskilled laborer. One of the women was "dans la plus excessive misère" and both were poorly nourished; in spite of being hideously swollen, both gave birth to live children and survived the ordeal, although in one of the cases "ce ne fut qu'après un très-longtemps, et beaucoup de souffrance" (*Médecine*, vol. 6, p. 761). Chambon (and his source Guillaume Mauquest de Lamotte) obviously consider the poverty of the women a circumstance that complicated their case.

"Grossesse ventrale ou abdominale" recounts a dramatic story where courage is rewarded. A pregnant woman endured labor without ever giving birth, and gradually became weaker over the following months. Near death, she finally consented to an operation, in which the doctor removed a dead fetus from her right Fallopian tube—21 months after conception. The mother later had three more children.

Another woman who seemed to be suffering from an inflamed uterus or bladder was cured when fragments of rotted cork were spontaneously expelled; they came from a ring she had used for 18 years to support her prolapsed uterus ("Descente de matrice," *Médecine*, vol. 5, p. 404). Chambon's point in this story[34] was the importance of cleanliness.

"Délivrer" summarizes a recent case history, a woman who gave birth in April 1791 but without expelling the placenta. The presiding doctor preferred to wait, but the family, "inquiétée par le préjugé habituel, sur la nécessité d'une prompte deliverance," called in Chambon; he also counseled patience, and twenty-three hours later the placenta was expelled (*Médecine*, vol. 5, pp. 361-362). Chambon seems here to be encouraging patients and their families to trust both good physicians and Mother Nature.

Finally, a heartening story concerning a patient of Chambon's father in 1766, recounted in "Mort-né en apparence." A healthy woman gave birth without incident to a baby that showed signs of life *in utero* but emerged still-born. This was the third child the couple had lost in similar circumstances. When the fourth child was born, also apparently lifeless, the elder Chambon left the umbilical cord attached for a short while and placed the baby between its mother's thighs for warmth. Little by little the infant began to move and whimper. Without going into the theoretical explanation Chambon gives of this singular case (it involves, as one might expect, the effect of excess fluids in the mother's system), we shall note only the aptness of this image of a dormant life becoming a vigorous life.

It represents medicine at a time when it was on the threshold of its own vigorous new life, open to new methods, marked by discoveries and successes thanks to the empirical spirit that was now valued, and practiced by physicians like Chambon eager to share knowledge with a large audience of both professional colleagues and readers of encyclopedias.

Notes

[1] For information on known subscriber groups to the *Encyclopédie méthodique*, see Suzanne Tucoo-Chala, *Charles-Joseph Panckoucke et la librairie française, 1736-1798* (Pau and Paris: Marrimpouey Jeune and Jean Touzot, 1977), pp. 402-403. My personal copy of the octavo edition of Diderot and d'Alembert's *Encyclopédie, ou Dictionnaire raisonné des sciences, des arts et des métiers*, 39 vols. (Bern and Lausanne: Sociétés typographiques, 1778-1779) contains various material proofs of consultation such as mathematical calculations scribbled in the margins, a spa ticket, and a dessicated cherry pit.

[2] The original edition is *Encyclopédie, ou Dictionnaire raisonné des sciences, des arts et des métiers*, eds. Denis Diderot and Jean Le Rond d'Alembert, 17 vols. of text, 11 vols. of plates (Paris: Briasson, David, Le Breton, Durand, 1751-1772). For an introductory overview of the complex history of this famous work, see Madeleine Pinault, *L'Encyclopédie* (Paris: Presses universitaires de France, 1993).

[3] *Encyclopédie méthodique ou par ordre de matières*, 203 vols. (Paris and Liege: Panckoucke and Plomteux; Paris, Panckoucke, Henri Agasse, Pauline Agasse, 1782-1832). Basic works on the *Méthodique* include Christabel P. Braunrot and Kathleen Hardesty Doig, "The *Encyclopédie méthodique*: An Introduction," *Studies on Voltaire and the Eighteenth Century* 327 (1995), pp. 1-152; Martine Groult, *Savoir et matières: pensée scientifique et théorie de la connaissance de l'Encyclopédie à l'Encyclopédie Méthodique* (Paris: CNRS Editions, 2011); and Claude Blanckaert and Michel Porret, with the collaboration of Fabrice Brandli, *L'Encyclopédie méthodique (1782-1832): Des Lumières au positivisme* (Geneva: Droz, 2006). The "Vocabulaire universel" that was to unify the different dictionaries was never published.

[4] Prospectus, reprinted in *Beaux-arts*, vol. 1, p. lxxx.

[5] Because of the lengthy publication span and the piecemeal delivery of sections from various dictionaries, there is variation among sets of the *Méthodique*. For a recently established list of the "ideal" *Méthodique*, see Groult, *Savoir et matières*, pp. 331-350. Panckoucke was succeeded as general editor by his son-in-law Henri Agasse, who in turn was succeeded at his death by his widow, Panckoucke's daughter Pauline.

[6] The first half of volume 1 of *Médecine* appeared on 14 May 1787; the second half was published in 1790. The remaining twelve volumes appeared as follows, with the date of the second half in brackets: volume 2, 1790-[1792]; volume 3, 1790-[1792]; volume 4, 1792-[1794]; volume 5, 1792-[1794]; volume 6, 1793-[1794]; volume 7, 1798-[1799]; volume 8, 1808-[1814]; volume 9, 1816-[1819]; volume

10, 1821-[1823]; volume 11, 1824-[1825]; volume 12, 1827-[1828]; volume 13, 1830-[1832]. Future references to *Médecine* will be given in the text. There are no plates specifically for *Médecine*, although the companion *Chirurgie* has 113, including a series on gestation.

[7] The bibliography on this transformation is extensive. Useful studies include Erwin H. Ackerknecht, *Medicine at the Paris Hospital, 1794-1848* (Baltimore, MD: Johns Hopkins Press, 1967); Toby Gelfand, *Professionalizing Modern Medicine: Paris Surgeons and Medical Science and Institutions in the 18th Century* (Westport, CT: Greenwood Press), especially chap. 8, "The Emergence of the Hospital Medical School"; Sergio Moravia, "Philosophie et médecine en France à la fin du XVIIIe siècle," *Studies on Voltaire and the Eighteenth Century*, 89 (Oxford, 1992), pp. 1089-1151; Matthew Ramsey, *Professional and Popular Medicine in France 1770-1830* (New York: Cambridge University Press, 1988); Ann F. Laberge, *Mission and Method: The Early Nineteenth-Century French Public Health Movement* (Cambridge, UK: Cambridge University Press, 1992); and Laurence Brockliss and Colin Jones, eds., *The Medical World of Early Modern France* (Oxford, UK: Oxford University Press, 1997).

[8] Two examples of these distinguished contributors: Philippe Pinel, the mental health pioneer; and Louis René Villermé, author of many works on military medicine and public health, among other areas of medicine. The list of the team of collaborators identified in volume 13 of *Médecine* is given in Braunrot and Doig, p. 24, n.1.

[9] A possible explanation for the separate designation for military and veterinary medicine: military officers and landowners were among the probable intended readership of the *Méthodique*. Both these areas of medicine were also covered to some extent in the series *Art militaire* and *Agriculture*.

[10] On the *Méthodique*'s contribution to pediatric health care, see Daniel Teysseire, "Une étape dans la constitution de la pédiatrie: l'*Encyclopédie méthodique,*" *Dix-huitième siècle* 23 (1991): 159-169.

[11] Chambon does not seem to have contributed any articles after volume 9, published in 1816 but much of it quite possibly prepared long before. One can speculate that Chambon's political involvement in the Revolution and the dangers he faced subsequently, as we shall see below, prevented him from continuing to collaborate on *Médecine*.

[12] *La Vie et les œuvres de Nicolas Chambon de Montaux (1748-1826)* (Paris: G. Steinheil, 1906), p. 45.

[13] *Des maladies des femmes*, 2 vols. (Paris: rue et Hôtel Serpente, 1784); *Des maladies des filles*, 2 vols. (Paris: rue et Hôtel Serpente, 1785); and *Des maladies de la grossesse*, 2 vols. (Paris: rue et Hôtel Serpente, 1785).

[14] Chambon edited the texts from his books by adding introductory material or re-organizing the paragraphs, by inserting the articles in a larger discussion, and by deleting most of the extensive documentation given in the books. One example of the latter: the third through eighth paragraphs of "Lochies" (*Médecine*, vol. 8, pp. 292-293) are taken from *Maladies des femmes*, vol. 1, pp. 69-75; a four-line quotation in Latin from Albrecht von Haller, *Elementa physiologiae corporis*

humani, vol. 3, p. 298 (8 vols., Lausanne: Société typographique, 1757-1766) is deleted from the seventh paragraph.

[15] See Gelfand, *Professionalizing Modern Medicine*, pp. 141-144, and Génévrier, pp. 14-15.

[16] In 1814 Chambon wrote a letter defending himself against various accusations concerning his mayoralty, especially that of having voted the death penalty for the king. See Génévrier, pp. 19-28 for the text of the letter.

[17] Chambon's efforts included a humiliating request to Napoleon, whom the physician detested, for a post. See Génévrier, pp. 37-39.

[18] To Galen and Hippocrates, among others. The latter's ideas on medical treatment for girls and women, to which Chambon refers frequently, were developed in two treatises (in French, "Des maladies des femmes" and "Des maladies des jeunes filles," in *Œuvres completes d'Hippocrate*, ed. Françoise Kourilsky, Paris: Union littéraire et artistique, 1955). On humoralism in the eighteenth century, a useful source is Elizabeth A. Williams, *The Physical and the Moral: Anthropology, Physiology, and Philosophical Medicine in France, 1750-1850* (Cambridge, UK: Cambridge University Press, 1994), pp. 57-62.

[19] *A Cultural History of Medical Vitalism in Enlightenment Montpellier* (Burlington, VT: Ashgate, 2003), pp. 7-8.

[20] Among the treatments for the opposite problem, excessive breast development, which presents "un aspect desagréable" and can affect breathing, are leeches ("Gonflement douloureux des seins," *Médecine*, vol. 6, pp. 661-662).

[21] As we shall see below, Chambon broaches this subject in "Matrice." He also refers here to the companion article, "Masturbation," by Jean Joseph de Brieude.

[22] Chambon is clearly more concerned in these articles with upper-class young women of leisure, mainly from an urban environment. The same phenomenon of illnesses manifesting hysterical symptoms was also increasingly observable in working women in the countryside as well as the city. See Lindsay Wilson, *Women and Medicine in the French Enlightenment: The Debate over Maladies des Femmes* (Baltimore, MD: The Johns Hopkins University Press, 1993), pp. 130-157.

[23] Description of an illness in a novel-like narrative was characteristic of certain medical writings of the period. See Alexandre Wenger, " La Lecture hygiénique: formes narratives et épistolarité dans la médecine des Lumières," *Études Épistémè* 13 (Spring 2008): 108-120. Chambon is among the writers studied (114-116).

[24] Titles of articles often have parenthetical explanatory phrases, especially when there are several sub-articles under a term.

[25] See for example "Hydropisie des ovaires," *Médecine*, vol. 8, p. 360.

[26] This case is an example of the additions Chambon made in the *Médecine* articles to sections carried over from his *Des maladies des filles*. The "sedition" to which he refers may have been connected with unrest during the Revolution. See Wilson, *Women and Medicine in the French Enlightenment*, pp. 134-135, for a brief discussion of illnesses brought on by the stress of political events.

[27] A "vinaigre de Vénus" and another commonly called "Courier de Cythère" were associated with retaining the appearance of virginity. The former was often

marketed as a remedy for the vapors. The famous distiller Antoine Claude Maille sold them, along with many other types of distillations, in his Paris shop. Elie Fréron mentions visiting the shop and laughing at a "Vinaigre de Pucelle pour les Dames" (*L'Année littéraire*, 1767, p. 136). The "vinaigre de Vénus" was particularly expensive. Maille was selling it by the pint for 96 livres in 1753 (*Mercure de France*, July 1753, p. 214). We are grateful to Morag Martin for information on this point.

[28] In a companion article, "Fausse grossesse," in a section attributed to a letter by the eighteenth-century anatomist and physician Giovanni Battista Morgagni, Chambon recounts many examples of genuine pregnancies in spite of indications that there was no pregnancy, including some cases in mothers aged 60.

[29] This article is a good example of Chambon's extensive use of the literature on a subject. The authorities cited are Hippocrates; Morgagni; Aëtius of Amida, a disciple of Galen who wrote in the late fifth century; a certain Slevogt; and Nicolas Puzos, a French obstetrician who died in 1753.

[30] Another country practice is criticized in "Lochies": the excessive use of cordials to re-energize women during labor, to the point that many were drunk when the baby was born. Chambon does not exclude allowing alcoholic refreshment in some cases, but holds that its use requires "tant de réserve, une prudence si consommée & une sagacité réelle, qu'on ne peut guère l'attendre du grand nombre des personnes qui se mêlent de guérir" (*Médecine*, vol. 6, p. 299).

[31] See, for example, Mahon's "Avortement," classified under "Médecine légale," and his "Grossesse," classified under "Police médicale." In the latter article, among Mahon's suggestions is an appeal to authorities to reconsider harsh laws that dishonor unwed mothers, which can cause them to attempt abortions (*Médecine*, vol. 6, pp. 725-726).

[32] The article "Allaitement," 33 pages, by Michel Augustin Thouret, is the major entry in *Médecine* promoting maternal nursing.

[33] Wilson notes the appeal of the many case histories that appeared in both scientific and popular journals: the stories "mingle science with literature, the real with the bizarre, instructing as they entertained" (*Women and Medicine in the French Enlightenment*, p. 7).

[34] Which he attributes to François Rousset, an early seventeenth-century physician and author of several works in Latin on obstetrics.

PART II:

WOMEN AS MEDICAL AGENTS

Chapter Four

'Augustine Debaralle, insensee, folle, charlatane, et enfin tout ce qu'il vous plaira': A Female Healer's Struggle for Medical Recognition in Napoleonic France[1]

Morag Martin

Augustine Debaralle, first a student midwife and science writer, then an inventor of remedies and healer extraordinaire in her home region of the Nord, and finally a fugitive from the law, greatly desired to be recognized for her medical genius, not just by patients and local authorities, but also by the national medical profession. The male physicians in Paris who labeled her insane were thankful that she never got this wish. In many respects, her story resembles those of other unofficial healers and inventors of remedies who hoped to make a living during the Empire. She stands out due to her desire for greater recognition and for her aggressive self-promotion, traits that were unusual for a woman healer. Physicians, *officiers de santé* and local administrators, concerned with the protection of the newly professionalized monopoly on healing, responded with excessive vehemence to a young, single woman operating publically outside the norms of female healing. Due to the post-revolutionary fear of disruptive women (after the years of women violently protesting in the streets), Debaralle's actions eventually led to her imprisonment and subsequent silencing of her medical endeavors. Nevertheless, the bureaucracy of medical permissions and lack of coherent policing temporarily left her with space in which to operate and express her frustrations regarding the limitations imposed on women healers.[2] From her point of view, her genius for curing disease was denied and then ignored by official channels. She did not wish to be simply a midwife (even one trained at the most elite school by the best physicians and surgeons). Her strong, angry and defiant voice vividly illustrates the constant recreations of self a woman in medicine had to perform: she labeled herself mockingly "insensée" and "sorcière," in addition to "oculiste," "cultivatrice des hautes sciences" and "femme de lettres." Unable to obtain any positive response from those in power, she became increasingly paranoid and delusional. Debaralle was a daughter of the Revolution sure of her duties to heal humanity; her insistence on national recognition of her skills illustrates the impossibility in the post–revolutionary climate for women to participate in either the debates or practices of healing outside the limited spheres reserved for them.

As historians, we have little direct knowledge of the personalities, struggles and minds of female healers, midwives and matrons from this period. Elite, urban women who overcame many obstacles to succeed in the medical world, usually on the margins, published scientific works or were written about. Women, usually widows, were present in large numbers among sedentary rural empirics, but their goal was to stay invisible to the authorities, not wanting to gain larger recognition. Most self-promoting traveling charlatans were men, sometimes working with their wives. Both groups of healers show up briefly in the historical records as petitioners for patents and permissions or as defendants arrested for breaking the law.[3] Countless advertisements and petitions to woo the public survived in the archives. Debaralle left her mark by publishing a scientific tract as a midwifery student. She then waged an exceptionally aggressive and exhaustive battle over two years for permission to sell her remedies and, more broadly, for public recognition from the Parisian medical school, the Ministry of the Interior and local officials, for eight years. She also created an angry and very personal advertising campaign that was unlikely to sway the authorities in favor of a medical permission or leniency for her criminal acts. Her delusions of grandeur and her blindness to the futility of her cause make her a visible (and quite pitiable) figure in a world where female medical practitioners were mostly silent if not invisible.

Augustine Georgette Joseph Debaralle was born on 30 March 1782 in Valenciennes to the ranks of the artisanal class. Her father was an *amidonnier*, a profession that had only recently been incorporated into a guild and whose main clients were perfumers who fabricated hair powder for wigs. Her own godmother was a nun and her younger sister's was a *marchande à la toilette*, a job that allowed women to sell rouge and other cosmetics outside the more powerful perfumers' control. Debaralle's family and friends within the lower ranks of the luxury trades or the church would see their worlds upended by the Revolution. With the subsequent decline in demand for wigs and powder, starch merchants lost their most lucrative and respectable outlet. Food shortages led to a public outcry against the use of wheat for starch, which discredited a profession now open to all comers.[4] Additionally, in 1793, the British bombarded Valenciennes for forty-three days, destroying large parts of the city, including the Debaralle's parish church.[5] Understandably, Debaralle claimed her father lost his fortune due to circumstances beyond his control.[6] She grew up during a period of rapid change that created not just professional instability but also vocational malleability. Tellingly, a relative identified himself as "entrepreneur et fournisseur de médicamens" to the local military hospital. This grand title appropriated the functions of apothecaries and sprang, in essence, from the same creative impulse that Debaralle would later act on.[7]

In 1804, as a twenty-two year old orphan, Debaralle was chosen by the prefect of the Department of the Nord to attend, through a generous scholarship, the brand new midwifery-training program at the Hospice de la Maternité in Paris.[8] Jean-Antoine Chaptal, Minister of the Interior, opened the school in 1802 in order to elevate the knowledge of midwives and save the lives of mothers and children. To fill the school with students from all of France, and not just the Parisian region, Chaptal encouraged the local prefects to send students chosen for their intelligence and moral standing. Few departments responded enthusiastically due to the cost of such a program. Most preferred to create their own training schools or certify women who were already experienced in birthing. Luckily for Chaptal, the prefect of the Nord, Christophe Dieudonné, took the call seriously because he realized that his local resources were meager. Between 1804 and 1809 the Nord sent eighty-four young women to Paris, by far the most of any region. Amazingly the 1809 census listed eighty as actively practicing midwives, indicating the success of the program for the region.[9] Over time the program would provide thousands of young women throughout France with a chance to gain professional standing, the only means by which women could enter medicine virtually coequal to male practitioners in their field.[10]

The school was looking for women between the ages of eighteen and thirty-five, of any marital status, but the average age was twenty-four and most were single as Debaralle was.[11] Exceptionally older practicing midwives could be admitted for further study, but they were not considered the ideal recruits. It proved difficult initially for the Nord administrators to fulfill their goal of thirty new students a year. In 1804,

Dieudonné bemoaned that despite the availability of fairly cheap training for midwives in Paris, no young woman from the countryside had been willing to attend because of the distance to Paris, the ties of rural people to the land and an unwillingness to sacrifice for a greater cause. Dieudonné overcame this reticence by offering well-funded scholarships and targeting urban daughters of the artisanal class, rather than solely rural girls, as well as promising to pay returning midwives for working with the indigent.[12] As an urban girl, Debaralle may not have been the ideal midwife (the authorities were hoping for rural placements), but she had the requisite literacy, proper moral character confirmed by a local priest, and was willing to move to the capital, as she had no family to constrain her choices.

Moral rectitude was central to the running of a reputable midwifery school, since most of the students were single, young and new to the temptations of the city. The Maternité enforced strict rules of conduct meant to keep students virtuous and fully occupied. The main midwife, Marie Louise Lachapelle, and the *Filles de la Charité* who ran the hospital, jointly oversaw the students' comportment. Students were not allowed to leave the building unless they were accompanied by family members, turning the school into a form of penitentiary, albeit one with abundant food and clean rooms.[13] The administrators expected students to be "douces, actives, patientes, calmes, modestes, prudentes, courageuses, discrètes, probes, et surtout désintéressées."[14] These mostly well-worn feminine adjectives reinforced the role of a midwife as an ally to local authorities in the battle against infanticide and illegitimacy. The midwife should be all ears, not gossiping or sympathizing with her patient's plight. The school taught their students to be strong and active, but ultimately wished them to be reactive to the commands and expectations of the local authorities.

The students were to learn both the practical and theoretical sides of birthing, as well as general lessons in vaccination, phlebotomy, hygiene and herbal medicine, subjects useful to the health of their future rural patients.[15] However, the goal was not to train them as general medical practitioners, but as advisors in maternal health who knew their limitations. The head midwife stepped in during difficult births and forbade students from using forceps or participating in caesarean sections. Jean Louis Baudelocque, the head surgeon and professor-in-chief, stressed the importance of allowing nature to take its course and encouraged a non-interventionist method of birthing for midwives, in contrast with the aggressive method for surgeons.[16] In his manual aimed at rural midwives, first published in 1775 and revised for the Maternité, he clearly laid out the parameters within which midwives should operate alone.[17]

Yet, much about the school opened up new vistas on medicine for these young women, which is likely to have encouraged Debaralle to think big. Students had the privilege of being lectured on anatomy and gynecology by two eminent *accoucheurs en chefs*: first Baudelocque and, after 1810, Antoine Dubois.[18] The students read not just Baudelocque's manual for country midwives, but also his more complex and scientific manual intended for physicians, in which he described the use of forceps in detail.[19] The *médecin en chef*, the anatomist François Chaussier, gave thrice-weekly theoretical courses and demonstrated the anatomical dissection of cadavers. Both Baudelocque and Chaussier promoted the use of clinical medicine at the Maternité. They instructed students to take notes on their patient's conditions and medications. At graduation, the instructors commended students who were especially skilled at clinical observations. They praised a student who entered the same year as Debaralle, Mme Pacaud, for assisting the doctors in their anatomical research.[20] And in his graduation speeches, Chaussier lectured about complex medical cases and his research findings.[21]

The male instructors clearly thought that their students were superior to rural matrons and could practice at a level of expertise that approached that of the "meilleurs accoucheurs, les égaler, les surpasser même à quelques égards."[22] The male medical professionals in charge believed in the new science and techniques of birthing, but also believed that women were as well, if not better, suited than men to learn and practice these techniques in the provinces.[23] Women, unlike men, would more likely let nature take its course and would not choose to operate immediately. Baudelocque saw midwives as an essential part of medicine, not just replacements for missing obstetricians.[24] The school emphasized that women could gain clinical skills, anatomical knowledge and total competence when it came to so-called natural births. The main role model for these female accomplishments was the head midwife Lachapelle. Though Chaussier lectured regularly, it was Lachapelle who gave hands-on instruction and translated his complex ideas into simpler terms.[25] Lachapelle strongly promoted women's right to a professional vocation and refused to allow male medical students to learn alongside her charges.[26]

Both the strong female leadership at the Maternité and the depth of medical knowledge taught there clearly had an impact on Debaralle. While still a student, she researched and wrote a medical tract. Having observed at least two dissections performed on deceased mothers and infants, and likely having read on the subject, she put together a pamphlet on the circulation of blood to the fetus. She wrote it in medical jargon that corresponded with the description Baudelocque gave in his manual for doctors, although her account was more detailed. Neither she nor Baudelocque included the theories published by Raphaël Bienvenu Sabatier in 1774, but instead they stuck to the traditional view of fetal blood circulation proposed by William Harvey in 1628. To write such a pamphlet Debaralle immersed herself in the anatomy of the heart and circulatory system. Her purported purpose for this tract was to explain what happened at birth if the blood flow to the fetus was cut off too early, but her main focus lay in anatomical details with little practical use at the bedside of an expectant mother.[27]

That Debaralle had grander ambitions for this pamphlet was obvious. She promised that

> si le public accueille favorablement ce traité, je me ferai un nouveau plaisir de lui en offrir plusieurs autres, dont l'un est aussi curieux pour la nouveauté de son espèce, qu'il est instructif; et les autres très-utiles à l'humanité.[28]

Debaralle later claimed to have written other tracts on diverse medical topics, but due to a lack of funds never published them.[29] In her advertisement for her tract she gave herself the grandiose title of "cultivatrice des hautes sciences, professant actuellement l'état d'accoucheuse."[30] Her studies at the Maternité gave her the confidence to define herself as a scientist, only temporarily practicing a female art, a clear sign of her greater ambition.

Debaralle was a barely educated student midwife. What sort of career could she have had as a medical writer? Prominent female midwives, such as Angélique Marguerite de Coudray and Lachapelle published birthing manuals written in an accessible style that were meant to teach rural women the best practices of midwifery. With greater scope and ambition, Marie-Anne Boivin, who had been a student at the Maternité and then worked alongside Lachapelle, published an ambitious handbook in 1812 that covered topics, such as the use of forceps, which went beyond the scope of a country midwife's training manual. In her conclusion, Boivin included the aphorism of an Italian doctor that advised midwives to learn to call for help and leave the difficult cases to surgeons.[31] Boivin herself never followed this advice. She published numerous works on gynecology and performed operations that were usually limited to surgeons.[32] So it appears that Debaralle's act of writing and publishing a scientific tract was not unusual at the Maternité. In fact, according to Boivin, some of the Maternité students spoke Greek and Latin, and there was even a request from a surgeon for one of the students to translate English obstetrical manuals.[33]

But Debaralle was not from this class of educated women. Most female writers of scientific medical literature were upper-class or bourgeois women, raised in a world of Enlightenment science that accepted a limited number of women as long as they remained feminine in their pursuits. A few women of the urban upper-artisanal class did find public acclaim, such as Marie Catherine Biheron, daughter of a Parisian apothecary, who was known across Europe for her anatomical models, her lectures on internal organs and even her sex education for young women.[34] Biheron, Boivin and others like them spent years proving their skills while still coming under fire from male medical professionals. Debaralle neglected to build up her education, patronage or ties to institutions such as the Maternité by publishing without permission an ambitious scientific tract. During the shift in the early nineteenth-century toward a stricter separation of the sexes and professionalization of medicine, such a tract by a barely educated midwifery student would have been dismissed by anyone she wished to impress. Like her enlightened predecessors, however, Debaralle desired recognition, publishing under her own name and adopting titles that represented the scope of her ambition.

Despite (or most likely because of) her foray into scientific writing, Debaralle did not graduate with honors. Only thirty-three of the ninety-three students admitted that academic year presented themselves for the examination in June 1805, the others preferring to stay another year with the approval of their prefect.[35] Though only a handful passed with distinction, the rest showed themselves to have "manifesté de l'intelligence et du jugement, et des connaissances suffisantes tant dans la théorie que de la pratique […]."[36] All except Debaralle. While the official documents do not go into details about her failing, Debaralle claimed that Baudelocque, Chaussier, and Dubois wanted to disgrace her for having "tenu tête" to them.[37] It is possible that when facing a panel of distinguished professors she made claims and judgments they would have considered inappropriate for a midwifery student. While other students declaimed on proper birthing positions or the moral rules of midwifery, Debaralle may have chosen to lecture the panel on the circulation of fetal blood.[38] Additionally, she had to leave the strict confinement of the institution unaccompanied to secure a printing of her self-published work. That she was not asked to stay another year suggests the administrators wanted to punish her for her behavior or attitude, rather than for academic reasons. Only five of 447 women failed the examination from 1802-1808 for "ignorance et inaptitude" because most stayed on until they passed or left early if they felt inadequate to the task. Debaralle clearly had the intelligence necessary to do well at the Maternité, but she lacked the willingness to conform to its vision of feminine behavior and medical training.[39]

Her failure was not the proper and moral response to the expensive education she received from the department of the Nord. But although she was in the minority to squander this opportunity, the school did not end up having the effect on infant mortality administrators had hoped for. Even though the instructors insisted that graduates obey the wishes of their prefect, once home, most ended up practicing in the cities or main towns of the department, rather than taking on the hard work of rural midwifery. In the countryside, their diplomas had no meaning, while most expectant mothers preferred the comfort of local matrons rather than young, overly educated *sages-femmes*.[40] The Maternité speakers at graduation, well aware of these problems, stressed that the profession was neither well paid nor stable, and did not promise the comforts expected in other medical fields.[41]

Debaralle's failing to graduate proved to be a key moment in her life. Up until that point, she had attempted to create for herself the identity of a female medical professional by working within the language and theories of the Parisian physicians she had encountered. Rejected for these endeavors, she could have probably returned to her home region and practiced midwifery unhindered. Though medical exam boards run by *officiers de santé* were supposed to register all midwives, mayors and local authorities hardly ever targeted midwives who failed to do so.[42] Debaralle did return to the Nord, but chose instead to openly advertise herself as a healer and an inventor of patent remedies, leaving behind the respectable titles of "midwife" and "scientist." If she succeeded, she could gain much greater wealth than as a rural midwife. By age twenty-four, she claimed that her remedies could cure just about any illness and was calling herself "une théologienne" who with "un seul coup d'oil [*sic*] […] embrasse l'univers."[43] In her public writings, she almost completely rejected the clinical medical terms and theories that she had learned and instead adopted the language of healers to persuade the public of her expertise. She called its attention to her study of alchemy, chemistry and the occult, rather than her training at the Maternité in anatomy and clinical medicine.[44] By speaking out against the theories of professional physicians, she put into words the fears and frustrations of local communities who were often suspicious of the new theories used by physicians and surgeons.

None of her actions were deemed legitimate or legal for women to partake in. One of the many disruptions brought by the Revolution was the elimination of regulations over medical care and pharmaceuticals, allowing anyone to practice, at least for a short time. In 1803, due to pressure from medical professionals, the Napoleonic government passed the Ventôse law to establish regulations that would define who would be allowed to practice medicine. The law instituted a two-tiered system to train medical practitioners: "doctors who could practice anywhere, and health officers, who would be able to practice only in rural areas."[45] A loophole in the law, section 23, allowed those who had practiced medicine for at least three years since the closing of the universities and who had local notable support, to receive a certificate equivalent to the diploma of an *officier de santé*. Local prefects in need of medical care certified "mediocre and little educated" health officers.[46] The Germinal law, passed a few weeks later, limited the sale of remedies to pharmacists and outlawed the advertising and hawking of patent medicines or their sale in pharmacies. But an 1805 decree allowed government permissions for remedies with the approval of a medical board that undermined the rigor of the earlier legislation.[47] Like many others at the time, these laws lacked clear means of enforcement. From the beginning, medical professionals complained that the new laws allowed non-professionals to continue practicing with little regulation, while unofficial practitioners complained that the law constrained them and stifled their innovations.

Women were not explicitly banned from practicing medicine under the original law of 1803, but the male medical committees in charge of approving medical practitioners as well as entrance to medical schools nevertheless rejected all requests by women.[48] In August 1803, Chaptal closed loopholes by specifically excluding women, empirics, those who had dishonored themselves and those who put on public shows, categories that described Debaralle well.[49] As for the selling of remedies, the law made it clear that women would not be allowed into the newly established profession of pharmacist.[50] As a creator of remedies, Debaralle did have the legal option of asking for a special permission and a government patent, but this had become increasingly difficult in the post-revolutionary climate of medical policing of outsiders.[51] Debaralle's illegal option was to quietly hawk her goods and heal the sick without attracting attention from the official competition, in her case the *officiers de santé* and pharmacists.

Debaralle had no intention of keeping quiet her resentment of men's prerogative to heal and save lives, especially their monopoly on innovations and techniques of healing. She did not wish to have the "appétit dévorant que j'ai pour ce charmant emploi si utile à l'humanité" denied.[52] She wondered incredulously “les lois civiles ont-elles exclu le sexe féminin du droit de l'art de guérir?” and answered “non” despite the clarification of the 1803 law.[53] In keeping with the traditional view of treatment as charity, she believed her practices fell into the category of humanitarian acts based in religious morality. During the Old Regime, charitable healers, especially women, were tolerated as imitating the work of Christ.[54] In 1805, however, the government made it clear that charitable healing applied only to priests and could not include remedies or fees.[55] Nevertheless, due to a lack of personnel, the government allowed orders of nuns and lay sisters to continue their Old Regime practice of running hospitals and their pharmacies, making diagnoses and administering bloodletting.[56] These orders reinforced the traditional association of women with wise medical advice and care.[57] Debaralle could have joined a lay religious order such as the sisters of charity to gain freedom in administering healthcare, but that would also mean the strict supervision she had lived under at the Maternité. Lay sisters, who did not wear habits or take vows, had to remain pure even as they ministered to society's most morally suspect populations, including prostitutes and criminals.[58]

Debaralle ignored the legal limitations imposed on her as a single businesswoman and persevered in her attempt to make a space for herself as a coequal to male medical practitioners. One way to do this was to prove she could debate medical and scientific theories with her aspirational peer group. Throughout her struggle for the right to practice and sell medicine, she attempted to engage Parisian professionals in discussion about medical theories, even as she stubbornly clung to ideas they had rejected. For instance, when the doctors in Tournay (in the nearby department of Jemappes, part of her territory) were asked to issue free vaccinations to the poor, she took the side of a local legislator, arguing strongly about their dangers. In this case, she was turning her back on her schooling at the Maternité, where she had been trained to administer vaccinations.[59] Another time, she included in one of her advertisements an “observation” on smallpox, in which she speculated on its link to illnesses related to old age such as arthritis and loss of hearing.[60] She also entered a medical contest on curing the croup open only to doctors.[61] Although her actual proposal is missing, her focus on humeral treatments indicates that it would not have met the standards of the day. The doctors administering the contest, including her old teachers Baudelocque and Chaussier, were put off by her stance against vaccines, her utter lack of propriety in entering the contest and her ineptitude in medical matters. Ultimately, they believed that even responding to her theories would give her too much attention.[62]

When it came to attention, Debaralle garnered much when she openly touted and sold her medicines and practiced healing on her clients. Calling herself a "dame consultante en médecine," she travelled (from the fifth to the twentieth of every month) to the homes of individuals who had been abandoned by medical professionals throughout the Nord and Jemappes. She promised results using only "remèdes doux" instead of harsh drugs or surgery. Customers could buy her remedies from her directly or from their local pharmacies (even though patent medicines could not be sold without a permission). Some remedies were for common ailments such as fever, cough, inflammation of the limbs and bladder infections. She listed remedies that pertained solely to women's ailments, specifically those related to pregnancy such as post-partum depression (she called it "aliénation d'esprit provenue par suite de couche") and difficult labor recovery.[63] Her main remedies, however, were aimed at treating the loss of hearing and sight, two time-honored charlatan cures. Promising miracles was a surefire way to gain the disapproval of the medical community.

Unlike many of the simpler recipes of this period, Debaralle's contained up to twenty-four different ingredients, though none that were widely considered dangerous. Many were the traditional ingredients of rural cures: milk, beer, herbs, vegetables and honey. She also listed the ingredients that she thought were ineffective, such as ink, bone powder, lemon juice and sugar. Her ministrations included instructions to her patients about what to eat while taking her remedies, an aspect of treatment common to humeral medicine but also practiced by the hospital sisters she worked alongside at the Maternité.[64] Women had played an important role in the science of medical cookery until the late eighteenth century, at which point the medical profession labeled chemistry and pharmacy distinctly male fields.[65]

Not surprisingly, by selling remedies, promising cures and healing the sick, Debaralle put herself at odds with the *officiers de santé* of the Nord as soon as she returned in 1805. These men alerted the authorities of the Nord and she was cited (and maybe fined) for practicing medicine without permission. Though she went into hiding for five months due to this first run-in with the law, she did not remain silent about the inadequacies of the *officiers*' training.[66] She clearly looked down on these men as not worth her time, especially since the Maternité had emphasized the student midwives' superiority in all things obstetric. Debaralle attempted to discredit the *officiers* by having local mayors write to the Minister of Interior about their ineptitude.[67] She also accused them of using mercury in their treatments, and needing the "lumières du sexe féminin pour s'enrichir."[68] Many physicians did not respect *officiers de santé*, whose education at second-tier medical schools was cursory, and probably agreed with these criticisms even while they defended their male colleagues against competition from midwives, healing sisters and empirics.

Wishing to bypass local judgments, Debaralle petitioned the Paris École de Médecine in 1806 for a patent and the right to practice medicine.[69] The latter request was not in their purview, but her patent request was sent to a special committee of physicians. The physicians took their job seriously so they might not overlook legitimate requests, but they suspected most inventors to be charlatans not worth their consideration. They rejected most on the grounds that they lacked originality or contained dangerous ingredients. The committee dragged its feet for years and insisted that inventors submit their recipes, going against the concept of a *remède secret*. It did so because it knew that a stubborn inventor could be issued a *brevet d'invention* by the government if they insisted and paid the fee. Revolutionary law put freedom of invention above government regulation and originality, which led to the issuing of patents to medicines that then had to be policed by local authorities because they had never been actually authorized by the medical committee. This state of affairs left the medical committee feeling cynical and frustrated, because they knew they had no real power to stop patented medicines from being sold.[70]

They rejected Debaralle's initial request for a patent on the basis that she had not submitted her recipes (a common complaint), but it is clear from the language in their notes and correspondence that they had no intention of granting her request no matter what her remedies were made of. The committee felt strongly that "la dame Debaralle peut être considérée comme une espèce d'insensée."[71] The male physicians who read her letters all came to the same conclusion: she was dangerous not because she posed a threat to the public (without her ingredients they could not judge that), but because she made outrageous medical claims about the causes and treatments of diseases. Their visceral response to her early requests (whose tone was not quite as assertive and grandiose as it later became) indicates that the committee would not listen to a woman whose adopted persona crossed the boundaries of what they thought proper and respectful for addressing their august body.

While most female petitioners mentioned their poverty, the loss of their husbands or their large families, Debaralle, single and orphaned, never used her personal life to plead for recognition.[72] Instead, she stood by her own genius as a woman and marshaled supporters for her cause, a ploy common to male petitioners. She named sixty-seven notables, mayors, ex-mayors, notaries, landowners, farmers, midwives and artisans who had seen her perform miraculous cures and could attest to her "sublime talent et ma grande jeunesse joint à mon courage entièrement dévoué pour l'art de guérir."[73] Like many empirics, she depended on the signature of a notary on her petitions to make her medicines appear more reliable. As Matthew Ramsey has argued, however, after the Revolution long lists of supporters no longer had a positive influence in the awarding of patents.[74]

From Debaralle's point of view, letting a panel of physicians control remedies and healing was excessive and would silence a medical genius, such as herself, who had the power to save the French people. Some inventors wanted to be allowed to test the market and to leave it to the public to accept or reject their products, rather than the corrupt state system. Essentially giving a monopoly to doctors and pharmacists meant ignoring other methods that had proven effective in the past. Despite the growth of clinical and experimental medicine in the late eighteenth century, the committee did not test the remedies or their ingredients before deciding if they worked or were dangerous. Instead they compared ingredients to the accepted pharmacopeia to judge a new remedy's efficacy.[75]

The patent committee members were routinely suspected of stealing the recipes of popular *remèdes secrets* and profiting from their sale.[76] Debaralle accused them of stealing her unguent and thus "crapuleusement [imitant] les véritables charlatans."[77] She had been reluctant to send the committee her recipe, and when she finally did, she became convinced that a certain Faltranck from the Swiss Alps was selling her invention. The male medical professionals' theft represented their own inadequacies in the face of a woman whose inventiveness was for "l'honneur de son sexe."[78] She wrote to the École de médecine to inform them that due to their injustice she would let humanity "souffrir et mourir" rather than treat any more patients with her cures, and she threatened to take her secrets to her grave if they did not grant her patent.[79]

Despite raging against the unfairness of the system, Debaralle, like most inventors, still wanted the benefits afforded by an official patent. Without the approval of the medical profession, an inventor was simply another untrustworthy charlatan. Many inventors hoped to use their permission (along with a government patent) to gain regional if not national customers through advertisements, which made the traditional travelling mountebank a thing of the past. The 1803 law allowed advertisements of *remèdes secrets* to be published only if they had the permission of the École de médecine (enforced by the local prefect), but the law had little effect in limiting the number of handbills and newspaper advertisements.[80] Yet, unlike the Old Regime when these sellers advertised alongside professionals in the pages of journals, by the early nineteenth century professional doctors and pharmacists had begun to disappear from advertisements in journals aimed at a general audience, while more specialized medical journals censored their content.[81] No longer able to position themselves next to more official names, inventors of medicines needed a patent now more than ever as proof of their official connection with the medical profession. But since most were not patented, it also provided a space where inventors could point to the inequalities of the new system of medical approval. This act of advertising was a direct challenge to doctors whose identity revolved around discrediting all challenges to their standing. These would-be inventors did not realize that the increasing discredit of advertising meant that these tracts could only further antagonize those who controlled medical permissions.

Debaralle avidly advertised in local *affiches* and the *Gazette de France* in addition to publishing leaflets and tracts. Like most advertisements for remedies, Debaralle promoted her products and their benefits, and included the names of patients who could attest to her successes. When published solely as tracts, advertisements for remedies were typically florid, over-the-top claims for miracle cures. When published in respectable journals, advertisements for *remèdes secrets* tended to be short and discreet, and often did not name the seller, depending instead on the public's recognition of the cure and the legitimacy of its patent or permission. In contrast, Debaralle's inserts and tracts were clearly her weapons to publicize her long struggle for a permission. They were long, angry missives that focused as much on her victimization by the ministry and the individual doctors in Paris as on her actual remedies. She mocked these "imbeciles" for calling her "insensée, folle, charlatane […]."[82] She accused the doctors in Paris of being "assassins privilégiés" whose only motivation was "lâche cupidité." She publicly challenged them to a cure-off of sorts to prove who was the better healer. None of her attempts to publicly humiliate the medical professionals of Paris were likely to have gained her any sympathy.[83]

Debaralle hoped, however, that her advertisements would garner her public support, transforming her struggle into a *cause célèbre*. She urged her patients to use the press to publish their opinions of her work, especially regarding invitations to work in their community. Her campaign extended from the Nord to Jemappes, and she even asked readers from as far as the Corrèze to corroborate her claims.[84] She wanted her readership to be actively involved in her struggle against the medical community and urged them to ignore "tous les sarcasmes que l'on a fait circuler contre elle."[85] She eventually included all of these advertisements in her petitions to the Minister of the Interior so that he might see both what the "cabaleuse ignorance" of her enemies was doing and to show him that she was capable of fighting back using public opinion.[86] Debaralle informed readers of her advertisements that they could request a copy of her correspondence with the Minister if they wanted proof of the conspiracy to quash her genius and livelihood.[87]

Over time, Debaralle's crusade for recognition took on a very personal and increasingly paranoid quality. In her advertisements, she publicly expressed her anger at the treatment she had received from Baudelocque and Dubois.[88] At the heart of her rancor was her failure to receive a midwifery certificate as well as the persecution of her medical practices she believed this engendered. She accused Dubois of profiting from the theft of her recipes, simply because a Sieur Dubois was selling Faltranck's Swiss unguent (the medicine she claimed was stolen from her). This Dubois was a pharmacist, but the name alone was enough to raise Debaralle's suspicion and she ended many of her advertisements with the following lament: "c'est sous le nom du sieur Dubois que la faculté de médecine veut recouvrir son honteuse misère à mes dépenses."[89] Having once stood up for herself against the men of the Maternité, she was sure that they had a personal vendetta against her righteous claim for medical recognition.[90]

Despite her many tracts and inserts, Debaralle had little success disseminating her advertisements to medical journals aimed at a more professional readership. In May of 1807, P. J. Marie de Saint-Ursin, editor of the *Gazette de santé*, received Debaralle's advertisement/complaint. He published only part of it to show the great lengths to which charlatans would go and was especially angered that she attacked the local *officiers de santé* by name. The reason he did not publish her entire advertisement was because

> la plume se refuse de continuer la suite de telles ordures […]. Bon dieu, est-ce de bonne foi qu'une intrigante, sans missions comme sans titre, ose se porter accusatrice contre des médecins investis par la loi du pouvoir de la dénoncer devant les tribunaux […]. Nous invitons, au nom de l'honneur et de la sureté publique, les personnes qui ont des renseignements sur cette Canidie [sorcière], à nous les faire parvenir et à notre tour nous en composerons son acte d'accusation.[91]

Marie de Saint-Ursin juxtaposed the legal status of *officiers de santé* to Debaralle's status as a witch to make clear the gender component of his distrust. Debaralle was not just any charlatan, but a woman whose remedies were akin to black magic and who deserved to be punished like other women who had stepped outside their traditional roles. Instead of a witch burning, however, Marie de Saint-Ursin hoped for a public hearing in front of a medical jury, a more enlightened solution.

Marie de Saint-Ursin believed strongly that one of his responsibilities as the editor of a medical journal was to warn the public about charlatan tricks. He published lists of contraband medicines to protect legitimate patented remedies. He also listed the prison sentences of charlatans who sold or practiced medicine, making special note of those who had killed innocent children. The fates of these criminal inventors were intended as a warning for patients and would-be charlatans. The *Gazette*'s main readers were urban, educated men and women, who would have read the lists more for their shock value. While he blamed gullible patients who patronized healers, Marie de Saint-Ursin also hoped to energize physicians to better protect their monopoly.[92]

The doctors in Paris, like Marie de Saint-Ursin, responded viscerally to Debaralle's petitions and advertisements, above and beyond her influence and possibility for harm. Her medicines were not actually dangerous in terms of contemporary notions. Many other similar remedies were simply rejected by the committee without further action. Debaralle's case, however, required constant responses from a frustrated medical committee who insisted that she be treated as a madwoman rather than as a legitimate petitioner. The complex system of patents and medical permissions instituted after the Revolution had to be constantly protected and reinforced from within to stop such an individual from gaining access. But despite their rejections, Debaralle did not desist in her requests because she desired fervently not only to practice her activities unbothered (illegal as they were), but also to be given credit for them and recognized by male physicians as their equal. In a climate when inventors of remedies were unlikely to gain an official permission and healers were automatically defined as charlatans, Debaralle's delusional mindset allowed her to create a space for her ideas and remedies that would not have been at all possible if she had been the mild-mannered, discreet and obedient midwife student the Maternité expected.

Debaralle's accusations and increasingly delusional behavior served only to anger further those she wanted to sway. After a year of correspondence, in December 1807, the committee members decided that Debaralle could not be dissuaded. Despite their desire to institute a "repressive program," these physicians spent a lot of ink and time responding to Debaralle before they decided to involve physical forms of policing.[93] They asked the Minister of the Interior to stop forwarding her letters and to police her actions.[94] Because this was her second offense, authorities could now impose three to ten days in jail for a repeat offense.[95] However, instead of an immediate arrest order, the Minister asked the new prefect of the Nord, François de Pommereul, to make sure she could not sell or advertise her remedies. In turn, the mayor of Lille was to supervise her movements so as to take necessary police action if she was caught selling medicines.[96] Thus, despite direct evidence that she was practicing medicine, the authorities did not immediately act, preferring instead to issue a warning hoping she might cease her activities without the use of force. Since Debaralle also practiced in Jemappes, these constraints could only be partially effective.

Debaralle garnered more attention and policing than most patent requests, but her case illustrates the tension between local authorities and the Parisian establishment on the matter of unlicensed healers. Over the two years since her first citation, despite her continued public advertising of her skills and criticisms of the *officiers de santé*, the authorities of the Nord and Jemappes did little to stop her until the Parisian authorities got involved. Typically, orders from Paris led to infrequent police action against empirics and few prosecutions. Low fines and short jail sentences were also not strong enough deterrents to stop recidivism among healers.[97] Even if a prefect were enthusiastic about reforms, such as Dieudonné had been, he would not have been able to control local support for the more traditional health care systems in the department's towns and villages. Mayors and even prefects were accused of protecting charlatans or of ignoring the problem.[98] Public protests against arrests of well-known healers also stymied official efforts.[99] Rural patients were not transformed by the revolution in medicine overnight. Most did not have access to trained physicians or even *officiers de santé*, and more importantly could not afford to pay their fees. They were also more likely to trust a well-known empiric or village matron than an outsider.[100] Inventors and healers often evaded the law because of the law's protection of intellectual property, the support of local communities, the need for rural health care and the lack of effective policing.

Debaralle's assertiveness, her delusions of grandeur and her gender made her an easier target for repression, but she did initially have local support for her practice. She most frequently mentioned as a protector the mayor of Tournay, Charles Henri Derasse, whose city lay outside the jurisdiction of the police asked to monitor her activities.[101] She accused her enemies, specifically the *officiers de santé*, of having

> la bassesse de ramper après la protection du pauvre Derasse [...] afin que son autorisation de Maire les seconde dans les intrigues criminelles qu'ils

> ont injustement tramées contre cette dite demoiselle, au préjudice de ses talens et de sa personne [...].[102]

While Debaralle waged her fight from Paris to Tournay, she was sure her opponents worked behind the scenes to turn her supporters against her. Mayors of small towns may have been willing to look the other way because she provided a public service, in direct contrast to the medical establishment that was failing to provide citizens with affordable and available healthcare. Debaralle's local patrons could only have protected her if she had limited her advertising and her activities, and remained quietly within the area they controlled as a sedentary empiric. She, of course, was not quiet and spread her practices to three departments, as well as advertising nationally. As a single woman struggling to enter a male profession, Debaralle would have been in a precarious position if she no longer had the support of small town mayors.

By the fall of 1807, Debaralle appears to have lost Derasse's support. She wrote to the Minister of Justice to plead for his protection against "des gens de l'art qui voudraient de nouveau me plonger dans le milieu d'un gouffre d'abime éternelle."[103] It was soon after that the commission requested that she be policed, and we can assume from her later hints that this policing eventually led to a short incarceration.[104] She continued between 1808 and 1812 to write and petition the government, even claiming to have asked the Baron de Montesquiou Fezensac, *aide de camp* to Marechal Ney, to deliver a request for a passport to practice medicine to Emperor Napoleon himself. Due to the delivery of this passport, she claimed the police commissioner and a magistrate broke into her house to steal it. She blamed for her predicament the incompetent prefect of the Nord whom she labeled "ivrogne."[105]

By the end of 1812 she was, in her own words, "robespierristement séquestrée" by the authorities of Lille, this time for a lengthy sentence. It is not clear what the authorities charged her with, but she claimed it was for criticizing the government and petitioning for the rights of prisoners. During the harsh climate of repression of civil rights under Napoleon, a claim such as this would have been plausible, though her illegal medical practices were likely to have played a role. If it was due to her medical practices, her sentence of over six and a half months indicates it was her third offense and the authorities in Lille felt harsh punishment was necessary.[106] The ineffectual nature of her previous punishments (be they fines or short jail time) and the six years she was allowed to mostly freely practice highlight the difficulty officials had in actually policing the practices of medicine, despite their stated intentions of doing so. This final attempt to silence her, however, had a significant effect on her physical and mental health. Her incarceration was humiliating and exposed her to the horrors of Napoleonic prisons. She was convinced her female keepers were poisoning her food, she had partial sight loss and her jealous fellow inmates accused her of witchcraft because "ce n'était pas possible [...] qu'une demoiselle eut naturellement autant d'esprit."[107]

In July 1813 she escaped and, fearing pursuit by the authorities of Lille, hid herself in Paris, only to expose herself by petitioning the Imperial court to go after those in Lille who had abused her and to hopefully be awarded monetary compensation for her hardship in prison.[108] The court was unlikely to welcome her case, but the fact that she identified herself in the petition as an "altesse," great-granddaughter of a made-up sovereign Debarallecom, convinced the secretary in charge to jokingly suggest she be locked up in the insane asylum at Charenton.[109] The new emphasis at Charenton on "moral means" for treating the mentally ill meant that this fate would certainly not have been as horrendous as during the Old Regime or her own stay in prison. Still in their infancy, mental health hospitals had not yet turned their focus to a mass incarceration of the insane, and it would not be until the last decades of the nineteenth century that female hysteria took center stage. In this climate, Debaralle's delusions of grandeur and persecution were not sufficient cause for pursuing her and the case was ignored.[110]

What happened after this is unclear. In her 1813 petition to the court, she claimed she would petition for the release of inmates that she believed were unfairly imprisoned in Lille. Despite her empathy for others being "inné en moi," she realized this might lead to "mon malheur" since these petitions would put her at odds once again with her enemies in the Nord. Though she still called herself "oculiste" and "doctoresse," the literary accomplishments she presented to the authorities as proof of her genius included a memoir of her early life and two comedies. These new endeavors might prove less controversial if no more remunerative than medical practice. In Paris she could disappear and remake herself once more, having already traveled from midwifery student to science writer to healer and now to human rights activist and "femme de lettres." Despite her declining mental and physical health, her belief in her own untapped talents remained strong. Nevertheless, she signed her letter to the Imperial court "Debaralle l'infortunée," a far cry from her opening title of "altesse."[111] Whatever fragile mental state she had before her arrest was made much worse by her incarceration, which opened the door for the first time for desperate self-pity rather than triumphant bravado.

The doctors and administrators who encountered Debaralle's tracts and petitions saw her as an insane, dangerous con artist (charges undoubtedly partly true).[112] But she was also a young woman sure of her own medical skills (however unscientific they may have been) who was lured by the promise of a medical education. She learned first-hand about the limited possibilities for women in the Parisian medical world, and returned to the provinces disgusted and prepared to challenge its authority. Unlike Boivin and other women who persevered on the periphery of a male profession, Debaralle did not have the patience to submit to expectations of feminine spaces for healing, which limited freedom of movement and scope for inventiveness. Her growing delusions and paranoia were in many ways what made her efforts possible and even temporarily successful, fueling a blind obstinacy in the face of insurmountable odds. The Revolution she had grown up in opened up spaces for creative inventions of self that Debaralle clung to as a means for survival despite the increasingly strict Napoleonic legislation. She, like others, found temporary spaces to practice her skills where official medical personnel were lacking and authorities, both national and regional, were slow to respond. But it was clear that eventually Debaralle's voice and mission would be silenced (at least when it came to her medical practices and theories), not just because she challenged the official medical world's monopoly but because she insisted on speaking louder than those who opposed her.

Notes

[1] Augustine Debaralle, advertisement (1807), Archives Nationales (AN), F/8/149. I would like to thank Cathy McClive, Colin Jones, Jennifer Davis and Carl Almer for help with various versions of this paper; to Rebecca Geoffroy-Schwinden for her research assistance at the Archives Nationales; to the archivists at the Archives de l'Assistance Publique et Hôpitaux de Paris, the Archives de la Seine and the Miner Medical Library at the University of Rochester.

[2] On the medical theories about proper female behavior after the Terror see Sean Quinlan, "Physical and Moral Regeneration after the Terror: Medical Culture, Sensibility and Family Politics in France, 1794-1804," *Social History* 29.2 (May 2004): 152-157. The policing of medicine as part of the larger social control studied by Michel Foucault and others after him is at the center of this work, but as Matthew Ramsey and others have shown, this policing was not as normalizing or disciplinarian as the newly professionalized doctors envisioned it in the eighteenth or early nineteenth centuries. See Michel Foucault, *Birth of the Clinic*, trans. A.M. Sheridan (New York: Pantheon Books, 1973); Matthew Ramsey, "Medical Power and Popular Medicine: Illegal Healers in Nineteenth-century France," *Journal of Social History* 10 (1977): 560-587.

[3] Matthew Ramsey, *Professional and Popular Medicine in France 1770-1830* (New York: Cambridge University Press, 1988), pp. 140, 158, 220.

[4] On the history of *amidonnier* see Morag Martin, *Selling Beauty: Cosmetics, Commerce and French Society, 1750-1830* (Baltimore, MD: Johns Hopkins University Press, 2009), pp.162-164; Catherine Lanoë, *La Poudre et le fard: une histoire des cosmétiques de la Renaissance aux Lumières* (Seyssel: Champ Vallon, 2008), pp. 188-203.

[5] The city lost almost 5000 people during the Revolution, from a high of 24,000 before the Revolution. See Christophe Dieudonné, *Statistique du département du Nord*, vol. 1 (Douai, 1804), p. 144.

[6] Debaralle letter to the Cour Impériale (14 September 1813), AN BB/18/798, case 8578.

[7] Augustine Debaralle, born 30 March 1782; Romaine Debaralle born 31 December 1784; Amélie Debaralle marriage to Louis François Baltazar Isanbard 3 November 1781. See Paroisse de St. Nicolas, Canton de Valenciennes, Registres paroissiaux, AD Lille, BMS, volumes l-lxi, 1737-1794, microfilmed by the Genealogical Society of Salt Lake City Utah, film #1172372.

[8] By 1813 she mentioned that both her parents were dead, but since they do not show up in the Valenciennes *état civil* after 1802 or in the parish records pre-1789, they must have passed away during the Revolutionary years. See Debaralle letter to the Cour Impériale (14 September 1813), AN BB/18/798, case 8578.

[9] Before the training started there were only sixty-one officially registered midwives and *accoucheurs* in the *Nord*, so this extra group of eighty was much needed. See Dieudonné, vol. 3, p. 156; *Recueil des procès verbaux de distribution de prix aux élèves-sages-femmes,* vol. 1 (Paris, 1816), tables attached at back; *Annuaire du département du Nord pour l'an 1809* (Lille, 1809), pp. 31-40.

[10] Olivier Faure, *Les Français et leur médecine au XIXe siècle* (Paris: Belin, 1993), p. 25. Medical students were not trained in obstetrics until the 1850s, while *officiers de santé* were only given cursory training in birthing. For historians who stress women's professional development see June Burton, *Napoleon and the Woman Question* (Lubbock: Texas Tech University Press, 2007); Scarlett Beauvalet-Boutouyrie, *Naître à l'hôpital au XIXe siècle* (Paris: Belin, 1999).

[11] Beauvalet-Boutouyrie, pp. 135-136.

[12] Dieudonné, vol. 3, p. 156; S. Bottin, *Annuaire statistique du department du Nord pour l'an 1806* (Lille, 1806), p. 340.

[13] Beauvalet-Boutouyrie, p. 121.

[14] Speech by M. Alhoy, membre de la commission administrative, "Procès verbal de la distribution des prix" (25 Prairial, An XIII) [14 May 1805], 6, in *Recueil des procès-verbaux*, vol. 1.

[15] Beauvalet-Boutouyrie, p. 158.

[16] Speech by Baudelocque, "Procès verbal de la distribution des prix" (27 Frimaire An XIII) [18 Nov. 1804], pp. 24-25, in *Recueil des procès-verbaux*, vol. 1. Dubois had similar concerns. See Paul Delauney, *Maternité de Paris* (Paris: Rousset, 1909), p. 215.

[17] Jean Louis Baudelocque, *Principes sur l'art des accouchemens, par demandes et réponses, en faveur des sages-femmes de la campagne* (Paris: Méquignon l'aîné, 1812).

[18] Both served as the Imperial family's obstetrician. Baudelocque is best remembered for inventing a type of caliper that allowed doctors to decide if surgery was necessary. Dubois travelled with Napoleon to Egypt, delivered the King of Rome and invented a type of forceps. June Burton implies that both of these men spent much time teaching midwifery students, but Beauvalet-Boutouyrie claims they were too busy with other responsibilities to do so. See Burton, pp. 95-97; Beauvalet-Boutouyrie, p. 124.

[19] Baudelocque, *L'art des accouchemens*, 2 vols. (Paris: Méquignon l'aîné, 1781).

[20] The midwife in question was present at the dissection of two patients who presented interesting cases for science, according to Chaussier. See speech by Chaussier, "Procès-verbal" (25 Prairial, An XIII) [14 May 1805], pp. 35-37 and (29 June 1807), pp. 26-27, both in *Recueil des procès-verbaux*, vol. 1.

[21] "Procès-verbal" (29 June 1807), p. 21, in *Recueil des procès-verbaux*, vol. 1. He also thanked students who followed him on rounds and took copious clinical notes. See "Procès-verbal" (December 1806), p. 26 in *Recueil des procès-verbaux*, vol. 1.

[22] Speech by Baudelocque, "Procès-verbal" (1808-1809), p. 57 in *Recueil des procès-verbaux*, vol. 1; Louis Piesse, *Les Médecins français contemporains*, vol. 2 (Paris: 1828), p. 129.

[23] Baudelocque and Chaussier are not the only male physicians who supported women's right to dominate the profession. For examples of early modern doctors and scientists who argued for the feminine dominance of the profession see Leigh Whaley, *Women and the Practice of Medical Care in Early Modern Europe 1400-1800* (NY: Palgrave MacMillan, 2011), pp. 106-111.

[24] Speech by Baudeloque, *Procès-verbal* (29 Frimaire, An XII) [20 Nov. 1803], p. 25, in *Recueil des procès-verbaux*, vol. 1.

[25] Pierre Huard, *Science, médecine, pharmacie de la Révolution à l'Empire* (Paris: Editions Roger Dacosta, 1970), pp. 221, 223; Beauvalet-Boutouyrie, pp. 124-125.

[26] Beauvalet-Boutouyrie, p. 108.

[27] Baudelocque, *L'Art des accouchemens*, vol. 1 (Paris, 1796), pp. 175-177. For a description of Sabatier's discoveries and subsequent theories about fetal blood circulation, see Geoffrey S. Dawes, "Physiological Changes in the Circulation after Birth," in *Circulation of the Blood: Men and Ideas*, ed. Alfred P. Fishman and Dickinson W. Richard (New York: Oxford University Press, 1964), pp. 747-750.

[28] Augustine de Baralle, *Fruit de la récréation de l'auteur* (Paris: l'auteur, 1805), p. 3.

[29] Debaralle, letter to Cour Impériale (14 September 1813) AN BB/18/798, case 8578.

[30] *Catalogue des sciences médicales*, vol. 1 (Paris: Firmin Didot Frères, 1857), p. 367.

[31] Aphorisms of D'orazio Valota in Marie-Anne Boivin, *Mémorial de l'art des accouchements* (Paris: Méquignon père, 1812), p. 646.

[32] For her accomplishments the University of Marberg in Germany granted her a diploma of Doctor of Medicine. See Burton, pp. 103-105.

[33] Burton, n. 43, p. 223.

[34] Whaley, p. 142

[35] Of these thirty-three, an amazing twenty-two were from the *Nord*, with eight of their original thirty staying on another year. This obviously leaves out the failure of Debaralle, discussed below in the text. See *Annuaire statistique* (Lille: 1806), pp. 339-340.

[36] "Procès-verbal" (25 Prairial, An XIII) [15 May, 1805], p. 25, in *Recueil de procès-verbaux*, vol. 1.

[37] Dubois was not listed as being present at her exam. See Debaralle, letter to the Minister of the Interior (12 January 1807), AN F/8/149.

[38] See, for instance, examples of exam topics given to students the year before: "Procès-verbal" (29 Frimaire, An XII) [20 Nov. 1803], 27-28 in *Recueil des procès-verbaux*, vol. 1.

[39] "Procès-verbal" (1808-1809), p. 65 in *Recueil des procès-verbaux*, vol. 1. Guy Michel Razafindramboa found a vicious letter to Mme Lachapelle, head midwife, critiquing the methods of teaching. Though I was not able to locate this letter, his description of the tone, time period and handwriting make it likely to be from Debaralle. Guy Michel Razafindramboa, *Jean Louis Baudelocque, Pionnier de l'obstétrique* (Thèse en médecine, Université de Paris VII, 1978), p. 16.

[40] Jacques Gelis, *La Sage-femme ou le médecin: une nouvelle conception de la vie* (Paris: Fayard, 1988), pp. 214-215.

[41] Speech by Baudelocque, "Procès-verbal" (1808-1809), p. 45 in *Recueil des procès-verbaux*, vol. 1.

[42] Faure, *Les Français et leur médecine*, p. 28.

[43] "Extraits de registres des délibérations de l'assemblée des professeurs de l'école de médecine de Paris" (12 March 1807), AN F/8/149.

[44] "Extraits de registres" (12 March 1807), AN F/8/149.

[45] Ramsey, *Professional and Popular Medicine*, p. 77.

[46] Ramsey, *Professional and Popular Medicine*, p. 77. See also Faure, *Les Français et leur médicine,* p. 16.

[47] Ramsey, "Property Rights and the Right to Health: The Regulation of Secret Remedies in France 1789-1815," *Medical Fringe and Medical Orthodoxy 1750-1850*, eds. W.F. Bynum and Roy Porter (London: Crom Helm, 1987), p. 89.

[48] Ramsey, *Professional and Popular Medicine*, pp. 78-79, 86.

[49]Jacques Léonard, "Femmes, religion et médecine: Les religieuses qui soignent en France au XIXe siècle," *Annales, Economies, Société, Civilisation* (Sept-Oct 1977): 887.

[50]Jacques Léonard, "Women, Religion and Medicine," in *Medicine and Society in France*, ed. Robert Foster and Orest Ranum (Baltimore, MD: Johns Hopkins University Press, 1980), p. 24.

[51] Circulaire by the Minister of the Interior (16 April 1828) in Adolphe Trébuchet, *Jurisprudence de la médecine, de la chirurgie et de la pharmacie en France* (Paris: 1834), p. 367; Ramsey, *Professional and Popular Medicine*, p. 101.

[52] Debaralle, notes for letters, AN F/8/149.

[53] "Extraits de registres" (27 March 1807), AN F/8/149.

[54] Ramsey, *Professional and Popular Medicine,* p. 35; Faure, "Health Care provision and Poor Relief in 19th century Provincial France," in *Health Care and*

Poor Relief in 18th and 19th Century Europe, ed. Ole Peter Grell, Andrew Cunningham and Robert Jütte (New York: Ashgate, 2002), p. 313.

[55] Ramsey finds that priests were asked to take the same medical exams as other practitioners. See Ramsey, *Professional and Popular Medicine*, p. 99.

[56] Ramsey, *Professional and Popular Medicine*, p. 91; Faure, "Les Religieuses dans les petits hôpitaux en France au XIX siècle," in *L'Hôpital entre religions et laïcité: du moyen âge à nos jours*, ed. Jacqueline Lalouette (Paris: Letouzey et Ané, 2006), p. 71; Whaley, p. 127.

[57] For instance the physician Jean Liébault felt women had the knowledge to practice medicine, especially herbal remedies. For other examples see Whaley, pp. 58-59.

[58] The sisters of charity were also not allowed to care for pregnant women in most provincial hospitals, so as to protect their innocence. See Colin Jones, *Charitable Imperative: Hospitals and Nursing in Ancien Regime and Revolutionary* France (London: Routledge, 1989), p. 190; Marie Claude Dinet-Lecomte, *Les Soeurs hospitalières en France au XVIIe et XVIIIe siècles: la charité en action* (Paris: Champion, 2006), pp. 355-356, 405.

[59] Debaralle, *Observations* (s.d.), AN F/8/149; *Réflexions critiques et analytiques sur quelques passages de l'essai chronologique pour servir à l'histoire de Tournay par M. Hoverlant, ex-législateur* (Lille: V. Leleux, 1809), pp. 3-7.

[60] "Napoléon et les médecins," *Toute l'histoire de Napoléon*, vol. 8 (1951), p. 26.

[61] Debaralle knew about this contest by reading a local newspaper, which had copied an advertisement from the more prestigious *Gazette de santé.* Hoping to be awarded the grand prize of 10,000 francs and not wishing to look greedy, she asked that it be given to five orphans of the city of Lille and its mayor who supported her. See *Bulletin de l'école de médecine de Paris*, 8 (1807): 106; Debaralle, letter to the École de médecine (1807), AN F/8/149; *Gazette de santé* (11 August 1807): 23.

[62] "Extraits de registres des délibérations de l'assemblée des professeurs de l'école de médecine de Paris" (3 December 1807), AN F/8/149.

[63] Debaralle, advertisement (27 March 1807), AN F/8/149.

[64] Debaralle, "Invitation sommaire qui a été signifiée à messieurs les professeurs de l'école de médecine de Paris," (1 October 1807); letter to the Minister of the Interior (12 January 1807), AN F/8/149; Daniel Hickey, "To Improve the Training of Nurses in France: The Manuals Published as Teaching-Aids, 1775-1895," *Canadian Bulletin of Medical History* 27.1 (2010): 166.

[65] Londa Schiebinger, *The Mind Has No Sex? Women in the Origins of Modern Science* (Cambridge, MA: Harvard University Press, 1989), pp. 112-116.

[66] It is unclear if she was fined the 25 to 600 francs the law allowed. See Debaralle, letter to the Minister of the Interior (12 January 1807), AN F/8/149; André Narodetzki, "Le remède secret: législation et jurisprudence de la loi du 21 Germinal an XI au décret du 13 juillet 1926" (unpublished PhD thesis, University of Paris, 1928), p. 13. See also Ramsey, "Property Rights," p. 89.

[67] "Lettre du maire et son adjoint, défense de Mme Debaralle" (11 November 1806), AN F/8/149.

[68] Debaralle, advertisement (27 March 1807), AN F/8/149.
[69] Many empirics petitioned the government for the right to continue practicing their trade after 1803 believing it still had the Old Regime power of granting privileges. See Ramsey, *Professional and Popular Medicine*, p. 96.
[70] For a description of the work of the committee see Ramsey, "Property Rights," pp. 90-91; Morag Martin, p. 113.
[71] "Extraits de registres" (12 March 1807), AN F/8/149.
[72] Ramsey, *Professional and Popular Medicine*, p. 222.
[73] Debaralle, advertisement from *Gazette de France* (14 July 1806) and letter to the Minister of the Interior (12 January 1807), AN F/8/149.
[74] Ramsey, *Professional and Popular Medicine*, p. 101.
[75] Georges-Christophe Würtz, *Sur la police des remèdes secrets et sur les mesures les plus avantageuses au public à prendre à leur regard* (Amsterdam: l'héritier Guérin, 1807), pp. 10, 5, 12, 14, 51, 75.
[76] *Sur la police des remèdes secrets,* pp. 10, 5, 51, 75.
[77] Debaralle, "Invitation sommaire" (1 October 1807), AN F/8/149.
[78] Debaralle, "Invitation sommaire" (1 October 1807), AN F/8/149.
[79] Debaralle, scraps of notes, AN F/8/149.
[80] Louis Faligot, *La question des remèdes secrets sous la Révolution et l'Empire* (Toulouse: E.-H. Guitard, 1924), p. 56; Faure, *Les Français et leur médecine*, p. 68. On the Old Regime, see Colin Jones, "Great Chain of Buying," *American Historical Review* 101.1 (February 1996): 30-31. These advertisements grew in number after the Revolution. Laurence Brockliss and Colin Jones, *The Medical World of Early Modern France* (Oxford: Oxford University Press, 1997), p. 806.
[81] From a sample I took over nine years of the *Affiches de Paris* from 1800-1811 for the month of January (the busiest month in the advertising sector due to the New Year's festivities and the cold weather) only eleven pharmacists placed advertisements, none frequently. See *Affiches, annonces ou avis divers* 1800-1802, 1805-1807, 1810-1812. The *Gazette de santé* banned advertisements for secret remedies in 1778. Pharmacists officially made advertising illegal for themselves by the middle of the century. See Ramsey, "Property Rights," p. 84; *Atteinte à la liberté individuelle des médecins et pharmaciens, examen de la question des remèdes secrets* ([Paris]: les marchands de nouveautés, 1829), p. 12; Marc Martin, *Trois siècles de publicité en France* (Paris: Odile Jacob, 1992), p. 163.
[82] Debaralle, advertisement (July 1807), AN F/8/149.
[83] Debaralle, "Invitation sommaire" (1 octobre 1807), AN F/8/149.
[84] Debaralle, advertisement from *Gazette de France* (14 July 1807) and advertisement pamphlet (1807), AN F/8/149.
[85] Debaralle, advertisement (11 April 1807), AN F/8/149.
[86] Debaralle, letter to the Minister of Interior (10 April 1807), AN F/8/149. She also included an advertisement in her letter to the Minister of Justice. See "Napoléon et les médecins," p. 261.
[87] Debaralle, advertisement in *Gazette de France*, AN F/8/149.
[88] Though Baudelocque had good relations with the women at the *Maternité*, Dubois was not sympathetic to outspoken women according to his sister-in-law.

Dubois was said to treat his third wife as his property, wanting her to "think and say like him, laugh when he laughed, sleep when he slept [...] always available." See Mme Cavaignac, sister-in-law, quoted in Paul Busquet, *Les Biographies médicales: Dubois, Antoine le Baron*, vol. 1 (Paris: J.-B. Baillière et fils, 1930), p. 265.

[89] Debaralle, advertisement (July 1807), AN F/8/149.

[90] Debaralle, letter to the Minister of the Interior (12 January 1807), AN F/8/149.

[91] *Gazette de santé* (1 May 1807), p. 109.

[92] *Gazette de Santé* (11 March 1807); (11 December 1807); (1 Vendémiaire, An XIII) [23 Sept. 1804].

[93] Ramsey, "Medical Power," p. 579.

[94] École de médecine correspondence to the Minister of the Interior (3 December 1807), AN F/8/149.

[95] André Narodetzki, "Le remède secret: législation et jurisprudence de la loi du 21 Germinal an XI au décret du 13 Juillet 1926" (unpublished PhD thesis, University of Paris, 1928), p. 13. See also Ramsey, "Property Rights" p. 89.

[96] Debaralle, letter to the Minister of the Interior (12 January 1807); "A Mr le Préfet du Nord" (11 April 1807), "Préfecture du Nord au Maire de Lille" (17 April 1807), AN F/8/149; Faure, *Les Français et leur médecine*, p. 57.

[97] Faure, *Les Français et leur médecine*, pp. 19-20.

[98] Ramsey, *Professional and Popular Medicine*, p. 104. In 1810 when departments were asked to judge the number of charlatans selling remedies in their region, the Nord responded they were "répandus," but only listed a father and son team selling remedies. This points to the continued ability of especially sedentary rural healers to practice, with only certain more visible inventors, like Debaralle, gaining enough attention to be prosecuted. See Ramsey, "Sous le régime de la législation de 1803: trois enquêtes sur les charlatans au XIXe siècle," *Revue d'histoire moderne et contemporaine*, 27.3 (July-September 1980): 487.

[99] Ramsey, "Medical Power," pp. 576-577.

[100] The department of the Nord started a school to train health officers in 1806 to fill the gaps in medical care (taking students as young as fifteen). The Nord still had a low density of doctors and health officers. In 1804 there were 390 health officers for the whole department and Matthew Ramsey calculates that in the 1830s there were only 4.64 medical practitioners for every 10,000 occupants. *Annuaire statistique* (Lille, 1806), p. 390; Dieudonné, vol. 3, p. 157; Ramsey, *Professional and Popular Medicine,* Appendix A, p. 304.

[101] Derasse was son of a *chaufournier* who was made Chevalier de l'Empire and given the Légion d'Honneur in 1809. Tournay (or Tournai) in the Department of Jemappes today is part of Belgium. *Remarques véridiques sur le mémoire de MM, les chaufourniers de Tournai, adressé au Roi le 21 novembre 1821* (Tournai, 1821), p. 66; *Revue tournaisienne: histoire, archéologie, art, folklore*, 1 (Tournai, 1905): 72.

[102] Debaralle, advertisement (27 March 1807), AN F/8/149.

[103] Debaralle, letter to the École de médecine (October 1807), AN F/8/149; "Napoléon et les Médecins," p. 21.

[104] Debaralle letter to the Cour Imperiale (14 September 1813) AN BB/18/798, case 8578.

[105] The Prefect was now Jean-Marie Valentin Duplantier. Debaralle letter to the Cour Impériale (14 September 1813) AN BB/18/798, case 8578. Debaralle's belief that a "passport" (a form of permission) from the Emperor would allow her to practice medicine was a common assumption made by empirics who often carried with them "passports" written by local authorities that had no real legitimacy. Ramsey, "Sous le régime de la législation de 1803," p. 490.

[106] It is unclear how long her sentence was since she escaped. I have not been able to find documents on her arrest in Lille. Debaralle letter to the Cour Impériale (14 September 1813), AN BB/18/798, case 8578.

[107] She does not tell us at which prison she was held. Neither revolutionary ideals of hygienic and comfortable prisons, nor Bentham's panopticon cellular approach, were realized visions in this period. Despite some reforms in the prison system by Napoleon, locally run prisons remained untouched, while Napoleon's criminal code greatly increased the number of detainees and their length of stay. See Bernard Schapper, "Compression et répression sous le Consulat et l'Empire," *Revue historique de droit français et étranger* 69.1 (1991): 26. Michelle Perrot, *Les Ombres de l'histoire: crime et châtiment au XIXe siècle* (Paris: Flammarion, 2001), pp. 86-87, 186-187. For a detailed overview of the prison system in the region, see Christian Carlier, "Les Prisons du Nord au XIXe siècle," *Histoire pénitentiaire*, vol. 1 (Paris: Direction de l'Administration pénitentiaire, 2004), pp. 70-105; Nicole Garcin, *Justice criminelle, police et médecine légale dans le district de Lille sous la Révolution et la Iière République, 1789-1804*. Mémoire pour diplôme d'études supérieures faculté de droit et de sciences économiques de Lille, 1969.

[108] Criminals were kept in the *dépôt de mendicité* if their crimes were light but the *dépôt* was known for being easy to escape from. Dieudonné, vol. 3, p. 203.

[109] AN BB/18/798, case 8578.

[110] If the famous reformer of mental health studies Philippe Pinel had taken Debaralle's case, he would likely have diagnosed her as having only partial mania, and his follower Jean-Étienne Dominique Esquirol may have labeled her as suffering from "monomania." Hysteria was not yet a recognized form of mental instability, though it was used to describe Debaralle's behavior. For a discussion of classification of the mentally ill in this period, see Laurent Sueur, "Les Classifications des maladies mentales en France, dans la première moitié du XIXe siècles," *Revue historique* 289.2 (1993): 482-509. Many works treat the development of asylums, including of course that of Foucault. For a broad nineteenth-century view on women and incarceration, see Yannick Ripa, *La Ronde des folles. Femmes, folie et enfermement au XIXe siècle* (Paris: Aubier, 1986).

[111] Debaralle letter to the Cour Impériale (14 September 1813), AN BB/18/798, case 8578.

[112] Mathew Ramsey has found that professionals often judged empirics as insane, and many did show signs of paranoia. See Ramsey, *Professional* and *Popular Medicine*, p. 293.

CHAPTER FIVE

THE LABORATORY, THE BOUDOIR AND THE KITCHEN: MEDICINE, HOME AND DOMESTICITY

VALÉRIE LASTINGER

The process of barring access to the medical professions from women in France was slow but efficient. Started in the Middle Ages, it culminated in 1707 with the Treaty of Marly. Louis XIV sealed the complete exclusion of women from the medical profession by requiring that physicians have university degrees, while gaining entrance to a French university required one to be a Catholic male. After the Revolution, non-Catholic individuals would be admitted.[1] Women, Catholic or not, would have to wait until 1875 to see the first French woman physician, Madeleine Brès (1842-1925),[2] successfully defend her thesis. The admission of women to universities, legalized in 1866, had become a *cause célèbre*, and it was only because of Empress Eugénie's intervention that Brès was allowed to matriculate at the Paris Faculté de Médecine. In some ways, the Treaty of Marly was pointless, as universities had little to teach aspiring physicians, and few students enrolled and graduated. Academic standards, especially outside of Paris, were often low. In his *Professional and Popular Medicine in France, 1770-1830,* historian Matthew Ramsey cites the extreme example of a young medical student who, in 1785, "received his baccalaureate on the 18th of July, the *licence* on the 21st, and the doctorate on the 26th."[3]

For women though, the treaty marked their official exclusion from a profession where they had held significant roles until the end of the Middle Ages. In her *Histoire des femmes médecins* (1900) Mélanie Lipinska notes three dates that mark the progressive limitation of women's access to the medical profession, leading to the Treaty of Marly. In 1484, Charles VIII's edict made it more difficult for women to be surgeons. In

1694, even surgeons' widows were forbidden to practice, unless they had a male child or servant who could practice in their stead. Finally, in 1755, women were prohibited from practicing any field related to medicine, such as dentistry, except for midwifery.[4] The exclusion of women from the medical guild is not unique; it parallels what happened in all the other guilds.[5] It is particularly intriguing however that although women were expected to provide medical care as part of their growing domestic responsibilities, they were not permitted to practice medicine outside the home, or to be educated in the healing arts. As they were pushed away from the commercial practice of medicine, women were seated as the ultimate guardians and preservers of domestic life, increasingly accountable for the well-being, comfort, and health of their husbands and children.

Although in the seventeenth and eighteenth centuries, no woman practiced professional medicine, no one would ever suggest that Enlightenment women did not shape modern medicine. The work of cultural historians studying professional women can serve as a template for those seeking to understand their contributions. Before Geraldine Sheridan's pioneer study of women's participation in hard physical labor in her *Louder than Words*, the idea of women miners during a period we associate with Madame de Pompadour would have seemed ludicrous. But through a close reading of the plates of Diderot's *Encyclopédie,* Sheridan clearly demonstrates that many women of the Enlightenment were engaged in hard physical labor, which we typically associate with men laborers. Similarly, I would like to offer a brief analysis of how women of the long eighteenth century, while unable to become physicians, contributed to the advancement and the dissemination of medical and scientific knowledge. It is as though women, as they became more and more excluded from the commercial practice of medicine, took on an ever greater role in the dispensation of care through charitable work, and in the dissemination of basic medical knowledge through the writing of domestic manuals. Analyzing women's contributions to medicine between the Renaissance and the mid-nineteenth century, medical historians have commented on this very phenomenon:

> Mais nulle part, les femmes ne sont admises à la Faculté. On les laisse pratiquer les accouchements? Elles se distinguent en obstétrique. On les laisse secourir les blessés sur les champs de bataille? Elles s'y couvrent de gloire, comme Florence Nightingale, envoyée par l'Angleterre en Crimée, en 1854. Le taux de mortalité s'effondre spectaculairement. À son retour, elle peut ouvrir la première école d'infirmières et marque l'histoire de l'hygiène en écrivant *Notes on Nursing.*[6]

It is widely recognized that women, such as Louise Bourgeois and Angélique du Coudray, made important contributions to the field of obstetrics throughout the seventeenth and eighteenth centuries. However, this essay will focus not on midwives, but rather on women who contributed to medicine as researchers and teachers, or within the sphere of their everyday lives; women who made little distinction between their kitchen and a laboratory. At a time when pharmacy[7] was still in its infancy, and limited to a handful of medicines extracted from plants—quinine, aspirin, opium—preventive medicine, with hygiene and health maintenance, was far more important than curative medicine. Of all the places in the house, the kitchen, more than any other, was the locus of hygiene and health maintenance. Authors of manuals of domestic economy, who up to the end of the seventeenth century had transmitted recipes that owed little to the new emerging science of pharmacy, were becoming more selective when including cures. With the exception of obstetrics manuals, often authored by midwives, domestic economy manuals and medical manuals written for women were penned by men of science. Whereas the mid-Enlightenment had known so many brilliant scientific women, from Émilie du Châtelet (1706-1749) to Marie-Geneviève-Charlotte Thiroux d'Arconville (1720-1805), none of them authored domestic manuals. By the end of the long eighteenth century the situation was reversed. Although there were no more prominent women scientists, Armande Gacon-Dufour (1753-1835), a well-respected botanist and agro-scientist, claimed the field of domestic economy. By the middle of the nineteenth century, women were well accepted as legitimate scientific writers. With Gacon-Dufour, every home could become a laboratory; every woman had the opportunity to become a scientist. Cooking, cleaning, and the preparation of remedies required women to have basic knowledge of chemistry, physics, botany, mathematics, medicine, economy, and politics, and her books would give them that knowledge in a scientific context. Soon, domestic economy would become the only socially acceptable outlet for women with an interest in science.

Through the example of Marie Marguerite Biheron (1719-1795), an acclaimed anatomist who trained and later taught at the Jardin du Roi, and that of Armande Gacon-Dufour, readers will understand how women of science, who had been able to contribute openly to their field during the Enlightenment, slowly retreated to the kitchen, but then subverted this new space and made it an acceptable outlet for scientific curiosity.

The Jardin du Roi and the Laboratory

The scientific passion that swept through France and much of Europe during the long eighteenth century contributed to the development of loci where men—and *women*—could satisfy their intellectual curiosity and creative drive. Whereas the salons continued to play a central role in the creation of new knowledge, some of the medical sciences were not easily practiced in a salon. The growing interest in dissection and anatomy for example,[8] did not lend itself to home demonstration. To see dissections in action many went to the Jardin Royal des Plantes Médicinales. As Yves Laissus so clearly demonstrates, the Jardin du Roi as it was often called, became an institution that played a crucial role in establishing France as a scientific nation. It became a place that worked both with and against the teachings of the university. Built during the reign of Louis XIII with the original purpose of providing royal physicians with remedies, the garden became the Muséum d'Histoire Naturelle in 1793. The garden's role soon extended beyond growing medicinal plants; those who had an interest in medicine, botany, or chemistry, sometimes in addition to attending classes at the university, gathered at the garden. Learned laymen and women as well as university students and professors frequented the institution, and it is there, for example, that Louis XIV eagerly attended the dissection of an elephant in 1681,[9] an opportunity that certainly could not have taken place in a salon. The Jardin du Roi's faculty included two chairs each in anatomy, chemistry, and botany, chairs occupied by some of the most prestigious scholars of the time, who sometimes also taught at the university, as did, for example, Félix Vicq d'Azyr (1746-1794), Marie-Antoinette's physician. For contemporaries, the work of the scientists who conducted research and taught at the Jardin du Roi was neither marginal, nor considered to be on a lesser level than the research and teaching done in the university. Rather than placing the exclusively male university at the center, with the Jardin du Roi and the salons (which had both male and female members) lying at the margins, we should think of the two institutions as working sometimes in harmony, but sometimes clashing,[10] with a resulting synergy that allowed for a richer scientific community.

For women, the coexistence of the Académie des Sciences, the Faculté de Médecine and the Jardin du Roi meant access to scientific discourse. Though barred from the Faculté de Médecine, women could attend classes alongside men at the Jardin Royal des Plantes Médicinales. Not only were classes free and open to all, they were also taught in French, rather than Latin.[11] We know for a fact that some women, such as Madame Thiroux d'Arconville, the famed anatomist and chemist, took anatomy classes there, and one can imagine that other women known for their interest in dissection and anatomy also attended the Jardin du Roi, including Marguerite Biheron (1719-1795), the Marquise Marie Jeanne Constance de Voyer d'Argenson (1734-1782), Germaine de Staal Delauney (1693-1750), and Anne-Josèphe-Michel de Coigny (1750-1775).[12]

As Enlightenment women had access to medical classrooms and sometimes taught medical subjects, it is crucial to understand that, although by our standards learning originates in universities, this was not necessarily the case during the Enlightenment. Being barred from the *facultés* did not mean that women could not learn medical subjects. In her excellent *The Mind has no sex?* (1989), critic Londa Schiebinger places Émilie du Châtelet and Madeleine de Scudéry in a section called "Women at the Periphery,"[13] because of the impossibility for them to attend university or join a royal academy. While that much is true, we should not overlook that most of the teaching, learning, and discoveries that took place during the Enlightenment occurred outside of universities and against the will of their faculty.

The Boudoir and the Laboratory

There is perhaps no better example of this than Marguerite Biheron, famed anatomist and ceroplastics master, who went from being at the center of the anatomy laboratory at the Jardin, to being a marginalized scientific figure during the nineteenth century. In her *Mémoires* (1825), Madame de Genlis (1746-1830) evokes the anatomy lessons she took with Biheron, who built her models "des cadavres qu'elle avait dans un cabinet vitré au milieu de son jardin, " noting almost disapprovingly "je n'ai jamais voulu entrer dans ce cabinet, qui faisait ses délices et qu'elle appelait son *petit boudoir.*"[14] Although Genlis's recollections might give the impression that Biheron was a demented scientist who relished deviance or the macabre, eighteenth-century scholars are well-aware that when first designed, the boudoir was more a study or a laboratory than a locus of sexual pleasures. In the first part of the eighteenth century, Biheron's generation, boudoirs had been created as a private space where women could think and study,[15] although, admittedly, probably not dissect human bodies. In the second part of the eighteenth century, the generation of Genlis, boudoirs, however, had become rooms equipped with daybeds and mirrors, and had come to represent "blatant advertisement for exhibitionistic sexual display."[16]

Marie Marguerite Biheron came from a Parisian family of apothecaries, which included Michel, her grandfather, and Gilles Biheron, her father.[17]

Little is known of her life; she and her three siblings were orphaned when Marguerite was only four and one-half years old. Her oldest brother became a surgeon, the younger one followed the family tradition and became an apothecary, while her sister entered the convent.[18] It is probable that her brother Étienne, the surgeon, gave Biheron access to public dissections performed at the Jardin du Roi. There she met Madeleine Françoise Basseporte (1701-1780), her first botany and art teacher.

A well-established botanist and painter, Françoise Basseporte achieved a status in the scientific community that is too often overlooked. After directing a drawing academy for girls, founded by her first teacher, Paul Robert de Sery (1686-1733), official painter of the Cardinal of Rohan,[19] Basseporte worked at the Jardin du Roi under the direction of Claude Aubriet (1665-1742), the garden's royal botanical painter. In 1731, he sold his royal office to Basseporte, but by the terms of the contract, she assumed the position for eight years while Aubriet continued to receive the salary.[20] In 1742, upon Aubriet's death, she at last occupied the role and title of official painter she had acquired so many years before, and remained in her position there until her death in 1780.[21]

Through her position at the garden, Basseporte developed a network among artists and scientists.[22] Scholars believe that she recommended her pupil Biheron to the surgeon Sauveur-François Morand (1697-1773). Under Morand, her anatomy teacher, Biheron went from drawing to sculpting, and became one of the best known practitioners of ceroplastics of the period,[23] acquiring a distinguished reputation throughout Europe.

Under Morand's direction, she sculpted her first important pieces, part of a larger order soon to leave for Saint Petersburg. In 1759, Morand gave a lecture at the Académie des Sciences, using Biheron's first major work, a full model of a human body with moving parts. This model clearly surpassed the works of her most famous predecessor, Guillaume Desnoues, who introduced in France the art he had learned in Italy.[24] The technical and scientific achievements of the model are worth noting:

> Les membranes y sont imitées de manière à tromper les spectateurs: on l'a particulièrement remarqué dans l'épiploon, avec ses bandes graisseuses. On a observé dans les viscères creux, tels que l'estomac et les intestins, la consistance, la souplesse et la légèreté des viscères naturels; l'estomac même peut s'enfler pour en faire voir le relief, la figure et les contours: de plus, les parties solides comme le foie, les reins, le cerveau, quoique de cire, sont faites avec un alliage tel que ces parties ne peuvent se casser par le froid ou par accident, non plus que se ramollir dans les grandes chaleurs. Le corps de cette anatomie est recouvert d'une vraie peau, qui, outre qu'elle imite bien mieux que la cire l'enveloppe extérieure du corps humain, n'est point sujette comme elle à se jaunir à la longue [...].[25]

The commentator admired both Biheron's anatomical knowledge and her unprecedented technique, allowing her to imitate nature "avec une précision et une vérité dont jamais personne n'avait encore approché."[26] Twelve years later, she was again asked to demonstrate her work during a special session of the Académie Royale des Sciences, organized to impress the Royal Swedish Prince Gustav during his visit to Paris in March 1771. It seems that by then, no enlightened European dignitary could stop in the capital without seeing Biheron. Grimm,[27] a great admirer of the anatomist, commented at great length on the second demonstration.[28] This time, Biheron presented a second anatomical model, which also became a sensation. The model was not a complete body, but a truncated parturient woman, along with several fetuses of various sizes, which could be inserted in the uterus. The moving parts allowed spectators to witness the delivery of a child (minus the blood, the pain and the screams),

> depuis le moment où l'enfant est au couronnement jusqu'à celui auquel la femme est délivrée; on peut aussi mettre l'enfant ou les enfants dans quelque position que ce soit, pour imiter tous les accidents qui peuvent traverser l'accouchement.[29]

This presentation at the Académie is a testimony to Biheron's climb in scientific circles. On the day of the Royal Swedish Prince's visit, d'Alembert opened the session, followed by a presentation by some of the most prestigious academicians: Pierre Henri Macquer, Balthazar Georges Sage,[30] and Antoine Lavoisier. Finally, Biheron introduced her model, performed her demonstration, and clearly outshone her fellow scientists. Grimm, not even commenting on the illustrious presenters, remarked that "[on] termina la scéance par plusieurs démonstrations anatomiques, et c'est sans difficulté ce qu'il y a eu de plus digne de l'attention de Sa Majesté."[31] Beyond the sensationalism of showing her technical prowess[32] and presenting several difficult deliveries on a state-of-the art mannequin, Biheron was also admired for her intellectual talents which were even more valued by the Encyclopedists. Biheron "a dans ses idées beaucoup de netteté, et fait ses démonstrations avec autant de clarté que de précision."[33] Clearly, the Encyclopedists were impressed by Biheron's abilities as a wax modeler, but also as an anatomist and as a teacher.

A household name in medical circles at the Jardin du Roi, and at the Académie Royale des Sciences, Biheron was also routinely mentioned in anatomy treatises.[34] While the use of mannequins by medical students for practice is taken for granted today, albeit with twenty-first-century technology, we should not forget the contributions that scientists such as Biheron made to medicine. With the art of ceroplastics and related techniques, the study of anatomy evolved from a static science of death to physiology, the dynamic study of life. The medical community was well aware of Biheron's importance, and after her death, famous anatomist and physiologist Félix Vicq d'Azyr inventoried her productions.

A very creative anatomist and ceroplasticist, Biheron also gave anatomy lessons, which were in great demand. Her pupils primarily consisted of medical students, scientists and philosophers, including Diderot, Grimm, Benjamin Franklin, to name but a few. Critic Shane Agin has provided excellent insights on how, because of her teaching, she indirectly influenced the education of young women.[35] Diderot was so taken by Biheron's teaching that he had his daughter Angélique take a few lessons when she married, to educate her about sex and childbirth. He began advocating the practice to all who would listen, from politicians such as John Wilkes,[36] to the enlightened monarch Catherine the Great. He never was able to enact his plan of sending Biheron to Smolny Monastyr, the elite school for aristocratic women in Russia, although in a couple of letters to the Russian General Betsky, he enthusiastically described the contribution the anatomist could have made to the school.[37]

From the Birthing Room to Frankenstein's Laboratory

Marguerite Biheron and other Enlightenment women anatomists, though in small numbers, reflected the general scientific landscape of the period, again because much of the education one received happened within an international European intellectual community who met in *salons* and other private locations rather than at universities. Forbidding women and non-Catholic men from matriculating was easy—preventing individuals with a passion for education from learning was impossible. All the women anatomists and scientists mentioned above belonged to the same web of eighteenth-century intellectuals, spread over the long eighteenth century: Diderot, Jussieu, Buffon,[38] Lavoisier, Franklin, Linnaeus, Parmentier.[39] Some of these admirers held positions at the Jardin du Roi, some at universities, some in both places, and some in none. Given this context, it is appropriate to emphasize Biheron's role in the scientific community of the Enlightenment, and to examine how through the years, her image evolved from that of a fine intellectual mind to that of a destitute old maid.

Because of Biheron's position in the limelight, scholars have at their disposal a wealth of documents that create a dotted line between the apex of her popularity with the Enlightenment scientific community to her fall into oblivion during the nineteenth century—or worse, to her transformation into the pathetic shell of a half-crazed woman. In a way, the demise of her legacy began with the very contemporaries who admired her talents. While hailing her knowledge and abilities, they also began to make petty, malicious comments about her appearance and marital status. Despite all his praise about her performance at the Académie des Sciences, Grimm also commented on Biheron's person with a benevolent condescension:

> Cette fille, âgée de plus de cinquante ans, pauvre, subsistant d'une petite rente de douze ou quinze cents livres, infiniment dévote d'ailleurs, a eu toute sa vie la passion de l'anatomie.[40]

He closed his report wishing that the government would give her a pension, as "cette pauvre Mademoiselle Biheron, n'ayant jamais été jolie, n'ayant eu ni protection ni manège, est restée négligée."[41] Grimm's comments shed a revealing light on his perception of women's access to scientific education. On the one hand, he is not surprised that a homely single woman without social connections should be asked by the Académie des Sciences to make a presentation in front of a foreign prince, alongside the sharpest minds of the land, as if ordinary women making anatomy demonstrations in front of royal princes were such a common occurrence that it did not merit a special mention. On the other hand, he clearly neglects to scratch the surface to learn more about a scientist who obviously dazzled him as much with the models she had built as with the intelligence of her comments.

However patronizing his comments, Biheron was, for Grimm, a master and a pioneer. Although ceroplastics was a well-established sub-division of anatomy, especially in Italy and in France during the second part of the eighteenth century, Grimm gives her credit for imagining the creation of a complete human body, "une chose unique en Europe."[42] Located between art and science, ceroplastics was an art form very much in demand.[43] Honoré Fragonard (1732–1799), surgeon, anatomist, and first cousin of Rococo painter Jean-Honoré Fragonard (1732–1806), attained international fame for his *écorchés*. Fragonard belonged to a different class of wax anatomists than Biheron, as many of his pieces represented scenes—a skinless man on a galloping skinless horse—so his pieces were snatched up by aristocrats eager to display them in their *cabinets de curiosité*.[44] Fragonard's work was more clearly germane to sculpture and artistic composition than to education.[45] Ceroplasticists were either artists who had later trained as anatomists, like Biheron, or surgeons who had put their artistic talents at the service of their scientific calling, and the discipline attracted the most talented physicians of the time. It appears then that in spite of Grimm's comments that Biheron was "neglected and forgotten,"[46] she did have peers in her profession, as well as a wide network of scientists. She was very well connected, as so many scientists and philosophers corresponded with her, visited her, took lessons from her or sent their children to take anatomy classes with her, although at the same time, Grimm was right to note that she never found a patron or a protector. As she grew old, because of her financial situation, she "eventually sold her entire collection to Marie-Antoinette in 1786 for 6,000 livres."[47]

In the nineteenth and twentieth centuries, Biheron acquired a new image, and emerged as a reluctant anatomist and a midwife, in an effort to normalize her "unfeminine" career choice. The changes started subtly in 1811, with an entry in the *Biographie universelle*, where Biheron, under Basseporte's recommendation, began working "à la préparation des pièces artificielles d'anatomie. *Quelque rebutant et quelque désagréable que ce travail fût pour une femme, Mlle Biheron s'y livra avec courage*" (emphasis mine).[48] The note implies that no woman would ever willingly take up anatomy. By 1861, Lacroix, another biographer, noted that when first encouraged to take up anatomy, Biheron had "la plus grande répugnance pour cette science qui semblait si peu faite pour une jeune demoiselle. À force de prières, Melle Basseporte vainquit ses dégoûts."[49]

Whereas many men and women during the Enlightenment had developed a passion for anatomy and dissection, the mood had clearly changed at the beginning of the nineteenth century. Although Genlis had taken several anatomy lessons with Biheron, and had had female friends with whom she discussed anatomy, she became slightly repulsed by the idea when she published her *Mémoires* in 1825. The wax models on which Genlis had trained enthusiastically in the 1770s, at the height of Biheron's fame, became "[de] tristes imitations" of life.[50] Women were now supposed to express only disgust and reluctance at the idea of performing a dissection; medicine had been neatly and cleanly confined within the walls of the Faculté de Médecine. Gone were the days when Genlis's friend, the countess de Coigny, could be so fascinated with science that, rumor had it, "elle ne voyageait jamais sans avoir dans la vache de sa voiture un cadavre!"[51]

The 1830s saw another dip in Biheron's reputation as Louis Marie Prudhomme drew a portrait of Biheron reminiscent of Mary Shelley's *Frankenstein*,

> Sa passion pour [l'anatomie] fut telle, qu'elle engagea des personnes à voler des cadavres de militaires, et de les lui porter pour en faire la dissection. Ordinairement ces cadavres entraient en pourriture lorsqu'on les lui portait, et, pour attendre l'occasion et le loisir de les examiner

anatomiquement, elle fut souvent obligée de les cacher dans sa chambre pendant plusieurs jours.[52]

In fact, the only scientific book to claim Biheron in the nineteenth century was, curiously, a *Biographie des sages-femmes célèbres* (1834) by Aloïs Delacoux.[53] The inclusion of Biheron in the volume, when she had never been a midwife, may have been an attempt to reduce her career to a label that Delacoux and his medical contemporaries could accept, as midwifery was the last medical profession where women could still practice—though they were slowly being eliminated and replaced by male obstetricians. Although the mannequin Biheron had presented to the *Académie* in 1770 had been the bottom half of a parturient woman, her contemporaries never associated her with the famous midwives of the eighteenth century, such as Angélique Le Boursier du Coudray,[54] who taught their art with the aid of mechanical bodies. Scholars tend not to differentiate Biheron's and du Coudray's mannequins, but their purposes could not be more distinct. Whereas du Coudray had been charged with teaching midwives basic anatomy and the mechanics of delivery, which she did with a static stuffed mannequin, with parts that could be taken out (the fetus, the uterus, etc.), Biheron's model aimed at an exact representation of the anatomy (bones, muscles, membranes, etc.) and the physiology of some of the processes of the delivery. Her model was much more sophisticated than du Coudray's, as explained in the report written for the *Histoire de l'Académie* for the year 1770:

> [...] ce fantôme représente le bas-ventre et la moitié des cuisses, il est formé sur un bassin dont le coccyx est mobile; [...] l'entrée du rectum, celle des grandes lèvres, l'orifice de la matrice, peuvent être resserrés ou dilatés à volonté ; le corps de la matrice et son fond, sont inclinés d'un côté ou de l'autre, selon qu'on le désire ; ils peuvent se contracter en se rapprochant graduellement vers l'orifice.[55]

Although this wax model could be used by medical students to practice various surgeries sometimes performed during a delivery, obstetrics was only one of the many aspects of anatomy and physiology that fascinated Biheron. She was also well known for her rendition of other organs, "imités avec tant d'exactitude jusque dans les plus petits détails, jusque dans les nuances plus délicates, que vous aurez de la peine à distinguer les limites de l'art et de la nature."[56] Her imitations of skeletons were so perfect that Louis-Sébastien Mercier, in his *Tableau de Paris*, exclaimed, "on croyait en voir de véritables. Les muscles, les nerfs sont rendus avec une vérité frappante."[57]

The Birthing Room and the Classroom

Soon after the first doctorate of medicine was awarded to Elisabeth Garrett in 1870, Biheron's fate was again about to change. In 1900, Mélanie Lipinska also received her medical degree, and the topic of her thesis was a thick volume entitled *Histoire des femmes médecins de l'Antiquité jusqu'à nos jours*. Breaking with the nineteenth-century tradition, Lipinska depicted Biheron as she had been known in her time: as a scientist and anatomist, rather than either as a midwife or an old maid, lurking on the battlefields in search of cadavers to steal.[58] In 1906, Dorveaux provided an even better researched article, *Notes sur Mlle Biheron*,[59] which would later help twentieth- and twenty-first century scholars slowly turn their focus to this important figure. Today, much of the interest seems to be not so much in Biheron's place at the center of a scientific practice that propelled medicine into the study of physiology, but as a teacher of Diderot's daughter Angélique. Shane Agin's meticulous study highlights and documents the importance of Biheron's teaching in the advancement of women's knowledge of their own anatomy and physiology,[60] but modern critics have to be careful not to reduce her work to that of the sex educator of a great man's daughter. For Agin, Biheron "clearly belongs to the tradition of midwives and matrons," while at the same time she breaks "away from the tradition of midwifery by treating women not only as mothers, but also as wives, that is, as sexual beings."[61] While continuing to appreciate Biheron's contributions to sexual education, critics need to reframe her work in the original context in which it was first conducted—in a scientific community composed of men and women.

Back to the Kitchen

Whatever work remains to be done on Enlightenment women of science in the medical field, the abundance of writing on women such as Biheron, Basseporte, du Coudray, d'Arconville and so many others, makes it easy to imagine an eighteenth-century woman in a laboratory. Anatomy, botany, chemistry, physics, mathematics—no branch of science seems to have been off limits, no laboratory seems to have been able to keep women out. But as we have seen with Genlis's shift of attitude, by the end of the long eighteenth century, maybe for fear of being accused of hiding cadavers under their bed, it was no longer socially acceptable for women to perform dissections.[62] One is left to ponder what scientific outlets were left for women with an interest in science and medicine. Universities, where women continued to be *personae non gratae*, had become the almost exclusive places where knowledge was pushed to new limits.

In her *Ladies in the Laboratory, West European Women in Science, 1800-1900, A Survey of their Contribution to Science*, Mary R.S. Creese chose a specific criterion for her anthology, exclusively including women who had authored "publications indexed in the Royal Society *Catalogue*."[63] Based on this analysis, she provides an alarming graph of scientific production for French women. Although Creese notes that "Frenchwomen and women working in France form one of the three most productive groups of nineteenth-century women scientists in continental Europe," the corresponding graph shows almost no activity until 1870,[64] with all the contributions in medicine, representing only 4% of the overall publications, confined to the second part of the century. Had French women's interest in medicine disappeared, or rather, had it metamorphosed into something else?

Building on Creese's work, I would like to propose that scholars expand the net they cast when searching for women involved in medicine between 1780 and 1840. Certainly, there exists a strong expression of women's interest in health through charitable work, beginning with the renewal of interest in working with the poor as a way of salvation during the Catholic Reformation,[65] in particular with the publication of Madame Fouquet's remedies. Madame Fouquet's situation is unique in the experience of women in any scientific field. Although she helped many people, she continues to this day to be given credit for something she actually never did. Marie de Maupéou (1590-1681), wife of François Fouquet, mother of Louis XIV's superintendent of finances Nicolas Fouquet, was a very religious woman who expended much energy and money in organizing care for and distributing medicine to the poor. Although she is often credited with the authorship of both the *Recueil de receptes choisies, expérimentées et approuvées* (1675),[66] as well as the recipes published, she neither wrote the book, nor developed the formulas. As Olivier Lafont notes, the book stemmed from Louis Fouquet's desire to honor his mother, and Fouquet asked his own physician, Delescure, to complete the work:

> C'est incontestablement Louis Fouquet qui a voulu et financé la publication des recettes [...]. Delescure les a mises en ordre et en a ajouté quelques-unes de son cru, ou qui lui ont été fournies par des personnes fiables.[67]

As for the recipes themselves, Lafont, a professor at the Faculté de médicine et de pharmacie de Rouen, demonstrates that they were "assez proches des formules contenues dans les pharmacopées officielles."[68] The question of authorship does not in any way take away from the importance of Fouquet's contributions to medicine, which went beyond the publication of her formulas.

Although Fouquet's work continued to be popular during the eighteenth century, it is only during the late 1770s that another Christian woman stepped in for the poor, this time from the Protestant quarter, Suzanne Necker (1737-1794), who, like Fouquet, was the wife of the King's superintendent of finances, Jacques Necker. In 1778, she opened the Hospice de charité des paroisses de Saint-Sulpice et du Gros Caillou; in 1802, the hospital took the name it has today, Hôpital Necker. Unlike Madame Fouquet or even Biheron, it seems that Suzanne Necker, although certainly interested in the care of the poor, shone more as an administrator[69] than a caregiver or as a scientific researcher.

Aside from charitable work, it is important to point out that the women scientists of the Enlightenment did have daughters who relayed the torch of scientific involvement to the pioneers who became the first women to enter the Faculté de Médecine by the end of the nineteenth century, whose genealogy can be traced back to Basseporte. Although the jump that Biheron made, from studying botany drawing with Basseporte to becoming one of the primary anatomist sculptors of her time, is unusual, it is very easy to document the link between botany, a science always seen as befitting women's delicate natures, and medicine. For our purpose then, *cherchez la femme* becomes *cherchez la femme botaniste*, in order to find women involved in the study (rather than the charitable practice) of medicine. In addition to the gentle pastime of flower-drawing and specimen collection, botany has provided many opportunities for individuals searching for ways to improve health, from time immemorial. Herbalists, apothecaries, midwives—and witches—made extensive use of the chemicals found in plants to cure various ailments. As a result, during the eighteenth century, many plant-based activities, aside from pharmacology, came under the realm of medicine. Perfume manuals, for example, obviously contained make-up and perfume recipes, but they also gave the medical attributes of plants used. Because of the medical establishment's outcry against the lack of regulation for the fabrication and sale of personal hygiene products and for the use and abuse of harmful ingredients such as mercury, such books were penned by three different groups: by botanists, because plants entered into the composition of most perfumes and cosmetics; by physicians, because of their concern for the safety of their patients; or by midwives, because they provided intimate advice to mothers. Medical advice, then, was often mixed with perfumes and cosmetics recipes, as plants affected both beauty and health.

In addition to perfume treatises, dictionaries and manuals of domestic economy also constituted a vehicle for medical advice. Although physicians were winning the academic and political battles that allowed them to exclude other health providers from practicing medicine,[70] the number of university-educated physicians remained very low during the long eighteenth century, while the aspiration to a healthy long life for infants, children and adults was growing. Fortunately, literacy levels were growing as well, and advice manuals multiplied. While several physicians wrote successful health manuals, women, barred from entering the university and from practicing medicine, turned to domestic economy manuals. Some of the best-known were written by Madame Gacon-Dufour (1753-1835).

A Woman of Letters

A descendant of the poet Gacon (1667-1725), Marie Armande Jeanne Gacon was born in Paris, but little is known about her life. She reveals surprisingly little about herself in her manuals, a genre that often led authors to share their personal experience. Only a few details surface: she was brought up in a convent in Monfort-L'Amaury, near Paris,[71] and she never had children, except for an orphan abandoned at her doorstep, whom she raised until he died in an accident at the age of four, while jumping from the second level of a barn into a hay stack below.[72] She also alludes here and there to a few years when she lived on her country estate during the Revolution, in the town of Brie-Comte-Robert, which she refers to as Brie-sur-Hyères, its revolutionary name. There, she managed an estate, and was intensely involved in agricultural research and experimentation. In the nineteenth century, biographers give a few additional details that are repeated in various forms, and often carry their obvious bias.

> Quoique destinée à la fortune, elle reçut une éducation soignée; passa une partie de sa jeunesse au couvent, comme c'était alors l'usage, et de retour dans sa famille, épousa, quelques années après, un propriétaire fixé en province. Elle vécut à la campagne [...] et se délassait de ses travaux champêtres dans la société de gens de lettres distingués, qui fortifiaient et épuraient son goût pour la littérature. Quoique très-instruite et douée d'une mémoire prodigieuse, elle s'est livrée à [...] [l'écriture de] roman[s], soit historique[s], soit épistolaire[s].[73]

Other biographers mention that she was "lectrice à la cour de Louis XVI,"[74] and it is while at court that she collected the details and anecdotes that would fill her historical novels. In addition, she befriended the atheist

Pierre-Sylvain Maréchal (1750-1803)—a friend of Robespierre and other revolutionary figures. During the last years of his life, Maréchal "quitta Paris pour aller habiter à Mont-Rouge" where he spent his last years, "avec son épouse et quelques femmes instruites qui formaient sa société habituelle."[75] It is during this period that Maréchal wrote his *Projet de loi portant défense d'apprendre à lire aux femmes* (1801). Gacon-Dufour retorted with her *Contre le projet de loi de S***. M***, portant défense d'apprendre à lire aux femmes* (1801).[76] Maréchal died in Gacon-Dufour's arms, and four years later, when she edited his *De la vertu* (1807), she wrote a notice about the author, where she described their friendship.[77] Gacon was married twice,[78] the first time to a man named d'Humières, and the second time to Jules Michel Dufour de Saint-Pathus (1757-1828), lawyer, jurist and judge, who died in Brie-Comte-Robert in 1828. During the last years of her life, Gacon-Dufour "était retombée en enfance," when she died in 1835, "plus qu'octogénaire, chez une de ses nièces qui l'avait recueillie."[79]

Although little is known of her life, at court or afterwards, it is easy to surmise that she had observed people of all social classes in the countryside, and probably had endured very difficult times herself. Admitted to the Académie d'Agriculture de Paris, in 1788,[80] only two of her papers have survived, and both show her creativity applied to the difficulty of surviving the extremely cold winters Europe experienced between 1784 and 1794. On 12 February 1789, the Academy's Secretary signed a written report of her presentation entitled "Moyens de faire éclore artificiellement et d'élever des poulets pendant les plus grands froids," which she reproduced in its entirety in her *Manuel complet de la maîtresse de maison*[81] in 1826, some thirty years later. Around 1795, she authored "Moyens de nourrir et de faire travailler les abeilles pendant les plus grands frois, et de les préserver des dangers de l'hiver," an article which, fortunately for us, she also republished in *Recueil pratique d'économie*[82] in 1806.

Her incredible ingenuity in substituting alternatives for scarce and expensive food staples during the Revolution, and in the difficult years that followed, made her an easy target in the nineteenth century. The conservative literary critic Charles-Marie de Feletz, intending to criticize her *Mémoires, anecdoctes secrètes, historiques et inédites* (1807), wrote some often quoted venomous words about her resourcefulness, beginning his article by noting that she had "des secrets admirables; elle fait du vin sans raisins, des confitures sans sucre, et des livres sans jugement, sans esprit, sans style et sans raison,"[83] and closing his piece with equally acerbic comments:

> Je conclus de tout cela que si madame Gacon-Dufour veut absolument travailler pour nous, elle doit se contenter de nous donner ces petites recettes économiques qu'elle nous indique de temps en temps pour faire des confitures et des liqueurs, car drogue pour drogue, j'aime encore mieux ses *ratafia* que ses livres.[84]

The British *Monthly Review*, although a fan of Gacon-Dufour,[85] predicts that her substitute for teas, the small sage, will not find many adopters in England: "here, we do not expect to make any converts."[86] Whatever fun one may poke at very practical solutions developed in a time of great impoverishment, it is clear that while living in Brie-Comte-Robert during the Revolution and in the first years of the Empire, she focused on means to relieve the poverty, poor health and ignorance she observed around her. Examples peppered her works. Speaking of the year 1797, she notes:

> nous touchions alors au moment d'une guerre redoutable; nous en sommes menacés de même aujourd'hui [1806]. Ce fut cette circonstance qui m'avait inspiré le désir de donner les moyens que j'employais pour se passer du café et du sucre, et pourtant de ne point priver la classe malheureuse du peuple de ses jouissances.[87]

In her non-fictional works about domestic economy, health or agriculture, she often recovers the political tone of her earlier pamphlet, *Contre le projet de loi de S***. M***, portant défense d'apprendre à lire aux femmes*, to decry the destitution of peasants. First a member, then, in 1810, secretary, of the *Athénée des Arts*, an association dedicated to science, she gave the society

> des mémoires et des opuscules dont les amis des lettres apprendraient avec plaisir la publication, et plus particulièrement ceux dont le cœur est tout à la patrie, car il est peu de femmes, et d'hommes peut-être, qui aient plus que Mme Gacon-Dufour, l'amour de leur pays et des sentiments plus libéraux.[88]

At every turn of the page, readers are moved by the shadow of terror and the hardships she and people around her endured during those years, but also by the swell of hope she felt as, through her books and her example, she did her best to give her countrymen and women the tools to vanquish hunger, poverty and ignorance. Her laconic tone and her lack of self-pity transform her commentaries on wheat or parsley or honeybees into a poignant testimony of the last years of the eighteenth century. Her research on honeybees for example, one of her favorite topics, coincides with the Terror. Jean Sylvain Bailly (1736-1793), Paris's first mayor from 1789 until 1791, president of the Assemblée nationale, and fellow scientist, had organized a contest for Parisians to come up with ways to establish "des manufactures nouvelles dans le département de la Seine. [...]. J'indiquai à M. Bailly le moyen d'établir un rucher [...] ce qui aurait procuré un travail aisé à des vieillards et à des enfans." Bailly liked her idea, but unfortunately, "les événemens malheureux qui l'ont enlevé à ses amis et aux sciences, ne lui ont pas permis de s'en occuper" ; the "événemens malheureux," as Gacon-Dufour so soberly puts it, refer to Bailly's death at the guillotine in1793.[89] By then, Gacon-Dufour was safely in Brie-sur-Hyères, where she was "propriétaire de terres que je me déterminai à faire valoir."[90] In addition to her noble humanistic and political aspirations, one may also gather that the prolific literary output of Gacon-Dufour and Saint-Pathus[91] may have been in part due to a precarious financial state and the necessity to generate income.

A Woman of Science

An extremely productive writer, Gacon-Dufour authored thirty-four books and numerous articles. Aside from her convent education, of unknown depth or breadth, Gacon-Dufour's training remains somewhat of a mystery. Her works of non-fiction include many references to the ancient Greek and Latin authors.[92] As noted above, she had the reputation of being extremely learned and of having a prodigious memory. The presentation of her work at the Académie Royale des Sciences, and her collaboration with Charles-Nicolas-Sigisbert Sonnini de Manoncourt (1751-1812), known as Sonnini, for the publication of the *Bibliothèque physico-économique*,[93] a memoir about honeybees, for which she received a prize,[94] make Gacon-Dufour's place in the scientific community of the later part of the eighteenth century obvious. In the introduction to her *Manuel complet de la maîtresse de maison* (1826), she refers to several articles she published in the *Bibliothèque*.[95] As all the contributions to the publication were anonymous, it is difficult to gauge the extent of her work there, but one of her biographers notes that "liée d'amitié avec le célèbre Sonnini, elle coopéra avec lui à la *Biobliothèque agronomique*, journal dont elle continua seule la rédaction pendant l'absence de son collaborateur."[96]

Although there are no records of her presence at the Jardin du Roi, it would seem reasonable that it is there that Gacon-Dufour mapped her extensive knowledge of botany, which is the basis of all of her contribution to science—health, veterinary science, and domestic economy. We may not know when, where, or why, but she managed to collaborate with naturalists (Sonnini),[97] chemists (Eugène Julia de Fontenelle),[98] and pharmacists

(Stéphane Robinet),[99] all of whom had either taught or studied at the Jardin du Roi, or contributed to its mission. When compared to Basseporte's or Biheron's open work at the Jardin, Gacon-Dufour's was hidden: there are no records of her studies or her teachings, but the importance of the lessons she learned there benefited many of her contemporaries and the generations that followed. Although many of her contemporaries ignored Gacon-Dufour's presence and work among scientists, she pursued knowledge and its dissemination with passion, and she often collaborated with male colleagues. In 1826, Pierre Blanchard was looking for authors who might prepare a third edition of Dr. Armand Havet's very popular *Dictionnaire des ménages* (1820, 1822), after the young physician died unexpectedly in Madagascar, while on a botanical expedition. He turned to Stéphane Robinet, a promising young chemist, and to Gacon-Dufour, a well-established and respected author. Similarly, Eugène Julia de Fontanelle, with his long pedigree as a chemist and botanist, was happy to play second fiddle to Gacon-Dufour when she published her *Manuel du théorique et pratique du savonnier* (1827). Twenty-five years later, seventeen years after Gacon-Dufour's death, in 1852, he even published a *Nouveau Manuel du théorique et pratique du savonnier*, which still bore Gacon-Dufour's name.

It is difficult for readers today to understand that Gacon-Dufour, as a writer of dictionaries of botany and domestic economy manuals, was an active member of the medical community. As medicine was still struggling to define its place and to expand its realm of influence, chemists, physicians, and pharmacists often authored the types of manuals in which she was to make a name for herself. While we may question why a famous and respected chemist, pharmacist, and member of several medical academies should author a two-volume *Manuel complet du blanchiment et du blanchissage* (1834), the contemporaries of Julia de Fontenelle would have welcomed his expertise, as readers not only expected recipes to keep linen white, but were above all concerned with hygiene, as dirty laundry was a well-known cause of the spreading of infectious diseases.[100] For Gacon-Dufour, who lived in a time when surgery and plants were the two main means of treating illnesses, and hygiene the best way to prevent them, her role was important. She gladly shared her deep knowledge of botany, because plants, through agriculture, could ward off hunger, or, through various preparations, could cure ailments.

Every time a *ménagère* bought one of Gacon-Dufour's books, she could transform her kitchen into a laboratory, as she could cultivate and prepare plants, and treat members of her household, or even her neighbors.[101] For those who did not live in urban areas, cultivating and preserving plants was deemed essential, as "on est quelquefois obligé de faire une ou deux lieues pour se les procurer."[102] Influential groups in Paris may well have passed laws forbidding the practice of medicine by non-university graduates, but in reality, physicians were scarce around Brie-sur-Hyères, with only 5.19 physicians per 10,000 inhabitants in 1830.[103] Accordingly, all Gacon-Dufour's books on domestic economy devoted long passages to the preservation of health, and emphasized cleanliness and basic hygiene for men, women, and beasts. While Gacon-Dufour had a direct influence on women's health through her domestic economy book, no study of the role she played in this area would be complete without a brief survey of her *Manuel du parfumeur* (1825).

In *Selling Beauty*, Morag Martin comments that during the latter part of the eighteenth century, beauty manuals evolved into two types of books, as

> manuals written for the public primarily focused on teaching women how to apply products properly rather than how to make them, while recipe books transformed into commercial manuals to educate professional artisans.[104]

Gacon-Dufour's manual falls into the latter category. She restricted her ingredients to plants, excluding the use of chemicals, which, Martin notes, "were primarily the privilege of perfumers and distillers."[105] Gacon-Dufour emphasizes women's health, by-passing make-up to focus on hygiene, and redefining the role of perfumers: "il est peu d'arts dans la société qui soient plus utiles que celui du parfumeur. En aidant particulièrement à la propreté, il aide aussi à la bonne santé."[106] She has excluded all products reputed to cure skin imperfections, as she is convinced that "toutes ces recettes surannées sont nuisibles; qu'il entre même dans les matières qui les composent des choses plus malfaisantes qu'utiles."[107] She promotes the use of bathing in water lightly perfumed with herbs contained in sachets, much like our teabags, thus avoiding strong emanations, allowing baths that can "rafraîchir, délasser, donner de la circulation au sang." She willingly omits recipes preparing

> du *blanc,* des pommades pour teindre les cheveux, les sourcils, etc., etc.; cela était d'usage dans le siècle de Louis XIV, où la chimie et les sciences naturelles n'avaient point acquis le degré de perfection qu'elles possèdent maintenant; mais ne l'est plus aujourd'hui.[108]

Throughout the book, she also becomes an advocate for women's health. While instructing perfumers, she discourages them from fabricating and selling overpriced products, which can also be health hazards:

> Je me suis appliquée dans la série des pommades dont je donne ici les recettes, à éviter d'enseigner la manière d'en fabriquer pour le teint, pour la conservation des cheveux, étant persuadée, d'après l'observation de chimistes distingués, que ces pommades sont plus dangereuses qu'utiles. C'est autant dans l'intérêt du parfumeur que dans celui des dames que j'émets ces préceptes. Les dames raisonnables m'en sauront gré en ce qu'elles ne seront point forcées de faire un constant usage de ces pommades inventées par la cupidité, et qui un instant ont flatté des femmes avant qu'elles eussent la conviction que ces recettes ont plus nui qu'elles n'ont servi à la conservation de leur fraîcheur.[109]

Although she includes no recipes for make-up, hair dyes, or beauty cure-alls, her extensive knowledge of botany, combined with her desire to provide safe products made her book so successful that it was plagiarized by Elisabeth Celnart (1796-1865) in 1834, the year before Gacon-Dufour's death.

It would seem that Gacon-Dufour closed an era—that of the Enlightenment, of the Jardin du Roi—where women could learn freely. The *Athénée des Arts* would never have the influence that the Jardin had, and it would be a long time until women, like Marguerite Biheron, could make a career of anatomy, or, like Françoise Basseporte, could hold an official position in an institution of higher learning. It is not to say, however, that science, medicine and women parted ways at the end of the long eighteenth century. Rather, I would propose that we look in the domestic space to find the women scientists of the nineteenth century, as kitchens, dairies, stables, and fields could easily be transformed into laboratories. Indeed, one of the first articles listed in Cresse's inventory of women of science in the nineteenth century is no other than Cora Robinet, the younger sister of Gacon Dufour's collaborator, Stéphane Robinet. Many parallels can be drawn between the two women, including a passion for farming, honeybees, silkworms, but, above all, for the right of women to be educated. Author of the *Maison rustique des dames* (1845-1846), Madame Millet-Robinet, as she was known, was indefatigable when petitioning officials for the necessity of teaching girls scientific subjects, so that they could become productive members of France's agricultural economy. The success of her books—and those of other women—on agriculture and domestic economy during the nineteenth century is proof that French women were inspired to turn their homes into laboratories of domestic and scientific economy.

Works by Marie Armande Jeanne Gacon-Dufour

Mémoire pour le sexe féminin contre le sexe masculin. Paris:Royer, 1787.

L'Homme errant fixé par la raison, ou lettres de Célidor et du marquis de Tobers. Paris: Royer, 1787.

Les Dangers de la coquetterie. Paris: Buisson, 1787.

Le Préjugé vaincu, ou lettres de madame la comtesse de ... et de madame de ... refugiées en Angleterre. Paris: Royer, 1787.

Georgeana, ou la vertu persécutée et triomphante. Paris: Le Petit, 1797.

La Femme grenadier, nouvelle historique. Paris: Ouvrier, 1801.

Les Dangers d'un mariage forcé. Paris: Ouvrier, 1801. *Contre le projet de loi de S***. M***, portant défense d'apprendre à lire aux femmes, par une femme qui ne se pique pas d'être femme de lettres, ouvrage contenant des réponses argumentées remettant le sieur Maréchal à sa juste place de sot, d'esprit dérangé et de bouffon réactionnaire.* Paris: Ouvrier et Barnat, 1801.

Le Voyage de plusieurs émigrés, et leur retour en France. Paris: Buisson, 1802.

Mélicerte et Zirphile, roman historique et moral, suivi des sœurs rivales. Paris: Ouvrier, 1802.

Manuel de la ménagère à la ville et à la campagne, et de la femme de basse-cour; ouvrage dans lequel on trouve aussi des remèdes nouveaux pour la guérison des bestiaux, etc. Paris: Buisson, 1803.

Recueil pratique d'économie rurale et domestique. Paris: Buisson, 1804.

De la Nécessité de l'instruction pour les femmes. Paris: Buisson et Delaunay, 1805.

Les Dangers de la prévention. Paris: Buisson, 1806.

Correspondance inédite de Mme de Châteauroux avec le duc de Richelieu, le maréchal de Belle-Isle, MM. Duverney, de Chavigni, Madame de Flavacourt et autres. Paris: Collin, 1806.

Moyens de conserver la santé des habitants des campagnes et de les préserver des maladies dans leurs maisons et dans les champs. Paris: Buisson, 1806.

Mémoires, anecdotes secrètes galantes, historiques et inédites sur Mme de Lavallière, de Montespan, de Fontanges, de Maintenon et autres illustres personnages du siècle de Louis XIV. Paris: Collin, 1807.

La Cour de Catherine de Médicis, de Charles IX, de Henri III et de Henri IV. Paris: Collin, 1807.

Correspondance de plusieurs personnages illustres de la cour de Louis XV, depuis les années 1745 jusques et y compris 1774, faisant suite à la correspondance de Mme de Châteauroux. Paris: Collin, 1808.

Dictionnaire rural raisonné, dans lequel on trouve le détail des plantes préservatives et curatives des maladies des bestiaux. Paris: Collin, 1808.

Pièces inédites sur les règnes de Louis XIV, de Louis XV et de Louis XVI. Paris: Collin, 1809.

Les Voyageurs en Perse. Paris: Collin, 1809.

L'Héroïne moldave. Paris: Cogez, 1818.

Dictionnaire des ménages, ou recueil de recettes et d'instructions pour l'économie domestique. Paris: Blanchard, 1822.

Manuel du parfumeur, guide pour faire des parfums, lotions, sachets, vinaigres aromatiques, maquillages, poudres et dentifrices. Paris: Roret, 1825.

Manuel du pâtissier et de la pâtissière, à l'usage de la ville et de la campagne. Paris: Roret, 1825.

Manuel des habitants de la campagne et de la bonne fermière, ou guide pratique des travaux à faire pendant le cours de l'année, et où se trouve un grand nombre de nouveaux procédés d'économie rurale et domestique. Paris: Roret, 1825.

Manuel complet de la maîtresse de maison, et de la parfaite ménagère, ou guide pratique pour la gestion d'une maison à la ville et à la campagne; contenant les moyens d'y maintenir le bon ordre, et d'y établir l'abondance, de soigner les enfants, de conserver les substances alimentaires, etc. Paris: Roret, 1826.

Manuel théorique et pratique du savonnier, ou l'art de faire toutes sortes de savons. Paris: Roret, 1827.

Notes

[1] Matthew Ramsey, *Professional and Popular Medicine in France 1770-1830* (New York: Cambridge University Press, 1988), p. 49.

[2] Madeleine Brès was the third woman in the world to be awarded a doctorate of medicine from a university in France. Her predecessors were the British Elisabeth Garrett, who graduated in 1870, and the American Mary Putman in 1871.

[3] Ramsay, p. 50.

[4] Mélanie Lipinska, *Histoire des femmes médecins* (Paris: Librairie G. Jacques, 1900), p. 180.

[5] Geraldine Sheridan, *Louder than Words, Ways of Seeing Women Workers in Eighteenth-Century France* (Lubbock: Texas Tech University Press, 2009), pp. 74-75.
[6] Loriot Penneau, et al. "La femme médecin à travers les âges et les pays," *Histoire des Sciences Médicales* 15.4 (1981): 335-343, 339.
[7] The term pharmacy was first used in the middle of the century, and thus began a rivalry between herbalists, traditional healers, and the university-educated pharmacists.
[8] See for example Bernadette Bensaude-Vincent and Christine Blondel, *Science and Spectacle in the European Enlightenment* (Burlington, VT: Ashgate, 2008), pp. 144-145.
[9] Yves Laissus and Jean Torlais, *Le Jardin du roi et le Collège Royal dans l'enseignement des sciences au XVIIIe siècle* (Paris: Hermann, 1986), p. 316.
[10] The teaching and research stemming from William Harvey's discovery of the circulation of the blood, for example, were rejected by the Paris Faculté de Médecine, while they were embraced in the Jardin du Roi.
[11] Georges de la Faye, *Cours d'opérations de chirurgie démontrées au Jardin royal* (Paris: d'Houry, 1740), p. iv.
[12] Lipinska, pp. 187-190. Genlis, who also dabbled in anatomy, mentions Coigny, whom she had befriended during their years at the Précieux-Sang Convent. See Stéphanie Félicité du Crest de Saint-Aubain de Genlis, *Mémoires inédites de Madame la Comtesse de Genlis sur le dix-huitième siècle et la Révolution française depuis 1756 jusqu'à nos jours, Tome premier* (Paris: Baudouin Frères, 1825), pp. 337-338.
[13] Londa Schiebinger, *The Mind Has No Sex? Women in the Origins of Modern Science* (Cambridge, MA: Harvard University Press, 1989), pp. 26-30.
[14] Genlis, p. 339.
[15] Joan Dejean, *The Age of Comfort: When Paris Discovered Casual—and the Modern Home Began* (New York: Bloomsbury, 2009), p. 178.
[16] Dejean, p. 184.
[17] Paul Dorevaux, "Les femmes médecins, Notes sur Mademoiselle Biheron," *La Médecine anecdotique historique et littéraire* (1901-1904): 165-171, 166. Dorevaux's essay on Biheron is the best-documented account of her career. His careful documentation of his sources is extremely valuable.
[18] George Boulignier, "Une femme anatomiste au siècle des Lumières: Marie Marguerite Biheron (1719-1795)," *Histoire des sciences médicales* 35.4 (2001): 411-423, 414-415.
[19] Henry Bourin, *Paul-Ponce-Antoine Robert (de Sery)* (Paris: Picard et Fils, 1907), p. 9.
[20] "Nécrologe des artistes et des curieux, XXXII, Mademoiselle Basseporte," *Revue universelle des arts* 1861 (1861): 139-147, 140. The most detailed biography of Basseporte appears in the *Nécrologe* and is based on the recollections of Edme Mentelle (1730-1815). The account is highly influenced by the author's purpose—that Basseporte may have been a renowned artist, but that she was still

the embodiment of feminine virtues: abnegation, self-sacrifice, and domestic service.

[21] *Nécrologe*, 146. The *Nécrologe* states that although Basseporte kept the position, another artist was put in charge secretly, so as to spare Basseporte, then close to 80 years of age (147). Diderot had suggested as a replacement Marie Thérèse Reboul (1728-1805), spouse of Joseph-Marie Vien, one of the first women received at the Académie des Arts, also said to have been Basseporte's pupil. He noted: "Madame Vien: à nommer après Mademoiselle Basseporte au Jardin du Roy." See Denis Diderot, *Œuvres complètes*, ed. Jules Assézat and Maurice Tourneux, 19 (Paris: Garnier, 1876), p. 306.

[22] The Swedish botanist Carl Linnaeus remained in touch with Basseporte after he visited Paris in 1737. He makes a curious mention of her: "Faites toutes mes amitiés à Mlle Basseporte; j'en rêve; et si je deviens veuf, ce sera ma deuxième femme, qu'elle le veuille ou non, nolens volens." See Pierre Flourens, *Recueil des éloges historiques lus dans les séances publiques de l'Académie des Sciences* (Paris: Garnier, 1857), p. 78.

[23] Although it is easy to imagine why botany was a branch of science where women were readily accepted at a professional level, more surprising is their participation in the field of anatomy, and, in particular, in the practice of ceroplastics, or the sculpting of wax into anatomical representations. See Michel Lemire, *Artistes et mortels* (Paris: Chabaud, 1990).

[24] Dorevaux, p. 166.

[25] *Histoire de l'Académie Royale des Sciences*, année 1759 (Paris: Imprimerie Royale, 1765), pp. 94-95.

[26] *Histoire de l'Académie Royale des Sciences*, p. 95.

[27] Grimm seemed to have been smitten by Biheron, and was forever requesting that Diderot take Grimm's foreign friends to visit her while they were in Paris. This even caused a rift between the two men in 1768: "Je suis brouillé avec Grimm. Il y a ici un jeune prince de Saxe-Gotha. Il fallait lui faire une visite. Il fallait le conduire chez Mlle Biheron; il fallait aller diner avec lui. J'étais excédé de ces sortes de corvées." See Denis Diderot, *Œuvres complètes*, ed. Jules Assézat and Maurice Tourneux, 19 (Paris: Garnier, 1876), p. 296.

[28] Friedrich Melchior Grimm, *Correspondance littéraire, philosophique et critique*, 7 (Paris: Furne, 1770-1771), pp. 219-222.

[29] *Histoire de l'Académie Royale des Sciences*, année 1770 (Paris: Imprimerie Royale, 1773), pp. 49-50.

[30] Macquer (1718-1784), a chemist and a physician, was a professor of chemistry at the Jardin du Roi and an academician. Sage (1740-1824) was a chemist and mineralogist, who was received at the Académie des Sciences at the age of 30 in 1770.

[31] Grimm, p. 221.

[32] All anatomists kept their methods secret, as wax was only one of the products used to build their models. Scientists had to wait until the heat wave of 2003 for the secrets of anatomist Honoré Fragonard (1732-1799), the painter's first cousin, to be revealed. The heat caused some of his models to partially melt and an

analysis of the chemicals he used was then performed. See Christophe Maillot, "Honoré Fragonard et ses écorchés," N.p. (10 April 2009), Web. <http://www.art-et-science.fr/explorart/2009/ plastination2.html>.

[33] Grimm, p. 222.

[34] Boulignier, p. 416.

[35] See his "'Comment se font les enfants?' Sex Education and the Preservation of Innocence in Eighteenth-Century France," *Modern Language Notes* (2002): 722-739, as well as his "Sex Education in the Enlightened Nation," *Studies in Eighteenth-Century Culture* 37 (2008): 67-87.

[36] Denis Diderot, "Lettres inédites de Diderot," *Revue du dix-huitième siècle* 3-5 (1916): 113-114.

[37] Denis Diderot, *Œuvres complètes*, vol. 20, pp. 59-65.

[38] Biheron had made a cast of a baby girl born in October 1766 and suffering from cyclocephaly. The baby died a few hours later. From this cast was made an engraving, which Buffon included in his 1777 supplement to his *Histoire Naturelle*.

[39] Gacon-Dufour mentions that Antoine-Augustin Parmentier, another member of the Jardin du Roi, "avait la bonté de m'honorer de son amitié." See Marie Armande Jeanne Gacon-Dufour, *Manuel des habitans de la campagne et de la bonne fermière, ou guide pratique des travaux à faire pendant le cours de l'année, et où se trouve un grand nombre de nouveaux procédés d'économie rurale et domestique* (Paris: Roret, 1825), p. 9.

[40] Besides her involvement with anatomy, very few details are known about Biheron. Her name is mentioned in the depiction of a bizarre *séance* of *convultionnaires* as an active participant. See Georges Du Doyer de Gastel, "Conversations avec M. de la Barre et journée du Vendredi Saint 1760," in Maurice Tourneux, *Correspondance littéraire, philosophique et critique par Diderot, Grimm, Raynal, Meister, etc.*, vol.4 (Paris: Garnier, 1876), pp. 208-217. She also put an often-quoted question to a famous atheist, who was attending one of her demonstrations: "Eh bien, marchand de hasard, avez-vous assez d'esprit pour nous faire concevoir que le hasard en ait tant?" See *Biographie universelle, ancienne et moderne, supplément* (Paris: Michaud, 1838), vol. 65, p. 487.

[41] Grimm, pp. 221, 222.

[42] Grimm, p. 222. The most famous wax sculptor on anatomy, Guillaume Desnoues, only sculpted parts of the human body.

[43] The building of human bodies out of wax was many things to eighteenth-century Europeans: an opportunity to learn anatomy, an art form, a commercial activity, and one museum was even dubbed as "cours de morale" as its visit would soon scare young men away from prostitutes. See Louis Marie Prudhomme, *Miroir de l'ancien et du nouveau. Paris avec treize voyages en vélocifères dans ses environs*, 2nd in the ed. (Paris: Prudhomme, 1806), pp. 257-258. The pedagogical use of wax bodies for girls will be commented on below.

[44] For Biheron as a *cabinetière*, see Adeline Gargam, "Savoirs mondains, savoirs savants: les femmes et leurs cabinets de curiosités au siècle des Lumières," *Genre & Histoire* (2009), Web <http://genrehistorique.revues. org/ 899?lang=en>.

[45] See Maillot and cf. note 32 above.
[46] Grimm, p. 222.
[47] Bensaude-Vincent and Blondel, p. 144.
[48] *Biographie Universelle*, p. 487.
[49] Paul Lacroix, *Bibliothèque de la Reine Marie-Antoinette au Petit Trianon d'après l'inventaire original dressé par ordre de la Convention* (Paris: Jules Gay, 1863), p. 145. Lacroix seems oblivious to the contradiction of his assertions. A few pages later, he praises Basseporte for being a flexible teacher. Having taken under her wing Mlle Thouin, the penniless orphan daughter of the head gardener at the Jardin du Roi, she allowed the young Thouin to switch from drawing to geography, grammar, and history, since she did not like drawing (p. 146). Biheron's disgust for anatomy seems to exist more in the minds of her nineteenth-century critics than based on facts.
[50] Genlis, p. 338.
[51] Genlis, p. 338.
[52] Prudhomme, p. 363.
[53] Aloïs Delacoux, *Biographie des sages-femmes* (Paris: Trinquart, 1834). Delacoux's credentials on the cover include: "Docteur en médecine de la Faculté de Paris, Chef de service de santé de la dernière expédition en Lithuanie, médecin des épidémies; auteur de l'Éducation sanitaire des enfants et de l'hygiène des femmes."
[54] See the many names given by Nina Gelbart throughout her *The King's Midwife* (Berkeley: University of California Press, 1998); for an example of a midwife's advertisement for her mannequin, see Meusnier de Querlon (*Affiches, annonces, et avis divers: feuille hebdomadaire*, 24 février 1773: 30).
[55] *Histoire de l'Académie Royale des Sciences*, année 1770, p. 49.
[56] Grimm, p. 221.
[57] Quoted by Alfred Franklin, *Dictionnaire historique des arts, métiers et professions exercés dans Paris* (Paris: Welter, 1906), p. 116.
[58] Lipinska, pp. 187-190. Although Lipinska repeats some inaccuracies from Prudhomme and other nineteenth-century critics, she does bring her subject from out of the margins into the center.
[59] Dorevaux, pp.165-171.
[60] Agin, "'Comment se font les enfants?' Sex Education and the Preservation of Innocence in Eighteenth-Century France," footnotes, 732-735.
[61] Agin, "Sex Education in the Enlightened Nation," footnotes, 732.
[62] Genlis notes that her friend, the Comtesse de Coigny, died at a very young age in 1773, and that "on prétend que sa passion pour l'anatomie contribua à sa mort, en lui faisant respirer un mauvais air" (Genlis, p. 337).
[63] Mary R. S. Creese, *Ladies in the Laboratory, West European Women in Science, 1800-1900: A Survey of their Contribution to Science*, 2 (Lanham, MD: Scarecrow Press, 2004), p. 57.
[64] Creese, pp. 57, 58-59.
[65] For an excellent discussion of Fouquet and other charitable women's contributions to medicine in the seventeenth century, see Ramsey, pp. 35-38.

[66] For the sake of clarity, because libraries always catalog the many editions of the Fouquet book with Fouquet as the author, I cite her book in a similar way: Marie Fouquet, *Recueil de Receptes où est expliqué la manière de guérir* (Lyon: Jean Certe, 1676).

[67] Olivier Lafont, "Les remèdes de Madame Fouquet," *Revue historique de la pharmacie* (2012): 52-72, 59.

[68] Lafont, 67.

[69] Suzanne Necker left a *Hospice de charité, institution, règles et usages de cette maison*, which displays her superior administrative and financial acumen. See Suzanne Necker, *Hospice de charité, institution, règles et usages de cette maison* (Paris: Imprimerie Royale, 1780).

[70] In 1708, Philippe Hécquet (1661-1737), one of the most respected physicians of the seventeenth century and professor at the Faculté de Médecine, published *De l'indécence aux hommes d'accoucher les femmes et de l'obligation aux femmes de nourrir leurs enfants*; but by the end of the enlightenment, male obstetricians were slowly pushing midwives out of their art.

[71] Marie Armande Jeanne Gacon-Dufour, *Recueil pratique d'économie rurale et domestique* (Paris: Buisson, 1806), p. 2.

[72] Marie Armande Jeanne Gacon-Dufour, *Manuel complet de la maîtresse de maison, et de la parfaite ménagère, ou guide pratique pour la gestion d'une maison à la ville et à la campagne* (Paris: Roret, 1826), p. 20.

[73] Jay Arnault, et al., *Biographie nouvelle des contemporains, ou dictionnaire historique et raisonné*, 2 (Paris: Librairie historique, 1822), p. 402.

[74] *Biographie universelle*, pp. 11-12.

[75] *Biographie universelle*, pp. 27, 8.

[76] The complete title shows that she was not amused by her friend's text: *Contre le projet de loi de S***. M***, portant défense d'apprendre à lire aux femmes, par une femme qui ne se pique pas d'être femme de lettres, ouvrage contenant des réponses argumentées remettant le sieur Maréchal à sa juste place de sot, d'esprit dérangé et de bouffon réactionnaire.* In 1801, she published *La Femme grenadier, une nouvelle historique,* more likely as an answer to Pierre Sylvain Maréchal's *La Femme abbé* (Paris: Roux, 1801), published the same year, rather than as a biographical account (*Biographie Universelle*, p. 11). In addition, she authored at least two other feminist pamphlets: *Mémoire pour le sexe féminin contre le sexe masculin* (1787) and *De la Nécessité de l'instruction pour les femmes* (1805).

[77] Marie Armande Jeanne Gacon-Dufour, "Notice sur Sylvain Maréchal," in Pierre Sylvain Maréchal, *De la vertu* (Paris: Léopold Collin, 1807), pp. 1-72. Although Gacon-Dufour was the anonymous editor of Maréchal's work, her contemporaries knew that it was her work. See Rabbe, Wieilh de Boisjolin, Sainte-Beuve, eds., *Biographie Universelle et portative des contemporains*, 2 (Paris: Levrault, 1834). Interestingly, in her notice, also anonymous, she disguises herself as "un ami" rather than "une amie" of Maréchal.

[78] Although the dates of her marriages are not known, she was married to Dufour de Saint-Pathus in 1789, when she presented her report on chicken hatching to the Académie d'Agriculture. She was 36 years old. It appears that she continued using

the name d'Humières after her marriage to Saint-Pathus, as the first edition of her *Dangers de la coquetterie* of 1787 is catalogued under the name Madame d'Humières in Queen Marie-Antoinette's library (Lacroix, p. 123), while her *Préjugé vaincu* of the same year appears under the name Gacon-Dufour (Lacroix, p. 119).

[79] *Biographie universelle*, pp. 65, 11.

[80] Gacon-Dufour, *Recueil pratique*, p. 96.

[81] Gacon-Dufour, *Manuel complet*, pp. 127-130.

[82] Gacon-Dufour, *Recueil pratique*, pp. 97-102.

[83] Charles Marie de Feletz, *Jugements historiques et littéraires* (Paris: Librairie Classique de Perisse Frères, 1840), p. 454.

[84] Feletz, p. 459.

[85] The *General Index of the Monthly Review* inventories four articles about Gacon-Dufour's publications, from her works on domestic economy to her historical novels and medical works. See *A General Index of the Monthly Review from the Commencement of the New Series in January, 1790, to the End of the Eighty-First Volume, completed in December, 1816* (London, 1818), pp. 273, 277, 437, 761.

[86] *The Monthly Review or Literary Journal*, 46 (London: Stranban and Preston, 1805): 542.

[87] Gacon-Dufour, *Recueil pratique*, p. 121.

[88] Jay Arnault, et al., *Biographie nouvelle des contemporains, ou dictionnaire historique et raisonné*, vol. 6 (Paris: Letendu, 1827), p. 402.

[89] Gacon-Dufour, *Recueil pratique*, pp. 120-121.

[90] Gacon-Dufour, *Recueil pratique*, p. 90.

[91] Dufour de Saint-Pathus was even more published than his wife. In addition to numerous publications about the new *Code civil* he wrote various manuals, such as his *Manuel pratique des gardes-champêtres* (1822), and a philosophical work, *Diogène à Paris* (1787).

[92] Feletz mocks Gacon-Dufour for knowing Latin, and apparently writing to him in that language (Feletz, p. 461).

[93] The *Bibliothèque physico-économique instructive et amusante, ou Journal des découvertes et perfectionnemens de l'industrie nationale et étrangère, de l'économie rurale et domestique, de la physique, la chimie, l'histoire naturelle, la médecine domestique et vétérinaire, enfin des sciences et des arts qui se rattachent aux besoins de la vie* was a periodical published during the years 1782-1831, edited by Sonnini with Gacon-Dufour's collaboration. Many noted scientists collaborated in the *Bibliothèque physico-économique*, not the least among them Antoine-Augustin Parmentier (1737-1813).

[94] Joseph Jérôme le Français de Lalande, "Second supplément au dictionnaire des athées," in Pierre Sylvain Maréchal, *Dictionnaire des athées anciens et modernes* (Bruxelles: l'Éditeur, 1833), p. 62. More than likely, the prize in question is the one promised by Sylvain Bailly to stimulate the economic development of the city of Paris.

[95] Gacon-Dufour, *Manuel complet*, p. 6.

[96] Arnault, *Biographie nouvelle*, p. 402.

[97] During Buffon's tenure as "Intendant du Jardin du Roy," Sonnini had collaborated with the great naturalist (Laissus & Torlais, p. 298).
[98] Jean Sébastien Eugène Julia de Fontenelle (1780-1842), professor of medical chemistry at the Paris Faculté de Médecine, member of a long list of European scientific academies, published more than twenty-two manuals with Roret, the editor who also published some of Gacon-Dufour and Saint-Pathus' own manuals.
[99] Stéphane Robinet (1796-1869) started his career as a botanist and studied under the famous Louis-Nicolas Vauquelin, (1763-1829) at the Jardin du Roi. He then turned to chemistry and became a pharmacist. Member of the Légion d'Honneur, president of the Académie de Médecine, one of the founders of the *Journal de chimie médicale*, he became fascinated with hydrography during his later years, and at Haussmann's request, he directed a group of scientists in charge of solving the crucial problem of the water supply for the city of Paris. See Joseph Lefort, "Discours prononcé aux obsèques de M. Robinet," *Journal de pharmacie et de chimie*, 11 (1870): 257-261.
[100] At the beginning of the twentieth century, a study conducted by two physicians at the Laënnec Hospital concluded that "à trente ans, plus de la moitié des ouvriers et ouvrières du blanchissage meurent de la tuberculose [...] [et] près des quatre cinquièmes des décès chez les blanchisseurs et les blanchisseuses sont dus à la tuberculose." See M. A. Chapelet, "L'état actuel de la blanchisserie industrielle," *Revue scientifique* 4.2 (1910): 359.
[101] Gacon-Dufour, *Manuel complet*, p. 80.
[102] *Manuel complet*, p. 80.
[103] Ramsey, p. 304.
[104] Morag Martin, *Selling Beauty: Cosmetics, Commerce, and French Society, 1750-1830* (Baltimore, MD: Johns Hopkins University Press, 2009), p. 21.
[105] Martin, p. 21.
[106] Marie Armande Jeanne Gacon-Dufour, *Manuel du parfumeur, guide pour faire des parfums, lotions, sachets, vinaigres aromatiques, maquillages, poudres et dentifrices* (Paris: Roret, 1825), p. 1.
[107] *Manuel du parfumeur*, p. 4.
[108] *Manuel du parfumeur*, p. 5.
[109] *Manuel du parfumeur*, pp. 43-44.

CHAPTER SIX

FROM MOTHER MIDNIGHT TO DR. SLOP: UNDERSTANDING REPRODUCTION IN EIGHTEENTH-CENTURY LITERATURE AND CULTURE

PATSY FOWLER

Copulation, contraception, conception, and childbirth contribute to the plots of many eighteenth-century novels. Laurence Sterne's *Tristram Shandy* famously opens as Tristram contemplates his own conception and later details the debacle surrounding his actual birth; Raymond Stephanson even goes so far as to call Sterne's novel "one of the great eighteenth-century artifacts about conception."[1] Syrena Tricksey in Eliza Haywood's *Anti-Pamela* happily benefits from her experienced mother's knowledge of abortifacients, and Daniel Defoe's *Moll Flanders* offers the reader a menu of items and services available to women for their lying-in as well as their concomitant costs. To be sure, each offers valuable insight into and commentary on the reproductive practices in the period, but even with comprehensive footnotes, modern readers are often left with more cultural questions than answers as each answer sparks yet another question. It is impossible, of course, to anticipate and answer all those countless questions. Instead, I will employ the shifting role of the midwife, from knowledgeable crone armed with a wealth of experience to formally trained accoucheur with a bag of newfangled instruments, as a framework for understanding representations of reproduction in popular eighteenth-century novels.

Contextualizing the role of midwives—their knowledge, their skills and procedures, and the context in which they operated—offers a lens through which we can begin to understand women's sexual health and reproduction in the eighteenth century. The period witnessed a dramatic increase in use among the middle and upper classes of man-midwives or accoucheurs, men who had been trained by the College of Physicians or elsewhere in obstetrics. Judith Schneid Lewis estimates that there were several hundred practicing in London by mid-century.[2] The rise and acceptance of these man-midwives was complex, especially as they began to attend more commonplace births and not just those characterized by complication. Many "real" doctors, who as Roy Porter notes were already in the "least prestigious of learned professions,"[3] looked down upon these men for wasting their time on such frivolous matters. Sir Anthony Carlisle, a prominent surgeon, for instance, called midwifery a "humiliating office."[4] And not surprisingly, some questioned the judgment of husbands allowing other men so close to their wives' "privates," for as one pamphlet argued, the practice "gave the enemy direct access to the very citadel of female virtue."[5] Moreover, according to Porter, male midwives were viewed as "sexual infiltrator[s]" and "violator[s] of female modesty."[6] Using works such as Philip Thicknesse's *Man-Midwifery Analysed* (1764) and Francis Foster's *Thoughts on the Times* (1779), Porter demonstrates the degree to which at least some eighteenth-century men feared the sexual arousal that must arise during the manual manipulation of women's genitals by accoucheurs or "Touching Gentry" as Thicknesse called them.[7]

But, as Towler and Bramall note, "female modesty, which had hitherto excluded men from the birth chamber, was disappearing among the upper and middle classes and so the practice of male accoucheurs conducting the delivery became popular, especially since it was often done in imitation of the French aristocracy."[8] Indeed, in a time when fashionable status was often displayed, particularly in the rising classes, by the outlay of ready money, paying doctors or male midwives to do jobs previously done by women came to be viewed as a symbol of one's wealth.[9] And certainly, the eagerness of men to enter a predominantly female profession demonstrates that there was money to be made there. William Smellie, for example, claims that after they were put on half pay in 1748 many British army and navy surgeons began attending his lectures on midwifery as a means of securing more income.[10] Undeniably, some man-midwives became quite famous and wealthy because of society's new-found infatuation with them. In fact, status-seeking among the *beau monde* and the *nouveaux riche*s proved quite profitable for these men, allowing them to charge more for their services than their female counterparts; furthermore, publishing books and treatises on the subject became extremely profitable as well.[11]

The plethora of legitimate midwifery books published throughout the century, however, often competed with thinly-veiled pornographic texts published by men like Edmund Curll and passed off as medical books bearing titles such as *Aristotle's Masterpiece or the Secrets of Generation Displayed in all the Parts Thereof* (1684 and republished throughout the eighteenth century and beyond), *The Mysteries of Conjugal Love Revealed* (1703), and *Gonsologium Novum, or a new System of all the Secret Infirmities and Diseases Natural Accidental and Venereal in Men and Women* (1708).[12] Clearly, there was no shortage of men willing to offer expertise on women's sexual health and reproduction.

It is thus not surprising that the increase in male midwives resulted in a decrease in the practicing female midwives, many of whom were women with much practical experience but who lacked a formal education. The men, however, typically entered the profession with a formal education that included the study of anatomy and many had received specialized training and a bag of newly-fashionable, obstetric instruments—all things the female midwives weren't allowed. Among the tools of the trade were the forceps, and the vectis, which was a kind of long-handled shoehorn. There were also other instruments used for the gruesome job of removing dead fetuses, or even for killing infants stuck in the birth canal so they could be removed in pieces and the life of the mother could be saved—which, in the eighteenth century, was always the priority—as caesarians were not performed on live women at that point in time.[13]

The relationship between female midwives who brought with them years of practical experience and the new male midwives who had a bag of instruments and varying levels of book learning was indeed complex and often contentious. Certainly some male midwives and physicians such as William Smellie helped make huge advancements in midwifery by developing and refining instruments such as the forceps, and in educating both men and women in midwifery, albeit separately.[14] But, he and men like him drew the ire of female midwives for a number of reasons, including their reliance on and overuse of surgical instruments rather than more natural methods as well as for their condescending attitude toward women practicing the profession. Smellie, for instance, writes in his 1752 *Treatise on the Theory and Practice of Midwifery* that male midwives should come to the aid of female midwives who find themselves in difficulty; however, he warns that the men

> when called, instead of openly condemning her method of practice, (even though it be erroneous) ought to make allowance for the weakness of the sex, and rectify what is amiss, without exposing her mistakes.[15]

As Towler and Bramall and others have recognized, Smellie's assumption here is clear: if female midwives find themselves in difficulty, they, rather than some natural cause, are to blame. It is no wonder, then, that female midwives took issue with the attitudes that Smellie and other male practitioners had toward them. Elizabeth Nihell, one of the better-known and better-trained midwives practicing in mid-century, took Smellie to task for his condescension and his advocacy for and reliance on forceps and other instruments. In her book, one of the few written by a practicing female midwife, she calls male midwives "a band of mercenaries" made up of "broken barbers tailors or even pork butchers."[16] Similarly, Sarah Stone, a midwife practicing earlier in the century, admonishes the use of instruments and outlines the plight of women in the profession. Stone argues,

> I cannot comprehend why women are not capable of completing this business when begun, without calling in men to their assistance, who are often sent for when the work is near finished; and then the midwife who has taken all the pains, is counted of little value, and the young men command all the praise … I am certain that where twenty women are delivered with instruments (which is now become a common practice), that nineteen of them might be delivered without.[17]

It is no wonder that Stone, Nihell, and other female midwives reacted against this invasion upon their livelihoods, for they were at a distinct disadvantage. As Londa Schiebinger notes, scientific advancements in the understanding of pregnancy, labor, and delivery created the ultimate glass ceiling for them, and all their attempts to secure advantages (education, licensing, professional guilds and so forth) for themselves as professionals failed. Male midwives and doctors often refused to share new discoveries and newly developed techniques with their female counterparts, rather choosing to keep such information to themselves as a means of appearing more competent, increasing their clientele, and making more money. Lack of access to university and the simultaneously prohibitive lack of access to surgeons' instruments left female midwives in what Schiebinger calls a "double bind"[18] that unquestionably threatened their livelihood. Moreover, as Amanda Carson Banks notes, "Through guild membership and the concomitant persecution of nonmembers who attempted to practice medicine, physicians and surgeons controlled and regulated the medical profession as they saw fit";[19] hence, female midwives were left on the outside looking in.

The antagonism between the male and female midwives, then, was largely based on money and reputation as men encroached on one of the few professional domains available to women and demanded more money doing it, all the while claiming greater respect and prestige. This very real rivalry is perhaps best depicted in the novel *Tristram Shandy* (1760), where we see Dr. Slop with his fancified forceps replacing the trusty midwife who relied on manual dexterity to turn breech babies in preparation for birth. For as Dr. Slop says in defense of his profession: "What improvements we have made of late years in all branches of obstetrical knowledge, but particularly in that one single point of the safe and expeditious extraction of the foetus" (103).[20] And, of course, both Uncle Toby with his skinned knuckles and poor Tristram with his shattered nose pay the price of Dr. Slop's self-proclaimed expertise with forceps.[21]

With the success of these male midwives came a certain bravado—John Maubray, a London man-midwife, or "Andro-Boethogynist"[22] as he preferred to be called, wrote in his book, *The Female Physician, Containing all the Diseases Incident to that Sex. In Virgins, Wives, and Widows...The which is added, The Whole Art of New Improv'd Midwifery...* (1724), that the Obstetric "arts are so much improv'd and advanc'd that, they now seem to be arrived *at the very heights of perfection* (emphasis mine)."[23] Unfortunately, this perfection included the overuse of forceps by anxious man-midwives proving their mettle, and resulted in real-life cases mimicking Tristram Shandy's famous flattened nose. Furthermore, it is worth noting here that some of these early man-midwives perpetuated myths already endorsed by texts like *Aristotle's Masterpiece*, myths that ultimately proved harmful to women. For example, James McMath writes that a sign of conception in women was an orgasm, which he calls a "great itch," "her most voluptuous Tickle," "a light shivering of the Body as after pissing."[24] How he knew what a female orgasm felt like, he doesn't explain, but notions such as this imply that raped women do not conceive, and those who do, clearly must have participated willingly, experienced pleasure in the encounter, and therefore, were not raped.

Ultimately, as the century progressed, these more unscrupulous medical practices perpetuated by unqualified quacks seeking profit over professionalism, gave way to more serious research and medical advancements. Through the research and work of men like John Denman and the Hunter brothers, real strides were made in the knowledge surrounding pregnancy and childbirth, and the early work of man-midwives like Maubray was deemed quite archaic. It is worth noting here, that some of these advancements weren't "new" discoveries at all, at least for the female practitioners. For example, among the advancements claimed by man-midwife Bernard Pugh is the use of the hand on the abdomen to reposition the fetus, something that female midwives had perfected decades earlier. However, to be fair, there really were great leaps in the understanding of female anatomy and birthing as the century progressed. Denman's and Hunter's work, for instance, almost eliminated the use of forceps altogether; because of their research, it became common practice to wait six hours after the last contraction before employing forceps to aid in the birth, and William Smellie's invention of the curved forceps much improved their use when they did become necessary.[25]

There is perhaps, as Schiebinger notes, another way of reading this influx of men into the profession. Citing the work of Gunnar Heinsohn and Otto Steiger, she maintains that male midwives can be viewed as servicing the mercantile class by increasing the population of the middling and working classes.[26] That is, the new male midwives focused more on the delivery of babies and less on other aspects of women's sexual health such as the herbal remedies that so many counted on to prevent or end unwanted pregnancies. Hence, the practical contraceptive knowledge of Mother Midnight was replaced with the pronatalist policies of men taking over the profession and privileging their own agenda over the needs and wants of their female patients.

Although advancements in midwifery and obstetrics displaced many female midwives, they did not disappear altogether, and their ready knowledge of contraception and abortion proved necessary for many women who found themselves in need of such advice. Indeed, modern readers often find surprising the extent to which eighteenth-century women turned to midwives, prostitutes, servants, apothecaries, female relatives, and even family recipe books for information on the use of herbal remedies as birth control and abortifacients. And not insignificantly, many novels and other texts offered information to contemporary readers, albeit almost always in codified ways. In perhaps the most famous example, Moll Flanders explains that Mother Midnight in

> Discoursing about my being so far gone with Child, and the time I expected to come, she said something that look'd as if she could help me off with my Burthen sooner, if I was willing; in *English,* that she could give me something to make me Miscarry if I had a desire to put an end to my Troubles that way.[27]

The codified treatment of such things as purposefully induced abortions in novels becomes apparent when Moll claims to abhor the notion and explains that Mother Midnight hides the suggestion "so cleverly, that I cou'd not say she really intended it, or whether she only mentioned the practice as a horrible thing."[28] Even as Moll abhors, Mother Midnight retracts, and Defoe dodges, the suggestion that such things are possible and the hint on where to go for information would certainly have proved valuable knowledge for at least some eighteenth-century readers.

A less codified example occurs in Eliza Haywood's *Anti-Pamela,* although here, too, the author fails to actually provide details in the text. In this instance, it is the wise if unscrupulous birth mother rather than the midwife/Mother Midnight figure offering the advice. Finding herself pregnant, Syrena explains that she is willing to do "all that could be done to alleviate the Misfortune as much as possible." The narrator then explains, "[her mother] prepared a strong potion, which the girl willingly drank, and being so timely given, had the desired effect, and caused an abortion, to the great joy of both mother and daughter."[29] In her footnote, editor Catherine Ingrassia cites Angus McLaren's instructive book *Reproductive Rituals* to explain some of the different herbs used for this purpose. Similarly, John Riddle, in *Eve's Herbs: A History of Contraception and Abortion in the West,* traces the knowledge of such herbs and their uses from ancient times through the twentieth century. Like Schiebinger, and others, he, too, notes how different cultures sometimes attempted to eliminate the role of midwife and her vast knowledge, often, he explains, through accusations of witchcraft in attempts to increase the population. This "broken chain of knowledge"[30] as he calls it, fittingly traces the vital role women had in teaching each other how to prevent and eliminate unwanted pregnancies—which is exactly what we see Syrena's mother pass down to her, and Mother Midnight offer to Moll. These two examples demonstrate the passage of knowledge down from older, more experienced women to the younger generation and emphasize the importance of the mother or archetypal crone figure in perpetuating sexual knowledge; so, too, do they demonstrate patriarchal fear of that matrilineal progression of knowledge.

As described by McLaren, Riddle, and others, there were many herbs and plants used to manipulate fertility in the eighteenth-century, and they were administered in myriad ways. Rue, a strongly scented evergreen subshrub, was often taken by women as a means of preventing conception, apparently ingesting it regularly with food over prolonged periods of time. Nicholas Culpeper, who translated from Latin a popular, contemporary apothecary's guide, *The London Dispensatory*, wrote that "Rue or herb of grace [...] consumes the seed and is an enemy to generation."[31] Other plants such as calimant, cypress, agrimony, horehound, juniper, savin, and sassafras, taken alone and in various concoctions, were used as a means to "provoke the causes" as John Peachey, an Oxford educated physician, wrote in 1694.[32] The codification of this phrase, however, both reveals and hides how these plants were used. The phrase sounds innocent enough, but bringing on the menses implies they were not coming on their own, which for sexually active women meant they were likely pregnant. Peachey's semantics throughout, however, is not always so ambiguous, for he writes that the use of savin as an abortifacient is "too well known and too much used by Wenches" and can be used to "cause Miscarriage" and expel "a dead Child."[33] Additionally, herbs and plants such as wild sage, artemesia, penny royal, and marigolds were all used in this way as well. Ironically, James McMath, the Scottish physician, wrote in the *Expert Midwife* (1694) that menstrual blood smelling of marigolds demonstrated prime fertility;[34] marigolds apparently could function as both an abortifacient and a predictor of fertility.

There is no way of knowing how many early pregnancies ended because of these plants and herbs intended to "provoke menses," and there is certainly no way of knowing how many of them were used as more intentional abortifacients. And even then, there was disagreement among the herbalists about the morality of using these plants. Some writers, like Culpeper, wrote without judgment or even endorsed their use. Others followed their descriptions of herbs with warnings that a plant is "reckon'd injurious to women and occasions barrenness and hinders conception and causes abortion."[35] Whether these warnings were in earnest or intended as subtle advice is uncertain. What remains clear, however, is that eighteenth-century women of all classes would have had access to contraceptive information from these published materials and from women such as Mother Midnight. And, indeed, some of this information was almost certainly passed down in recipe books by women, thereby creating a network of matrilineal intelligence surrounding sexual health.[36]

For details on the lying-in experience of women in and around London in the eighteenth century, *Moll Flanders* and *Tristram Shandy* once again offer revealing literary examples of what those experiences might have been like for women in varying circumstances. As has been well documented, Mother Midnight offers Moll a menu of three different lying-in packages from which to choose. These packages range in cost from thirteen and a half pounds to fifty-three and a half pounds. Each includes three months room and board, a nurse for one month, the use of varying qualities of linens, the cost of a Christening, and fees for Mother Midnight's services as a midwife. Additional costs were tied to servants, food, and accommodations for the father and/or friends. Upon Moll's selection of the least expensive option, Mother Midnight points out that the entire cost to Moll will be only about five pounds above her regular living expenses, a fact that very much pleases Moll.[37]

While Defoe's text outlines the financial costs associated with the lying-in of a woman of Moll's class and circumstance, Sterne offers satirical insight into the event from a more privileged class perspective, criticizing the excessive use and often misuse of forceps by men like Dr. Slop. For, here, we learn that Dr. Slop overrules the midwife, uses his forceps, with which he has already injured Uncle Toby's fists in mock demonstration, and ultimately crushes Tristram's nose during delivery.[38] Mrs. Shandy's lying-in, the philosophical discussion of who should make decisions regarding it, and the conflict between Dr. Slop and the midwife are all revelatory, but the text does not provide real insight into what typically took place inside the woman's chamber during delivery, leaving readers to wonder about the details.

For the aristocracy, particularly in the second half of the century when sentimentality became more in vogue, lying-in was a ritualistic and somewhat public to-do, meant both literally and metaphorically to initiate women, especially those delivering for the first time, into their new roles as mothers. Additionally, male family members also became more involved, at least emotionally, in this ritual, something we see demonstrated in *Tristram Shandy*, as Tristram's father and Uncle Toby participate in the ceremony surrounding the birth. In her thorough treatment of the subject, Judith Lewis explains that most lyings-in were planned for London and required the family to relocate for four to six weeks.[39] And even families already in London would rearrange their homes for the lying-in. No expense was spared, particularly for the first birth or the birth of an anticipated male heir; this included expensive laces and linens as well as placing straw along the street outside in order to reduce noise from the horses traveling past. Several secluded rooms would be prepared including an inner chamber for the woman and an outer room for visitors; often rooms for the man-midwife and a nurse would be provided as well. Generally, nurses were hired for the month surrounding the lying-in, and their jobs were to look after both mother and child. Often secured months in advance, these nurses sometimes worked specifically with certain midwives, and some had been trained for delivery in cases where the male midwife might not make the birth in time. Additionally, a wet nurse might also be employed—although later in the century many aristocratic women, especially those who hoped to delay their next pregnancy, might nurse their own children. After the birth, colored ribbons were often hung on door-knockers as a means of publicly announcing the successful birth and sex of the child.

We often imagine that aristocratic births occurred in grand four post beds, the same beds where conception may have occurred, maybe even the same beds where titled heirs had been conceived and birthed for generations. But by mid-century, smaller, portable beds were often used, and they were designed to make linen changes and access to the mother easier. Interestingly, these birthing beds were often shared among the women in a family and seemed to create a homosocial bond among kinswomen—the matriarchal version of the ancestral bed passed down by the patriarchs.[40] Furthermore, these specialized beds allowed for a shift from the bed where conception had occurred, thus cleansing the birth of any sexual connotation and instead tying it to a more sentimental or spiritual transformation in the family dynamic.[41]

But, certainly not all births occurred in beds. Specialized stools and chairs had long been designed for the purpose of aiding in childbirth; Rueff's stool, dating back to the 1500s, and van Deventer's chair from the 1700s are two such examples. In fact, Dutch obstetrician Henry van Deventer's book, *The Art of Midwifery Improv'd*, had been translated into English in the 1740s, and in it he advocates using a birth chair of his own design and lists it among the recommended equipment that midwives should have. The chair, according to Towler and Bramall, was easily disassembled, thereby making it transportable, and it was intricately designed with a hinged back that allowed the mother to sit straight or at a more reclined angle. The seat was similar to a modern toilet seat with a large hole cut into it but with wider sides remaining to support the woman's thighs.[42]

Although Defoe does not provide specific information regarding Moll's lying-in with Mother Midnight, we can assume based on information contained in contemporary midwifery books that Moll would have been allowed to walk about, sit, lie down, or otherwise keep herself comfortable until her water broke; she would then be prepared to deliver with the help of Mother Midnight and several other women, who were there to comfort, encourage, and provide leverage as she delivered the child. According to Jane Sharpe, a late seventeenth-century midwife and the first woman to write a textbook on midwifery, "when the waters run forth the birth is near […] for when those skins are broken the infant can no longer stay there than a naked man in a heap of snow."[43] Sharpe also warns midwives against using their fingernails to break the placenta, instructs them on how to digitally determine the infant's position, and details how to stroke the abdomen to manipulate and encourage delivery. Interestingly, she reminds midwives that not all women deliver in the same position; that is, some prefer kneeling, some prefer sitting on birthing stools, and some prefer to lie upon their backs in a bed with a pillow under their buttocks with their legs held upwards.[44] Sharpe, like many of her contemporaries, also iterates the importance of delivering the afterbirth and instructs midwives on the best way to do so, although debate continued on just what was best practice.

Throughout the century women would remain quite active socially until they began contractions; at this point the midwife was summoned and the woman would begin what in the latter part of the century had become known fashionably as her *confinement,* a term that typically replaced phrases such as "brought to bed."[45] As delivery approached for the aristocratic woman, she no longer chose her delivery position; rather, according to Lewis, she would be placed on the left side of the bed and made to lie on her left side with her legs bent in front of her. This was to preserve the greatest amount of modesty so that neither she nor the accoucheur would see each other; it was also thought to provide the greatest access to the birth canal.[46] Also during the delivery, the woman would typically wear a shift pushed up under her arms and a short petticoat around her waist. After delivery, the petticoat was typically removed and the shift pulled down, again in an attempt at maintaining modesty; the woman and child were then placed in the more comfortable center of the bed. In the coming days and weeks as the fashionable woman healed and regained strength, she would begin to accept visitors and venture downstairs in the home. And after four to six weeks she would be ready to re-enter society. This was traditionally marked by a visit to her local church for what was called "churching," although some women chose to undergo the ritual in their chambers rather than formally visiting the church. While in some cultures this symbolized a kind of cleansing, Lewis explains that for British women it was more of a thanksgiving for the successful birth. The Christening would follow quickly thereafter. Anthropologically, Lewis notes, the lying-in ritual signified the changing status of the woman and the family. The move to London and subsequent confinement at birth was a move away from the site of conception, and the entrance back into society was a move back into the regular life of the woman and family.[47] This, not surprisingly, coincides with the increased sentimentality and changing familial attitudes taking place later in the century, notions Sterne ridicules in *Tristram Shandy*.

Mirroring these changes, Tim Hitchcock argues that sexual practices in the eighteenth century evolved, becoming more focused on traditional intercourse, achieving conception, increasing the population, and centering on the dynamics of family. He writes,

> At the beginning of the century [sex] was an activity characterized by mutual masturbation, much kissing and fondling, and long hours spent in mutual touching, but very little penal/vaginal penetration—at least before

> marriage. If penetration did occur, *coitus interruptus* was likely to be practiced, and if this failed and a pregnancy resulted, there was always recourse to abortion.[48]

According to Hitchcock's historical argument, as the century progressed, penetrative sex became more the focus. He continues,

> Forms of sexual activity which dramatically increased the risk of pregnancy generally reflected the interest of men over of those of women. [...]. The increasingly phallo-centric and penetrative sexual culture of the late eighteenth century both encouraged and made possible the denigration of female sexuality and perceived passivity. In the process it also reflected and contributed to women's increasingly restricted role in society as a whole.[49]

While Hitchcock's article delineates how the changing sexual practices of the period no longer coincide with women's interests, it also lays bare the more restrictive roles women began to inhabit in relation to their reproductive lives. The sexual agency of fictional characters, such as Defoe's Moll Flanders and Eliza Haywood's Syrena Tricksey, follows Mother Midnight off the proverbial stage. Just as the knowledgeable matriarch is replaced by the book-learned accoucheur, so too, the desiring, dynamic heroine with ready access to sexual knowledge and pleasure devolves into the passive Elizabeth Shandy, a woman who, at the moment of her son's conception, wonders if the clock has been wound and who, at the moment of his birth, endures Dr. Slop and his mishandled forceps. Unfortunately, the medical advancements in women's reproductive health seen throughout the eighteenth century were not necessarily indicative of improvements in the overall lives of women—sexual, professional, or otherwise.

Notes

1 Raymond Stephanson, "*Tristram Shandy* and the Art of Conception," in *Vital Matters: Eighteenth-Century Views of Conception, Life, and Death,* ed. Helen Deutsch and Mary Terrall (Toronto: University of Toronto Press, 2012), p. 93. Stephanson's essay offers a cogent and thorough treatment of the philosophical dialogue taking place in Sterne's novel as he traces many of the contemporary debates surrounding sex and childbirth.

2 Judith Schneid Lewis, *In the Family Way: Childbearing in the British Aristocracy, 1760-1860* (New Brunswick, NJ: Rutgers University Press, 1986), p. 94.

[3] Roy Porter, "A Touch of Danger: The Man-Midwife as Sexual Predator," in *Sexual Underworlds of the Enlightenment*, ed. G. S. Rousseau and Roy Porter (Chapel Hill: University of North Carolina Press, 1988), p. 206.
[4] Quoted in Lewis, p. 87.
[5] See *Profligacy of our Women* (1779); quoted in Lewis, p. 86. It is probably not surprising that the wives were often blamed for the perceived lasciviousness of male midwives.
[6] Lewis, p. 217.
[7] Quoted in Porter, p. 222.
[8] Jean Towler and Joan Bramall, *Midwives in History and Society* (London: Croom Helm, 1986), p. 101. Porter's essay also addresses contemporary fears surrounding lascivious and hypocritical women who would gain pleasure by allowing these men to touch them under the guise of assisting in childbirth.
[9] It is relevant to note here that the lyings-in of poor women were still largely attended by female midwives. One well-known female midwife, Elizabeth Nihell, claims to have delivered over 900 children without charge. See Londa Schiebinger, *The Mind Has No Sex? Women in the Origins of Modern Science* (Cambridge, MA: Harvard University Press, 1989), p. 110.
[10] Amanda Carson Banks, *Birth Chairs, Midwives, and Medicine* (Jackson: University Press of Mississippi, 1999), p. 40.
[11] Examples include John Maubray's *The Female Physician...The Whole Art of New Improv'd Midwifery* (1724), Henry Bracken's *The Midwife's Companion* (1737), Thomas Dawkes' *The Midwife Rightly Instructed* (1736), William Smellie's *Treatise on the Theory and Practice of Midwifery* (1752), and Benjamin Pugh's *A Treatise of Midwifery* (1754) among others. See Towler and Bramall, pp. 99-134.
[12] For a longer discussion of these pseudo-medical sex manuals see Peter Wagner, "The Discourse on Sex—or Sex as Discourse: Eighteenth-Century Medical and Paramedical Erotica," in Rousseau and Porter, pp. 46-68.
[13] See Lewis, p.180.
[14] Smellie is also credited with defining terms related to terminating pregnancies. According to him, *miscarriages* happened within the first 10 days, *expulsion* occurred up until the third month, and *abortions* happened in the following months. See John M. Riddle, *Eve's Herbs: A History of Contraception and Abortion in the West* (Cambridge, MA: Harvard University Press, 1997), p. 194.
[15] Quoted in Towler and Bramall, p. 103.
[16] Towler and Bramall, p. 104.
[17] Towler and Bramall, pp. 117-118.
[18] Schiebinger, p. 108.
[19] Banks, p. 26.
[20] Laurence Sterne, *Tristram Shandy,* ed. Howard Anderson (New York: W. W. Norton, 1980), p. 103.
[21] For a discussion of Dr. Slop and his use of instruments see Arthur H. Cash, "The Birth of Tristram Shandy: Sterne and Dr. Burton," in *Sexuality in Eighteenth-Century Britain,* ed. Paul-Gabriel Boucé (Manchester: Manchester University

Press, 1982), pp. 198-224. The article includes photos and drawings of several obstetric instruments.

[22] Schiebinger defines this as "man-helpers of women," p. 108.

[23] Quoted in Robert A. Erickson, "'The Books of Generation': Some Observations on the Style of the British Midwife Books, 1671-1764," in *Sexuality in Eighteenth-Century Britain,* ed. Paul-Gabriel Boucé, (Manchester: Manchester University Press, 1982), pp. 82-83.

[24] Erickson, p. 82.

[25] Lewis, p. 179.

[26] Schiebinger, p. 111. See also Riddle, pp. 168-169.

[27] Daniel Defoe, *The Fortunes and Misfortunes of the Famous Moll Flanders,* ed. G. A. Starr (Oxford: Oxford University Press, 1971), pp. 168-169.

[28] Defoe, p. 169.

[29] Eliza Haywood, *Anti-Pamela,* ed. Catherine Ingrassia (Toronto: Broadview Press, 2004), p. 84.

[30] Riddle, p. 167.

[31] Quoted in Riddle, p. 186.

[32] Riddle, p. 185.

[33] Riddle, p. 185.

[34] Erickson, p. 81.

[35] John Peachy, quoted in Riddle, p. 185.

[36] Phyllis Thompson, "From Still Room to Living Room: Recipe Books as Eighteenth-Century Social Media" (Paper presented at the Southeastern American Society for Eighteenth-Century Studies, Charleston, SC, 28 February-3 March 2013).

[37] Defoe, pp. 164-166.

[38] Sterne, pp. 103-156.

[39] Lewis, pp. 153-191.

[40] Lewis, p. 161.

[41] Lewis, p. 162.

[42] See Towler and Bramall, pp. 120-122. They also include illustrations of Rueff's (p. 83) and Van Deventer's (p. 122) birthing chairs. For a lengthy treatment, see also Amanda Carson Banks, *Birth Chairs, Midwives, and Medicine,* (Jackson: University Press of Mississippi, 1999).

[43] Quoted in Towler and Bramall, pp. 94-95. Sharpe's book was originally titled *The Midwives Book or the Whole Art of Midwifery Discovered*, published in 1671. Subsequent editions published in the eighteenth century, however, were called *The Compleat Midwife's Companion.*

[44] Towler and Bramall, p. 95.

[45] Towler and Bramall, p. 72.

[46] Towler and Bramall, p. 177.

[47] Lewis, pp. 193-217.

[48] Tim Hitchcock, "Redefining Sex in Eighteenth-Century England," *History Workshop Journal*, 41 (1996): 79.

[49] Hitchcock, p. 80.

PART III:

GENDERING OF DISEASE

Chapter Seven

Love and Disease: The Contaminated Letters of Julie de Lespinasse

Felicia B. Sturzer

The "Muse of the Encyclopedia," Julie de Lespinasse (1732-1776), *salonnière* and *grande amoureuse*, whose love letters to Jacques-Antoine-Hippolyte de Guibert (1743-1790) inscribe a woman's destiny in the epistolary tradition of the *liebestod*, was consumed not only by passion, but also by a devastating disease—phthisis, better known as tuberculosis. Critical efforts have mainly focused on situating the Lespinasse correspondence within the literary framework of the female victim's text, defined by love, absence, suffering and untimely death.[1] While there is justification for this view, it has obscured our vision of Julie de Lespinasse the woman, whose terminal illness predated her acquaintance with Guibert. The destiny of Julie, the romantic heroine, is created by a consumptive *épistolière* who enters the realm of literature by transforming disease into metaphor: "Il faut subir mon horrible destinée, souffrir, vous aimer, et mourir bientôt."[2] The creative process of writing enables Julie to inscribe and embellish the physical signs of a body ravaged by disease with the emotional manifestations of a mind consumed by desire. Her "contaminated" love letters provide a case study of a *salonnière* afflicted with the last stages of tuberculosis who perpetuates and problematises not only the myth of the *grande amoureuse*, but the relationship between a writing subject, the patient as objectified "other," and the shifting parameters of medical discourse during the Enlightenment.[3]

The life of Julie de Lespinasse, the illegitimate daughter of Julie d'Albon, parallels that of fictional heroines rendered vulnerable by circumstances of birth and gender. Introduced to society by M[me] du Deffand, Julie de Lespinasse became a lifelong friend of Condorcet

(1743-1794) and d'Alembert (1717-1783), sharing a house with the latter on the rue Saint-Dominique until the day she died. There, as head of a salon that attracted the leading intellectuals of Europe, she became the "Muse of the Encyclopedia." In 1767 she fell in love with the marquis de Mora, son of the Spanish ambassador to France. Although the love was reciprocated and Mora promised to marry Julie, he died of tuberculosis on 27 May 1774, en route to see her. Meanwhile, in 1772, at the age of forty, she met the Comte de Guibert, a 29-year-old colonel well-known as the author of the *Essai général de tactique*. Julie became his mistress, writing him frequent letters framed by expressions of love and hatred. Frustrated by his constant absence and insensitivity, she writes letters that are both passionate and ambivalent. Pressured by family considerations and his own ambition, Guibert married Mlle de Courcelles in 1775, and less than a year later, on 22 May1776, Julie de Lespinasse died—by her own claim, of a broken heart. In what was probably her last letter to Guibert, in May 1776, she invokes his love, transformed into poison, to facilitate her death:

> Mon ami, je vous aime; c'est un calmant qui engourdit ma douleur. Il ne tient qu'à vous de la changer en poison, et de tous les poisons ce sera le plus prompt et le plus violent. Hélas! je me trouve si mal de vivre, que je suis prête à implorer votre générosité pour m'accorder ce secours...Je m'éteins, adieu.[4]

Julie's letters are characterised by binary oppositions and a fragmented, metaphorical discourse that intertwines the erotic with the medical. While she invokes the ambiguous power of Guibert's love, which is both a balm and a poison, medications and opiates mask her mental anguish and deaden the pain of her physical deterioration. As Julie loses control of her body, an object consumed by disease and manipulated by others, she asserts herself as subject through the act of writing. This article focuses on the discursive interaction between the medical and the erotic, authenticity and fiction, that converge and diverge in the textual body of the Lespinasse correspondence with Guibert and Condorcet between 1770 and 1776. Catherine Blondeau has noted the incongruous and jarring mixture of medical bulletins and exalted passion that structures the correspondence. Readers who reduce the letters to merely medical and autobiographical facts fail to discern the textual complexity of their symbolic content.[5] It is precisely from such a blending of fact and metaphor, however, that Julie de Lespinasse the woman emerges:

> Mon ami, cette âme qui ressemble au thermomètre qui est d'abord à la glace, et puis au tempéré, et peu de temps après au climat brûlant de

> l'équateur, cette âme, ainsi entraînée par une force irrésistible, a bien de la peine à se modérer et à se calmer; elle vous désire, elle vous craint, elle vous aime.[6]

In this letter to Guibert, written in 1773, she expresses not only desire for her lover but the effects of hectic fever, identified by the physician William Cullen (1710-1790) as symptomatic of phthisis. Rising in the morning and evening, with periods of remission in between, such fevers drained Julie physically and mentally.[7] The thermometer, a recurring motif, registers not only her fluctuating fever but her unstable emotional state, alternating between depression and elation, anxiety and heightened sensitivity, all characteristic of various stages of tuberculosis:

> J'ai froid, si froid que mon thermomètre est à vingt degrés de Réaumur. Ce froid concentré, cet état de torture perpétuel me jettent dans un découragement si profond, que je n'ai plus la force de désirer une meilleure disposition.

Debilitating lethargy resulted from the opium she used to diminish her pain and calm the anxiety caused by Guibert's absence and his delay in responding to her letters:

> J'ai pensé en mourir, tant cela avait mis mes nerfs en contraction et en convulsion. Je n'obtiens après cela du calme qu'avec une dose d'opium, qui me jette dans un état d'affaissement qui ressemble à l'imbécilité.[8]

Thus, as the medical establishment was struggling to redefine itself within shifting scientific and religious ideologies, Julie de Lespinasse envisioned a subject in which body and mind struggled to achieve unity.

Although the history of disease during the Enlightenment is outside the scope of this essay, a few brief remarks are in order. Anne Vila's recent work on the concept of "sensibility" in French medical and literary discourses focuses on the ambiguous interpretations of *sensibilité*, a concept that encompassed both physiological (the body's reaction to stimuli) and psychological-moral meanings (feelings of compassion, virtue, sympathy and pity) that frequently intersected. Expanding the scope of their theoretical investigations, physicians extended their study of the sensual body into all aspects of knowledge, becoming *médecins philosophes* who "promoted both a holistic vision of the human being as a sensibility-driven organism, and a very precise set of techniques for observing, controlling, and correcting sensibility." The skilled physician excelled in the art of medical observation and interpretation of the patient's symptoms, using his own senses to refine his theoretical knowledge.[9] As John O'Neal points out, this was especially significant since it challenged the traditional separation between the surgeon, whose practice included observing and touching the patient, thus using a sensory approach to illness, and the physician-theoretician, who thought about the symptoms of a particular disease but did not touch the body in which it manifested itself.[10]

Amid discussions on the nature of sensibility and its effects on both mind and body, the meaning of "symptom" and "sign" in the pathology of disease has become problematic among literary critics and medical historians alike. O'Neal maintains that throughout the eighteenth century, physicians used *symptoms* to identify and "classify diseases," an indirect method resulting in confusing and often erroneous conclusions. This was consistent with the mind-body dualism of Descartes that characterised medical thinking and favored more abstract, unifying theories, rather than direct (i.e. sensory) observation of the physical signs of disease. The desire for greater diagnostic specificity was fulfilled in 1808 with Corvisart's translation from Latin into French of Leopold Auenbrugger's work on the percussion of the thorax, *Inventum novum* (1761). By emphasising the importance of the senses in diagnosing specific *signs* of disease, in this case the sounds perceived by the physician in the lungs as a result of percussion, Auenbrugger demonstrated the superiority of specific, internal, physical signs over external, observed symptoms that could indicate any number of different illnesses. "Authentic" medicine, O'Neal claims, could thus best be practised by "physicians who use their hands" and senses as diagnostic procedures, marking a decisive shift from the classification of symptoms to the observation of signs.[11]

Although Corvisart's popularisation of Auenbrugger's method may have resulted in improved medical diagnosis and greater awareness of the importance of sensory perceptions, I would suggest that the discursive distinction between *symptom* and *sign* was at best blurred throughout the eighteenth century, since such terminology and the medical practice it implied frequently merged. In the *Encyclopédie* article on "Médecine" we find the following discussion of how the physician reaches a diagnosis: "c'est par les effets seuls que nous pouvons juger des causes; la connaissance des effets doit donc précéder en nous le raisonnement."[12] Priority is given to observed "effects" of an illness over abstract theories, a view which seems to reject a holistic understanding in favor of direct and specific documentation of the pathology of disease. "Effets" is used as a synonym for the "symptoms" of various illnesses, which physicians are specifically encouraged to observe and carefully analyse in order to distinguish among them. This is best accomplished, the writer elaborates, by observing nature, referring to the wisdom of the past and incorporating the new information resulting from modern discoveries. While reactive, theoretical, and historical modes of thinking, characteristic of the *médecin philosophe*, are not totally rejected, the article emphasises observable phenomena rather than abstract systems in reaching a diagnosis. Furthermore, the *Encyclopédie* article on "Phtisie" specifically uses the terms *symptomes* and *signes* interchangeably in discussing the identification of this disease:

> *Symptomes.* La *phtisie* commence accompagnée d'une douleur légère, d'une chaleur modique, et d'une oppression de poitrine. Le sang qui sort du poumon est ordinairement rouge, vermeil et écumeux; plein de petites fibres, de membranes, de vaisseaux artériels, veineux et bronchiques; il sort avec toux et bruit, ou rallement des poumons. Le pouls est mol, foible et ondoyant; la respiration est difficile: tous ces symptomes sont précédés d'un goût de sel dans la bouche.
>
> Lorsque la *phtisie* est menaçante ou confirmée, on la peut reconnoître par les signes suivans.
>
> 1. Une toux sèche qui continue pendant plusieurs mois [...]. Le vomissement qui vient de cette toux après le repas, est un signe très-certain de la *phtisie.*
>
> 2. La fievre éthique, où l'on sent une chaleur à la paume de la main et aux joues, surtout après le repas.
>
> 3. L'exténuation des parties solides qui se remarque particulierement à l'extrémité des doigts, et qui cause la courbure des ongles.[13]

Symptoms, precursors to a possible case of phtisis, are followed by more definitive *signs*, which can be used to make a diagnosis.[14] Both signs and symptoms, however, result from direct observation by the physician (the kind and duration of the cough, for example, and the sounds emanating from the chest) as well as the active participation of patients who voice their complaints (heat in the palm of the hands, vomiting, a salty taste in the mouth).

The reference to pulse-taking, a physical sign of the sensitive body reacting to a stimulus, points to the growing importance of such sensory experience in eighteenth-century medical practice. Vila points out that the medical articles in the *Encyclopédie* invariably refer to the article on "Pouls" by Ménuret de Chambaud, who was influenced by Bordeu's treatise, *Recherches sur le pouls par rapport aux crises* (1747). Pulses, it was claimed, provided the link to all parts of the body, revealing subtle changes in the functioning of internal organs. Thus, the pulse "bears the signature of each organ, and thus allows the medical observer not just to translate physio-pathological phenomena into treatable terms, but to 'hear' the body's inner language directly."[15] I maintain that *sign* and *symptom* merge, as touching and listening, recording and observing physical sensations challenged traditional ideology on the relationship between the physical body and the stimulation of a sensory universe. I suggest, therefore, that the increasing emphasis on sensory perceptions shifted medical practice towards a more empirical approach as the eighteenth century drew to a close, while the terminology—*symptoms* against *signs* as observable phenomena—remained essentially unchanged. According to Roy Porter the human sciences complemented the emerging "sciences of nature." Thus, the Enlightenment eventually created competing discourses that sought to define the psychological as well as the physical existence of men and women.[16] Hence the interplay between mind and body that frames the Lespinasse correspondence emerges as a manifestation of the shifting parameters that defined medical discourse in the closing years of the eighteenth century.

Within this context, Julie, as both observer and patient, subject and object of her text, prisoner of a body consumed by desire and tuberculosis, constructs a textual bridge between contrasting and often conflicting modes of thought and expression. The descriptions, by herself and others, of the physical transformations her body undergoes constitute a catalogue of symptoms subject to interpretation, diagnosis and treatment. An astute observer, Julie the patient compulsively documents the signs of her disease. The interpretations of such signs by patient and physician facilitate their transformation into the literary metaphors that framed both Julie's passion as *romanesque* heroine and her illness. This occurred during two overlapping periods: Julie's relationship with Gonçalve de Mora, from 1770-1774, the year of his death; and the affair with Guibert, from 1772 to 1776, the year of her death.

For Sainte-Beuve, Julie de Lespinasse personified absolute passion, outside the bounds of time and space: a view adopted by scholars of her correspondence throughout the nineteenth century and into the present.[17] Jean-Noël Pascal argues that successive editions of Julie's letters to Guibert progressively transformed her original text into a literary work, particularly in the 1809 edition where "L'éditeur [...] a cherché à fabriquer de la littérature avec du réel authentique, à transformer la femme de chair en personnage de roman."[18] In his edition of Julie's correspondence with Condorcet, d'Alembert, Guibert and the comte de Crillon, Charles Henry argues that "mademoiselle de Lespinasse a conquis la postérité par son âme, par les intensités de sa souffrance, les élans de son désir, la force de sa raison. Elle dut la vie à l'amour: elle en vécut; elle en mourut."[19] Julie continued to die for love well into the twentieth century. Susan Carrell suggests that her letters perpetuate the literary tradition of the monophonic formula derived from Guilleragues' *Lettres portugaises* (1669). As communication with an absent lover became increasingly difficult, Julie creates "her own autobiographical myth," writing letters in which she redefines herself and marginalises Guibert.[20] François Bott refers to her as "probablement une des demoiselles les plus romanesques de France."[21]

These critical views are supported by numerous medical and fictional texts, framed by religious and political discourses. The causal agent of tuberculosis, the tubercle bacillus, was not identified until 1882 by Robert Koch, and debate regarding the origin and transmissibility of the disease continued throughout the eighteenth century.[22] Direct sensory observation of the patient had become more important by the nineteenth century, but the association of tuberculosis, particularly in women, with passion, anxiety and depression was prevalent in earlier medical literature. The English doctor Richard Morton (1637-1698), in his guide for the prevention of consumption, advised his patients, among other things, to avoid stress, "melancholy, and all poring of his thoughts, as much as ever he can, and endeavor to be cheerful."[23] In the volume on medicine in the *Encyclopédie méthodique* (1824), a lengthy article discussing the multiple forms of phthisis and their manifestations suggests that weight loss and lack of appetite, both of which are symptoms, can originate in "l'amour malheureux, une espérance déçue, un sentiment habituel d'inquiétude," resulting in a dangerous state of consumption.[24] Even René-Théophile-Hyacinthe Laënnec (1781-1826), a physician who, in addition to inventing the stethoscope, greatly contributed to contemporary knowledge of pulmonary diseases, suggested that "passions tristes" were a possible cause of pulmonary consumption.[25] It is not surprising, therefore, that the physicians whom Julie de Lespinasse consulted regarding her illness could only offer the observation that "nous n'avons point de remède pour l'âme."[26]

The idea that emotional and hereditary factors played a role in the onset of tuberculosis was promulgated by members of the Paris Faculty of Medicine as late as 1866.[27] Hence, in his discussion of real and imagined emotional and mental disorders during the eighteenth century, Robert Mauzi associates Julie de Lespinasse with fictional heroines whose unhappiness became a morbid destiny, characteristic of "une âme malade." But the misfortune and passion which characterised their existence set these women apart, their very marginalisation defining their "otherness": "Il ne faut donc pas s'étonner que la passion métamorphose les âmes. Entre l'âme autonome et l'âme passionnée s'établit une totale rupture.

L'âme passionnée devient *une autre*."[28] Julie, however, was aware not only of her "otherness" but also of the fact that she was terminally ill, and she transformed the symptoms of her illness into symbols of her passion: "[...] je suis atteinte d'une maladie mortelle dans laquelle tous les soulagements que j'ai voulu apporter, se sont convertis en poison, et n'ont servi qu'à rendre mes maux plus aigus." Physical suffering signalled not only her imminent death but heightened her sense of existence: "Je vis, j'existe si fort, qu'il y a des moments où je me surprends à aimer à la folie jusqu'à mon malheur."[29] Ultimately, to live passionately was to love and to suffer.

The mystery surrounding tuberculosis aroused interest in its pathological progression as well as its social and psychological consequences. As society's need to understand a disease lethal to large segments of the population in Europe increased, the medical significance of tuberculosis provided the narrative material for stories of suffering and sacrifice for a higher ideal. Critics have noted the large number of artistic and literary works throughout the nineteenth and twentieth centuries whose leitmotif is tuberculosis—Hugo's *Les Misérables*, Dumas's *La Dame aux camélias*, Turgenev's *On the eve*, Verdi's *La Traviata*, Puccini's *La Bohème*, Mann's *The Magic Mountain* and Gide's *The Immoralist* are but a few examples. Exemplifying uncompromising passion, sacrifice and the transcendence of the body to a more spiritual, purified state, such works romanticised disease, capturing the popular imagination and creating an idealised process of victimisation and suffering, followed by possible redemption through death.[30] Although there were male consumptives, it was females who were most frequently linked to the redemptive and purifying powers of tuberculosis. Women's dual roles of whore and virgin, already prevalent in preceding centuries, facilitated the creation of narratives that idealised the power of love. Tuberculosis redefined the very concept of womanhood, even as the lure of romanticism was fading. If medicine could not cure the disease, society's need to understand its destructive power was fulfilled by the narratives it inspired: "[...] making sense of life through tuberculosis—involved, above all, telling stories." The memoirs of Thérèse of Lisieux, who died in 1897 and was canonised in 1925, exemplify the transformation of disease into a catalyst for self-fulfillment and ultimate redemption. Destined, she believed, to die of tuberculosis, Thérèse played the role of the dying consumptive to its fullest, only this time love of man was replaced by love of God: "What she and the novelists had in common was the use of tuberculosis to express an age-old Christian attitude that exalted women's suffering as sublime, spiritual, and potentially redemptive."[31] A politically gendered discourse thus merged with religious ecstasy to form a narrative of female suffering and atonement.

For Julie de Lespinasse, love and disease likewise fulfilled a literary destiny that anticipated the heroines who were to follow her. Her letters create and promote a woman superior to all others:

> Vous ne savez pas tout ce que je *vaux*: songez donc que je sais souffrir et mourir; et voyez après cela, si je ressemble à toutes ces femmes qui savent plaire et s'amuser.

Heightened sensibility, symptomatic of tuberculosis, manifests itself in Julie's insistence on her superior ability to suffer. The true "story" of her extraordinary life is more fantastic, she claims, than that of *romanesque* heroines: "Mon histoire est un composé de circonstances si funestes, que cela m'a prouvé que le vrai n'est souvent pas vraisemblable. Les héroïnes de roman ont peu de choses à dire de leur éducation, la mienne mériterait d'être écrite par sa singularité." At the same time, Julie informs Guibert that she seeks differentiation from such fictional models:

> […] ne croyez point que […] je prenne mes modèles dans les romans de Mme Riccoboni: les femmes que la légèreté égarent, peuvent en effet se conduire d'après ces maximes et des principes de roman. Elles se font illusion […] elles n'ont point aimé […] leur âme n'a pu atteindre à la hauteur de l'amour et de la passion.

Unique in her capacity to suffer and to love, Lespinasse seeks an authenticity that rejects facile imitations—neither her life nor her text can be mimetic: "Dans tous les temps, dans toutes les circonstances, je vous ai dit vrai," she writes Guibert on 24 September 1775. Yet in the same letter she compares herself to the heroines in the novels of Prévost and Honoré d'Urfé's *Astrée*. References to Racine and Corneille likewise abound throughout her correspondence. Heightened sensitivity and lucidity alternate with periods of anxiety about her inability to express her thoughts clearly. Weakened by illness and various ineffective remedies, Julie's mind is imprisoned by her body. As early as 14 July 1773, she writes to Guibert: "[…] la durée des souffrances m'ont mise dans une espèce de stupidité qui m'ôte le pouvoir de penser [...] Mon âme a la fièvre continue avec des redoublements qui me conduisent souvent jusqu'au délire."[32]

While Julie claims her love for Guibert is authentic, it is also ambivalent, tainted by her guilt at betraying Mora. In a dialectic process that transforms the positive into a negative, desire is destroyed by the very object it seeks. As the memory of Mora informs the letters to Guibert,

Julie's delirious accusations, followed by excuses and justifications, are reinforced by the progression of her disease which she, the "malheureux malade," observes and describes in 1774:

> [...] j'avais le délire: mais c'était la dernière crise d'une maladie effroyable, dont il vaudrait mieux mourir que guérir, parce que la violence des accès de cette fièvre flétrit et abat les forces du malheureux malade, au point de ne pouvoir plus se promettre du plaisir de l'état de convalescence; mais en voilà assez, trop sans doute, sur ce que vous appelez mes *injustices* et votre *delicatesse*.

For Julie, death symbolised not only freedom from suffering but expiation through love for the betrayal of Mora. Her fragmented self seeks absolutes that shift with her rising and falling temperature. Her discourse thus alternates between contradictory assertions, reasoned discourse, emotional outbursts, regret and resignation, resulting in a series of oppositions. The same year, on 28 October, she writes to Guibert:

> J'ai offensé M. de Mora; et cependant je trouve une sorte de douceur à penser que lui seul m'aura fait connaître le bonheur; que ce n'est qu'à lui que je devrai d'avoir senti quelques moments tout le prix que peut avoir la vie. Enfin, quelquefois, je me crois moins coupable, parce que je me sens punie; et vous voyez bien que si j'étais aimée, tout cela serait effacé, renversé. Il faut du moins tenir à la vertu par le remords, et à ce qui m'a aimée, par le regret de l'avoir perdu.[33]

Love, life, and death are inextricably linked to pain and pleasure, as violent emotional upheavals were followed by calm and introspective reflection, the result of the power of love, the music of Gluck's *Orphée* and opium.

Existence becomes a madness that can only be relieved by death. As her tuberculosis progresses, Julie's concept of self becomes internalised, rejecting all exterior influences, focusing only on Guibert and her deteriorating body, even at the risk of existing in a void. In contrast to her lover, who takes pleasure in social pursuits, Julie wishes to withdraw from society, concentrating her attention on an idealised concept of love that condenses existence into a subjective reality of her own creation. For her, transfixed by the immediacy of passion, time is frozen in a non-evolving present: "[...] je suis bien loin de désirer d'être partout, car je voudrais bien n'être nulle part." In the context of Julie's salon activities and her extensive correspondence, this wish devoid of substance problematises the dichotomy between her private and public image. Time and space are condensed in the well-known letter to Guibert, dated "De tous les instants de ma vie, 1774," whose entire text reads: "Mon ami, je souffre, je vous aime, et je vous attends." Julie de Lespinasse's private space is nevertheless violated as Guibert's power to negate her subjectivity controls both her mental and physical states:

> Ce qu'il y a de sûr, c'est que, si quelqu'un pouvait être de mon secret, on connaîtrait à ma santé, à toute ma manière d'être, si j'ai reçu une lettre de vous. Oui, la circulation de mon sang en est sensiblement altérée, et alors il m'est impossible de prendre part à rien.[34]

For Julie, Guibert has the power to transform the communicative function of the letter into an act of aggression against a body already consumed by illness. As a contested space between health and sickness, between what is revealed and what is hidden, her body becomes a spectacle, observed, manipulated and recreated in Guibert's image.

Julie's anxiety, agitation, and suffering increase, especially after Guibert's marriage to Mlle de Courcelles in June 1775. In a lengthy letter to him, dated 23 September of that year, the discourses of passion and disease once more intersect. Realising that her feelings can never be reciprocated, Julie analyses her complicated relationship with Guibert, source of both the poison that consumes her and the balm that nourishes her will to live. Mora, who died proclaiming his love for her, and d'Alembert, whose devoted affection she belatedly recognises and profoundly values, exemplify ideals that Guibert can never hope to attain. She is humiliated by his marriage as an affront to her self-esteem, and his dual image of saviour and hangman evokes both love and hatred, destroying any illusions of happiness she may have had: "[…] je meurs de confusion en me rappelant ce que j'avais osé pretendre [...] Voyez, je vous prie, à quel degré d'illusion j'ai été menée!" But illusion dissipates as reality temporarily assumes the dominant role, with mind and body once more inextricably engaged in a struggle to the death. Referring to the letter she has just written to Guibert, Julie justifies the tension and confusion that characterise her discourse: "[…] je suis si malade, si abattue, que je n'ai pas eu la force d'y mettre de l'ordre […] Je le sens, les longues douleurs fatiguent l'âme et usent la tête."[35] Paralleling the tuberculosis invading Julie's body, Guibert exacerbates her mental and physical deterioration, as she writes on 17 July 1775: "Vous me faites mal; vous me tourmentez; vous m'avez fait une profonde blessure: mais je vous aime, et ce sentiment sera du baume ou du poison, selon votre volonté." References to the polarity of balm and poison are numerous, transformed into metaphors of heaven and hell: "Je n'ai connu que le climat de l'Enfer par-ci, par-là celui du Ciel; il n'y a plus moyen de façonner mon âme à une autre température."[36] Unable to satisfactorily communicate with Guibert, Julie is overwhelmed by her self-destructive passion. Her difficulty in expressing her emotions and Guibert's inability to understand her fully contribute not only to the anguish that characterises their correspondence, but also to its dialectical tension. On 10 July 1775 Julie writes: "Oh! mon ami, vous ne m'entendrez pas, vous me répondrez mal." Emotional outbursts characterise a voice progressively distant from the subject it addresses. On 9 November 1775 Julie complains to Guibert: "Je sens que je me meurs de n'avoir point de communication avec vous: cette privation est de tous les supplices le plus cruel pour moi."[37] Furthermore, the memory of Mora casts a shadow on any possibility for happiness. By writing of this deceased lover, Julie hopes to recapture his spirit and inscribe him in a text of her own creation. Her belief in the redemptive power of the written word seeks to transform illusion into truth and to invoke the promise of life after death.

Comments regarding Julie's health form a subtext in her letters not only to Guibert but to other correspondents as well, particularly her confidant, Condorcet. Julie's friend and personal secretary, the mathematician d'Alembert, and Condorcet also corresponded with Turgot (1727-1781) and his letters corroborate these references. Between 1770 and 1776, these letters constitute a tableau of shifting physical and mental symptoms and the treatments used to alleviate them. Six principal complaints characterise the pathology of Julie's illness: insomnia, lethargy with generalised muscular pain and stiffness, severe coughing spells, chest pain, high fevers and digestive disorders. Shortly before her death she told Guibert that she coughed

> à assourdir les vingt-quatre personnes qui étaient là. Je suis rentrée, j'ai eu des convulsions si violentes, qu'il ne m'est rien resté de mon dîner dans l'estomac. J'ai vomi avec des angoisses inexprimables; cette secousse m'a donné la fièvre, et beaucoup plus forte que celle d'hier.[38]

Although some of her symptoms were caused by rheumatism, the majority were primarily the result of tuberculosis:

> Pulmonary consumption [...] was long recognised as a clinical entity [...]. The important clinical signs were emaciation and wasting, cough, with the production of 'pus', and fever of the particular type known as hectic.[39]

References to depression and a morbid obsession with death alternate with periods of elated happiness. We should remember that Mora was also gravely ill with tuberculosis, particularly at the height of his affair with

Julie, between 1770-1774. The increased strain of her simultaneous love for two men, one of whom was dying and the other lukewarm in his affection, aggravated the symptoms of her physical deterioration and facilitated their transformation into metaphors of desire. Julie confides to Condorcet the damaging effects of her anxiety as she awaits the letters which bring news of Mora's health. Burning with fever, coughing, she awaits the mail. On 30 December 1770 Condorcet describes her state to Turgot: "Mlle de Lespinasse a eu avant-hier, pendant la nuit, une toux convulsive très violente […] elle a pris de l'opium […] elle s'est couchée hier avec la fièvre"; and again on 1 January 1771, "Mlle de Lespinasse a eu hier et avant-hier au soir un mouvement de fièvre et elle a toujours eu beaucoup de malaise et de courbature. Elle n'a point dormi cette nuit et est sans fièvre ce matin."[40] In June 1771, reacting to Mora's worsening condition, Julie suffered from recurrent fevers, for which she was advised to go to the spa at Seidlitz.[41] In September, discouraged by her worsening health, she wrote to Condorcet of her dejection and reported the disappointing advice of her physician: past the age of thirty one must have patience and not be deluded with vain hopes! References to her insomnia are followed by descriptions of a general aching and stiffness in the joints which limit her movements and make it difficult to think, a possible result once more of the abuse of opiates. On 18 November 1771 she wrote: "J'ai été toute la semaine dernière dans un état qui me permettait ni de penser, ni d'agir; il faut donc avoir pitié de moi." By 1772, the year she met Guibert, she was already preoccupied by thoughts of death and suicide: "Jamais ma santé n'a été si mauvaise. Je suis dans un état de souffrance […] qui m'abat et me décourage de vivre." [42] Inflammation of the lungs leads to complaints of oppression and heat in the chest area, particularly as Julie's illness reached a terminal stage in 1776: "[…] je meurs déjà de soif, et j'ai la poitrine et les entrailles brûlantes."[43] The temporary loss of her voice resulted from a possible ulceration of the larynx. As the intensity and tension of her relationship with Guibert rose, she characterised her illness as a living death. Exploiting the therapeutic effects of opium as well as its power to kill, she wrote to Condorcet in July 1772: "J'ai pris de l'opium qui m'a ôté la moitié de mon existence et enfin je ne puis pas obtenir le seul bien auquel je prétends, qui est d'être presque aussi heureuse que si j'étais morte." She thus proclaimed her passion for Guibert as her ability to feel sensations or respond to outside stimulation diminished.

The deterioration of Julie's lungs, combined with the effect of large doses of opium, led to serious digestive problems that special diets failed to cure, resulting in a loss of appetite and, ultimately, the inability to eat.

In October 1772 she informed Condorcet that she had obtained some relief by drinking ass's milk every evening as a digestive and sleeping aid.[44] Pain and exterior stimuli such as food ultimately became indistinguishable from each other: in September 1774 she characterised her health as “un état de souffrance qui m’a ôté le pouvoir de parler et d’agir. Je ne puis plus manger: les mots de nourriture et de douleur sont devenus synonymes pour moi.” By October of that year her condition had worsened, and she records one of the few occasions when a physician comments on a palpable sign of her disease: “toute espèce de nourriture me fait un mal égal. Mon médecin en conclut qu’il se forme un embarras au *pylore*; je ne connaissais pas cet étrange mot […]. Je prends de la ciguë.”[45] Her suffering is so intense that she wishes to drink hemlock not to conserve her life, but to end it. Increasingly severe coughing spells prevented her from sleeping, and she sought relief with “occimêle cilitique,” a cough-suppressing syrup consisting of squills steeped in honey and vinegar.[46] While providing temporary relief, it likewise was not a cure.

These details corroborate the failed attempts at prophylaxis or effective treatments, much less a cure for tuberculosis. The disease had reached epidemic proportions by the end of the eighteenth century.[47] The advised regimen of hygiene and diet had changed little throughout the seventeenth century, when horseback riding had been added to the list of recommendations. In the article “Phtisie” in Diderot's *Encyclopédie* (1765) a multitude of popular remedies was suggested, but all of them had already been recommended by Richard Morton. These included milk or a bouillon made from rice or barley, the extended use of large doses of balsamic medicines, diuretics and expectorants, warm liqueurs, bleeding, mild purges and diaphoretics of boiled wood in lime water to increase perspiration. Cauterisation of the patient’s shaved head or blistering the nape of the neck, between the shoulders, the thighs and the legs were also recommended.[48] Julie tried several remedies with varying degrees of success, in many cases disregarding the warnings on recommended dosages. While opium was used to calm coughing spells and as a sleeping aid, it was accompanied by the warning that it should only be used in moderation, since it can result in lethargy, difficulty in breathing and coldness in the extremities, thereby hastening the death of the patient. As we have seen, Julie’s disregard of this advice gave rise to precisely such symptoms. Among other popular remedies were quinine, herbal teas, coffee and cocoa; towards the end of the eighteenth century, fresh country air became popular. In addition to a regimen of riding or work in the fields, eating moderate quantities of easily digested food was also recommended. In the early stages of the disease, called the “inflammatory suffering, Julie's physician could only confirm the futility of his atment:

> Votre mal ne vient pas de vous, il est hors de vous; et je vois avec chagrin […] que les médecins et la médecine ne peuvent rien, ou presque rien, pour votre soulagement. L'opium que je viens de vous ordonner pour mettre sur vos entrailles, il faudrait le mettre sur votre âme.[53]

The issues raised by Julie's correspondence are important to our derstanding of women and disease in the eighteenth century, as well as broader issue of the relationship between the female body as text and instrument of literary inscription. Many, Julie herself included, have imed that she died of love—but a love, we might add, whose textual dy is transformed and contaminated by disease.

Julie de Lespinasse died of tuberculosis on 22 May 1776, at two clock in the morning.

Notes

This article first appeared in *SVEC* 08 (2000): 3-16. Reprinted by permission of Voltaire Foundation, Oxford University. A preliminary version of this paper s presented at the annual meeting for the American Society for Eighteenth-ntury Studies, Tucson, Arizona, 5-9 April 1995.

ndré Beaunier, *La vie amoureuse de Julie de Lespinasse* (Paris: Flammarion, 25); Janine Bouissounouse, *Julie de Lespinasse, ses amitiés, sa passion* (Paris: chette, 1958); Susan Lee Carrell, *Le Soliloque de la passion féminine ou le logue illusoire: Etude d'une formule monophonique de la littérature épistolaire* aris: Jean-Michel Place, 1982); Carrell, "Julie de Lespinasse and the *liebestod*: minine Passion and Literary Consciousness" (paper delivered at the annual eting for the American Society for Eighteenth-Century Studies, Williamsburg, rginia, 13-16 March 1986), p.16; Eve Katz, "The Contradiction of Passion in the ve Letters of Julie de Lespinasse," *American Society of Legion of Honor gazine* 43 (1972): 9-24; Jean-Noël Pascal, "Guibert ou le héros du roman de ie," in *Guibert ou le soldat philosophe*, ed. by J. P. Charnay et al., Travaux du ntre d'études et de recherches sur les stratégies et les conflits (Château de ncennes, 1981); J.-N. Pascal, "De la lettre au roman: sur l'entrée en littérature de ie de Lespinasse," *Dix-huitième siècle* 21 (1989): 381-393.

ulie de Lespinasse, *Lettres*, ed. by Jacques Dupont (Paris: Editions de La Table nde, 1997), p. 300.

See Susan Sontag, *Illness as Metaphor* (New York: Farrar, Straus & Giroux, 78). Sontag argues that in the "popular imagination," diseases difficult to cure or ose pathology is not well understood, have been transformed into metaphors t represent our ambivalence toward the realities of such devastating diseases as berculosis and cancer.

phase," purging, bleeding and blistering were advocated, wh stages, "ulceration, balsams, expectorants, lime water and used.[49] The volume on *Médecine* in the *Encyclopédie* discusses variations of these remedies for different forms of p scrofula (tuberculosis of the lymph nodes) or diseases relate "la phthisie catarrhale," which we call bronchitis.[50]

Throughout 1773 and 1774, at the height of her affair wit pattern of physical degeneration concurrent with emotiona instability continues, as she indicates to Condorcet: "[…] je t […] je ne dors point." Seeking meaning in a life that eludes control of both her textual and physical bodies:

> […] je sens aussi la destruction de ma machine [...]. Je me tro lasse et fatigué de ce voyage qu'on appelle la vie. Je n'ai poi force pour en terminer brusquement le cours; mais je vois avec que je m'achemine à sa fin.[51]

Thoughts of suicide can only be overcome by the power symbiotic relationship between love and death, a constant in Guibert, is reaffirmed in the Condorcet correspondence, an him in his letters to Turgot.

Because of her attempt to achieve "le vrai" and accurately depth and range of her emotions, the textual fabric of Juli doubly "contaminated"—symbolically by passion for th captivates her mind and concretely by the tuberculosis that c body. Writing defines both her authenticity and her ill anguished voice of the romantics who were to follow. Ove constraints of language, she attempts to reintegrate within system what is out of place, "hors de propos," in conventio As she tries to represent a fragmented yet differentiated se page of Julie's text can only anticipate new possibilities in me writes to Guibert on 24 June 1773: "nous n'aurons pas la n […]. Je n'entends pas la langue des gens du monde."[52] Invoki of truth, yet denying her ability to achieve it, Julie questione of the very text she created. In an age when the separation mind was questioned, epistemological boundaries became blu Lespinasse nevertheless sought a unity of voice which elude not diminish the strength of her will. Five months before h January 1776, she described to Guibert a night of high fever headache, and the profound sadness that consumed her e Unable to distinguish between the multiple signs of her illness

[4] Julie de Lespinasse, *Correspondence entre Mlle de Lespinasse et le Comte de Guibert, publiée pour la première fois d'après le texte original par le Comte de Villeneuve-Guibert* (Paris: Calmann-Lévy, 1906), p. 536.
[5] Catherine Blondeau, "Lectures de la correspondance de Julie de Lespinasse: Une étude de réception," *SVEC* 308 (1993): 223-232.
[6] Lespinasse, *Lettres*, pp. 75-76.
[7] Lester S. King, *Medical Thinking: A Historical Preface* (Princeton: Princeton University Press, 1982), p. 27.
[8] Lespinasse, *Lettres*, p. 348 and p. 264.
[9] Anne Vila, *Enlightenment and Pathology: Sensibility in the Literature and Medicine of Eighteenth-century France* (Baltimore: John Hopkins University Press, 1998), p. 39. The introduction discusses the various meanings of "sensibility" in eighteenth-century France and Part I is a historical treatment of the medical construction of the sensible body. For a discussion of Chambaud's article, "Observateur" in Diderot's *Encyclopédie*, see p. 40.
[10] John O'Neal, "Auenbrugger, Corvisart, and the Perception of Disease," *Eighteenth-century Studies* 31.4 (summer 1998): 473-489.
[11] O'Neal, "Auenbrugger, Corvisart, and the Perception of Disease," pp. 473-476 and p. 484.
[12] Denis Diderot, "Médecine," in *Encyclopédie ou dictionnaire raisonné des arts, des sciences et des métiers*, vol. 10 (Neuchâtel: Samuel Faulche, 1765), p. 265.
[13] Diderot, *Encyclopédie*, vol. 12, p. 532.
[14] The *Oxford English Dictionary* defines "symptom" as "a bodily or mental phenomenon, circumstance, or change of condition arising from and accompanying a disease or affection, and constituting an indication or evidence of it—a characteristic sign of some particular disease." "Sign" is defined as "a token or indication (visible or otherwise) of some fact, quality."
[15] Vila, *Enlightenment and Pathology*, p. 59.
[16] "Medicine and Enlightenment," *SVEC* 305 (1992): 1895-1898. Porter has also suggested that the Enlightenment bias toward the humanistic study of man resulted in an emphasis of "nurture" over "nature," "mind" over "brain" and a resistance to medicine as a biologically grounded science.
[17] Sainte-Beuve, "Portraits de Guibert" (from *Causeries du lundi*), reproduced in Charnay et al., *Guibert ou le soldat philosophe*, p. 24.
[18] Pascal, "De la lettre au roman," p. 387.
[19] Charles Henry, *Lettres inédites de Mademoiselle de Lespinasse à Condorcet, à d'Alembert, à Guibert, au Comte de Crillon, publiées avec des lettres de ses amis, des documents nouveaux et une étude* (Paris: E. Dentu, 1887), p. 1.
[20] *Le Soliloque de la passion*, pp. 105-122; "Julie de Lespinasse and the *liebestod*," p. 16.
[21] *La Demoiselle des lumières* (Paris: Gallimard, 1997), p. 72.
[22] For a history of tuberculosis, see King, *Medical Thinking*; Frank Ryan, *The Forgotten Plague* (Boston: Little, Brown and Company, 1993); David Barnes, *The Making of a Social Disease: Tuberculosis in Nineteenth-century France* (Berkeley: University of California Press, 1995).

[23] Quoted in R. Y. Keers, *Pulmonary Tuberculosis: A Journey Down the Centuries* (London: Baillière Tindall, 1978), p. 25.
[24] Louis Jacques Moreau de la Sarthe, "Médecine" in *Encyclopédie méthodique* : *Médecine*, vol. 11 (Paris: Agasse, 1824), p. 745. I am grateful to Ann K. Doig of Georgia State University for making me aware of this source.
[25] See King, *Medical Thinking*, pp. 34-35; Barnes, *The Making of a Social Disease*, p. 25.
[26] Lespinasse, *Lettres*, p. 316.
[27] Barnes, *The Making of a Social Disease*, p. 25.
[28] Robert Mauzi, "Les maladies de l'âme au XVIIIe siècle," *Revue des Sciences Humaines* (1960): 477.
[29] Lespinasse, *Lettres*, p. 45 and p. 70.
[30] Sontag, *Illness as Metaphor*, pp. 14-23; Barnes, *The Making of a Social Disease*, pp. 50-62.
[31] Barnes, *The Making of a Social Disease*, p. 50 and pp. 68-69.
[32] Lespinasse, *Lettres*, p. 46, p. 117, pp. 247-248, p. 291 and p. 44.
[33] Lespinasse, *Lettres*, p. 126 and p. 176.
[34] Lespinasse, *Lettres*, p. 312, p. 77, and pp. 178-179.
[35] Lespinasse, *Lettres*, p. 289 and p. 290.
[36] Lespinasse, *Correspondance entre Mlle de Lespinasse et le Comte de Guibert*, p. 354 and p. 389.
[37] Lespinasse, *Lettres*, p. 259 and p. 319.
[38] Lespinasse, *Lettres*, p. 347.
[39] King, *Medical Thinking*, p. 43.
[40] Henry, *Lettres inédites de Mademoiselle de Lespinasse*, vol. 4, p. 261.
[41] Jean Lacouture and Marie-Christine d'Aragon, *Julie de Lespinasse: Mourir d'amour* (Paris: Ramsay, 1980), p. 200.
[42] Julie de Lespinasse, *Lettres à Condorcet: suivi du portrait de Condorcet rédigé par Julie de Lespinasse en 1774*, ed. Jean-Noël Pascal (Paris: Desjonquères, 1990), p. 51 and pp. 67-68.
[43] Lespinasse, *Lettres*, p. 329.
[44] Lespinasse, *Lettres à Condorcet*, p. 60 and p. 65.
[45] Lespinasse, *Lettres*, p. 137 and p. 147.
[46] Lespinasse, *Lettres à Condorcet*, pp. 69-70.
[47] Keers, *Pulmonary Tuberculosis*, p. 33.
[48] Diderot, *Encyclopédie*, vol. 12, pp. 532-533.
[49] Keers, *Pulmonary Tuberculosis*, p. 65.
[50] Louis Jacques Moreau de la Sarthe, *Encyclopédie méthodique: Médecine*, vol. 11, pp. 747-752; King, *Medical Thinking*, pp. 24-25.
[51] Lespinasse, *Lettres à Condorcet*, pp. 69-70 and p. 71.
[52] Lespinasse, *Lettres*, p. 259 and p. 37.
[53] Lespinasse, *Correspondence entre Mlle de Lespinasse et le Comte de Guibert*, pp. 502-503.

CHAPTER EIGHT

SILENCE RECONSIDERED: BRITISH LITERARY WOMEN AND BREAST CANCER

ELIZABETH KUIPERS

The Age of Enlightenment brought about significant advancements in the medical field. At the beginning of the century, most doctors upheld the humoral theory for illness, and breast cancer was no different. Although the earliest treatments of breast cancer, including those of Hippocrates, were recorded in ancient Egyptian papyri, the humoral theory that he espoused was the dominant science for about 2000 years. The humoral theory posits that breast cancer is a systemic disease caused by an excess of black bile in the body. Accordingly, breast cancer was treated with pharmaceuticals like castor oil, sulphur, opium, and even licorice.

As medical science progressed, so did the theories. The French physician Jean Astruc disproved the humoral theory about breast cancer by roasting a piece of breast cancer tissue and a piece of beef and comparing their taste. Since the breast tissue did not taste any different than the beef, he concluded that it did not have unusually high amounts of black bile or acid. In 1713 Bernardio Ramazzini concluded that the cause of breast cancer was linked to sex. Nuns who contracted the disease got it because they did not have sex and their reproductive organs decayed. Friedrich Hoffman of Prussia refined this theory, positing that women who were sexually active but still got cancer did so because they were practicing "vigorous sex" that resulted in lymphatic blockage. Johannes de Gorter argued that pus-filled inflammations in the breast mixed with blood, lodged in milk glands, and dried into tumors. Claude-Nicolas Le Cat blamed depression, which constricted blood vessels and trapped coagulated blood. He argued that the only way to cure breast cancer was to remove the infected breast.[1]

In the course of the eighteenth century, more and more physicians understood that breast cancer was a localized disease and began experimenting with surgery as a cure. The approaches varied vastly. In 1721, Gerd Tabor presented his thesis on "a new way to extirpate cancer of the breast."[2] His approach demanded that the surgery be as quick as possible, so he developed a kind of "guillotine machine" for the expeditious removal of the breast: the device compressed the breast tissue at its base and employed a curved knife for amputating the breast in one swift motion. This device is pictured, along with other surgical tools, in Diderot's *Encyclopédie ou dictionnaire raisonné des sciences, des arts et des métiers.*[3] Plate XXVIII focuses on the placement for incisions while Plate XXIX highlights various tools, among them the guillotine machine and a two-pronged fork used to lift the breast from the chest wall before cutting.

Other doctors understood that the cancer sometimes involved the lymph nodes and underlying tissues. Jean Louis Petit of Paris was widely recognized as a master surgeon and greatly influenced the direction of surgery as treatment of breast cancer by training doctors from all over the world and publishing his own textbook regarding surgery for breast cancer. Ultimately, the experimentation of the eighteenth century led to the radical mastectomy, but until anesthesia was introduced in 1846, surgery was considered the last option. Sakorafas and Safioleas note in the article "Breast Cancer Surgery: An Historical Narrative" that

> surgical treatment was widely considered worse than the disease itself due to the intense pain that the women had during and after surgery. Operations [...] must have been performed rapidly in a noisy and distracting atmosphere, and speed was a particularly desirable trait in a surgeon, who should have had a stout heart and an unquenchable optimism.[4]

Most of the documentation that exists from the eighteenth century is from the perspective of the physician and is, therefore, very clinical. There seems to be a vast silence from the women themselves. Audre Lorde, in discussing her own battle with cancer, argues that this silence is used in our society as a tool to separate women from the dominant discourse about cancer which is a public, medical discourse rather than a private one; the suppression of women's discourse about breast cancer results in a powerlessness for women which is reinforced by the ways in which our culture uses "cancer" as a metaphor for culturally unacceptable ideas like pollution, communism, and corruption.[5] This essay will examine three eighteenth century accounts of breast cancer in order to explore how Lorde's assertions hold up in a different time and place: a biography of

Mary Astell who died of breast cancer in 1731; Maria Edgeworth's *Belinda* (1801), a novelistic account of a woman's struggle with breast cancer; and finally, the earliest known account written by the patient, Frances Burney's 1811 letter to her sister recounting her mastectomy without anesthesia.

Mary Astell was born in England on 12 November 1666. She earned her reputation as a philosopher and rhetorician with works like *A Serious Proposal to the Ladies, Parts I and II. Wherein a Method is Offer'd for the Improvements of their Minds* (1694, 1697), and *Some Reflections Upon Marriage* (1700). Although she lived a fairly secluded life, her patrons included Lady Mary Chudleigh and Lady Mary Wortley Montague. She corresponded with the Archbishop of Canterbury, William Sancroft, who assisted her financially and by introducing her to her publisher. She has long been considered an early feminist based on her insistence that women should be educated, as is reflected in "A Serious Proposal," a plan for an all-female college. She bases her argument on Descartes's idea of the dualism of the mind and body; improving women's rational engagement with the world by way of education was merely an attempt to fulfill God's plan for creation, since women's minds are separate from their bodies and are thereby not innately weaker than men's.[6] Most of what we know about Astell's life is drawn from a short biography by George Ballard written in 1752. In *Memoirs of Several Ladies of Great Britain Who Have Been Celebrated for their Writings, or Skill in the Learned Languages, Arts, and Sciences*, Ballard recounts her professional life and contemporary opinions about her, as well as her death on 11 May 1731, shortly after her mastectomy. He writes,

> She seemed to enjoy an uninterrupted state of health till a few years before her death, when, having one of her breasts cut off, it so much impaired her constitution, that she did not long survive it. This was occasioned by a cancer which she had long concealed from the world in such a manner, that even few of her most intimate acquaintances knew any thing at all of the matter. She dressed and managed it herself, 'till she plainly perceived there was an absolute necessity for its being cut off: and then with the most intrepid resolution and courage, she then went to the Rev. Mr. Johnson, a gentleman very eminent for his skill in surgery, (with only one person to attend her) entreating him to take it off in the most private manner imaginable: and would hardly allow him to have persons whom necessity required to be at the operation. She seemed so regardless of the sufferings or pain she was to undergo, that she refused to have her hands held, and did not discover the least timidity, or impatience, but went thro' the operation without the least struggle or resistance; or even so much as giving a groan or a sigh: and showed the like patience and resignation

> throughout the [treatment] which that gentleman, to his lasting credit and honour, soon performed.[7]

Ballard paints Astell as the ultimate private woman who is courageous in the face of horrific circumstances. He expounds upon the idea of some of Astell's contemporaries that, apparently for religious reasons, Astell insists upon avoiding the public realm at every possible turn. Much like her insistence that she forfeited her "beloved obscurity" "not without pain and reluctancy," she does not debate or publicly disclose her ordeal.[8] She insists on the most privacy possible for her operation, even to the possible detriment of the success of the operation when she "hardly allows" the doctor to have the necessary persons assist him. Certainly this insistence on privacy is consistent with her desire to "most industriously shun a great Reputation."[9] It is also interesting, given her reputation as a highly devout person, that she chooses a religious man to conduct the operation; she can be assured that, if not for his medical obligations, certainly for his religious ones, he will deal with her treatment in the most private way possible.

Modern science tells us that early detection and treatment of breast cancer is essential to successfully battling the disease. Astell, afflicted with the disease in an era that did not know this, chooses, according to Ballard, to treat herself until it is painfully obvious even to her that her breast needs to be removed. One can only imagine how advanced her cancer must have been for her to have come to this conclusion. The narrative description reflects Astell's firm resolve as she not only demands that the doctor remove her breast but refuses to have anyone hold her down as she undergoes the radical amputation without anesthesia. The emphasis that Astell puts on the need to focus on the mental or spiritual rather than the material or physical might be an explanation, at least in part, for her courage in the face of surgery. She held that "dejected looks and melancholy airs were very unseemly in a Christian," and asserted that humans should always stay focused on the divine (p. 460). This attitude is certainly supported in Ballard's continued description of her decline:

> Soon after [the surgery], her health and strength now declined apace, and at length by a gradual decay of nature, being confined to her bed, and finding the time of her dissolution draw nigh, she ordered her coffin and shroud to be made, and brought to her bedside, and there to remain in her view, as a constant memento to her of her approaching fate, and that her mind might not deviate or stray one moment from God, its most proper object. Her thoughts were now so entirely fixed upon God and eternity, that for some days before her death, she earnestly desired that no company

> might be permitted to come to her; refusing at that time to see even her old and dear friend, the Lady Catherine Jones, purely because she would not be disturbed in the last moments of her divine contemplations.[10]

Her actions as described by Ballard reinforce her assertion that "Abstinence was her best Physick," for she not only carefully limits the interactions that would force her to contemplate her material losses and worldly friendships in death, she also embodies the Christian that she argues all should become by refusing to allow anyone to witness her dejection and melancholy. Indeed, it is unclear whether or not she even experienced any grief at her condition. However, I would suggest that her decision to actively pursue treatment for her very advanced breast cancer suggests a desire to at the very least postpone death. Elisa New, in a different context, has labeled this assertion of privacy as "feminist invisibility." In her discussion of Anne Bradstreet and Anne Hutchinson, she asserts that "such self-conscious, even cultivated unworldliness is, of course, the hallmark of Reformation theology [...]."[11] Ballard's account neatly reflects the mind-body split implicit in Cartesian dualism on which Astell based her own philosophy. Sadly, any discussion of Astell's personal attitude toward her fight with breast cancer must remain conjecture since she left no documents addressing the issue. This silence seems to support Lorde's assertion that the medical discourse about cancer is one that silences women, especially since Astell chose to participate in other discourses that were deemed masculine in her time.

In Maria Edgworth's *Belinda* (1801), we see a female who seems to react to the idea of breast cancer with silence in that, like Astell, she hides her presumed cancer as long as possible. Lady Delacour recounts her history to her protégée, Belinda, in an attempt to explain her public persona as a fashionable woman. She has not married for love, and the better part of her marriage has been a battle of wills between herself and Lord Delacour as each tries to outdo the other with financial extravagances and moral dissipation. Heike Hartung describes her narrative as a "self-reflexive display of the public persona in the aristocratic memoir" because of the distinction Lady Delacour insists on making between her public and private selves.[12] Seen by the public as an extravagant and fashionable woman who preys on others' weaknesses, Lady Delacour reveals her private self to Belinda by sharing with her the story of her maimed breast. In making this distinction, Edgeworth directly engages the notion of idealized feminine goodness and what it means for individual women. As Heather Macfadyen writes,

> The proper lady and the domestic woman are marked by their ability to regulate their own desires and the desires of other members of their circles. Such women privilege self-control over self-indulgence, the contained over the unbounded, order over chaos [...]. The fashionable woman, like the aristocratic woman with whom she is associated, thus becomes a threat to domesticity.[13]

This threat becomes obvious early in Lady Delacour's account of her history.

Before she recounts the accident which led to her cancerous breast, Lady Delacour establishes herself as outside the realm of "normal" womanhood. In the note that she sends to Belinda to summon her to her side, she calls herself an Amazon, hoping that Belinda can "admire [Amazons]."[14] The reference resonates on a number of levels. The tribe of Amazons were fierce warriors who removed one breast so that they would be better able to shoot bows in battle. A community made up solely of women, much like Lady Delacour's inner circle, the Amazons implicitly rejected essentialist notions about womanhood. Indeed, as Susan Greenfield points out, the term "amazon" is used in eighteenth-century literature, along with "sapphist" and "tommy" to describe lesbian characters.[15]

As Lady Delacour begins her description of her child-bearing years, she establishes herself as a non-maternal woman. She deems herself a prisoner at the hands of her in-laws who want to limit her activity during her pregnancy. She blames her refusal to oblige for the death of her first child. Her second child, she tells Belinda, she starved to death because of her inability to suckle the child adequately:

> My second child was a girl, but a poor diminutive, sickly thing. It was the fashion at the time for fine mothers to suckle their own children—so much the worse for the poor brats. Fine nurses never make fine children. There was a prodigious rout made about the matter; a vast deal of sentiment and sympathy, and compliments and inquiries; but after the novelty was over, I became heartily sick of the business; and at the end of about three months my poor child was sick too—I don't much like to think of it—it died. If I had put it out to nurse, I should have been thought by my friends an unnatural mother—but I should have saved its life.[16]

After her child's death Lady Delacour actively works to keep from being considered a maternal figure by repressing all evidence of emotional reactions to her loss, while she allows her mother-in-law to publicly mourn the child. However, Lady Delacour tempers the description of her callous attitude towards her children by explaining to Belinda that her suffering was greater than the outward show of those around her. Her "real" self is the private self rather than the public self. Indeed, she assures Belinda that she assumes the responsibility of the second child's death and would not "have the barbarity" to attempt to nurse another child.[17] Accordingly, when her third child, another girl, is born, she is immediately sent out to nurse. In doing so, Lady Delacour is openly admitting moral failure. Sangeeta Mediratta explains that the debate about employing wet nurses in the late eighteenth-century took on several layers of meaning:

> The breast became one of the most significant sites for the consolidation of national identity, gender difference, and (im)proper femininity. The widespread assault on the common practice of sending infants to wet-nurses is one instance of the period's deployment of women's breasts to construct notions of good and bad womanhood, true Englishness versus disloyalty to the nation, the good and bad breast. The popular middle- and upper-class practice of handing infants off to the wet-nurses…was seen as emerging from women's (and their husbands') desire to preserve the beauty of the breast by farming off the breast's 'real' nurturing function to lower-class women.[18]

Clearly, Lady Delacour understands that her inability or lack of desire to nurse her children results in a slur against her in terms of being a good mother. She accepts that her breast is sexual rather than maternal and, as her narrative will show, is outwardly marked as such.

This slur, however, is mitigated by Lady Delacour's recognition that much of her life has been tainted with folly. She accepts responsibility for her failure and mourns inwardly. Sending her daughter away, in her mind, ensures the daughter's survival, thus Lady Delacour's assertion that she could not be so barbaric as to ineffectively nurse this child as well. She acknowledges that the effect of sending her daughter away was that when she returned three years later, Lady Delacour could not recognize the child as her own. The absence of a fulfilled domestic life, she argues, becomes the impetus for her public life of folly. With nothing to engage her at home, she seeks fulfillment of the "'aching void' in [her] heart" outside the realm of domesticity in a time when the search causes her to be deemed morally degraded.[19] Her narrative makes it clear that she recognizes the error of her ways, thereby introducing the possibility of redemption for her.

In her friendship with Harriet Freke, Lady Delacour is led even farther away from the role of "good" wife and mother. Indeed, Susan Greenfield has argued that the relationship between Lady Delacour and Freke has homoerotic overtones.[20] Harriet persistently cross-dresses and leads Lady Delacour into socially unacceptable situations. Not the least of them is the duel in which Lady Delacour received the initial injury to her breast that she believes has turned cancerous. Always the puppet master, Harriet has manipulated Lady Delacour into fighting a duel to protect her honor and doing so in men's clothes. The duel becomes farcical when a mob of peasants demand the fight be stopped, not on the grounds that dueling is illegal, but because the participants have cross-dressed. The idea of Lady Delacour fighting for honor becomes more ludicrous when the handsome Clarence Hervey comes along driving a herd of pigs on a bet and asserting that losing the pigs will result in England being undone. The gravity with which they all undertake absurd tasks parallels the absurdity of the cross-dressing aristocracy fighting a duel of honor when none of the characters have ever exhibited any such virtue.

The duel is, however, integral to Lady Delacour's story because it is at that point that she is physically marked; her internal corruption is signified by the wound on her breast that results from the recoil of her own weapon. Edgeworth is not at all subtle in asserting that the wounds, literal and figurative, are of Lady Delacour's own making. Lady Delacour's marked breast becomes a site of struggle for her as she attempts to hide the wound and thereby maintain her position in the public eye. Until Belinda is let in on her secret, Lady Delacour only allows her servant Marriott to help her treat the wound. She meticulously hides her breast from her husband and seeks no treatment from physicians. She explains to Belinda,

> I could not—I never will consult a physician—I would not for the universe have my situation known.... Why, my dear, if I lose admiration, what have I left? Would you have me live upon pity? Consider, what a dreadful thing it must be to me, who have no friends, no family, to be confined to a sick room....[21]

She struggles to deal with her pain for two years, with help from Marriot to dress the wound and hide her condition.

The relationship that Lady Delacour has with Marriott is strange indeed. Lady Delacour regularly implies that Marriott, although a servant, has a great deal of power over her, even going so far as to say that Marriott rules her and will one day leave her. Marriott's care of the wounded breast and keeping Lady Delacour's most profound secret certainly give her power, but the relationship seems to have a homoerotic and, at times, even sadistic element to it. When Belinda is allowed into the boudoir, Marriott is angry and jealous, as her presence there threatens the homoerotic and gender-bending relationships between Lady Delacour, Marriott, and Harriet. Lady Delacour is under the sway of these influences for two years as she attempts to control her pain and hide her condition.

Lady Delacour's insistence on secrecy about her injury only removes her farther from the socially acceptable role of wife and mother. Her husband notes her locked boudoir and assumes that the secrecy is related to concealing a lover. Less than an overt rejection of her husband, her secrecy is a refusal to have her public image tarnished by public knowledge of her illness. Ironically, she seeks to maintain the public impression that she is promiscuous which is, in her opinion, less damaging to her reputation as a fashionable woman than her illness would be. It is only after a carriage accident that results in significant pain in her breast that Lady Delacour is convinced that a mastectomy is inevitable. But it is Belinda, in her purifying honesty, who plays a central role in convincing others of Lady Delacour's true situation. In addition to convincing Lady Delacour that a doctor should be called, she is instrumental in reuniting Lady Delacour with her husband and their daughter.

However, even after the doctor is called in, Lady Delacour continues to play the fashionable woman in that she manipulates and teases the doctors who have come to treat her. On the day they arrive to operate, Lady Delacour greets them enthusiastically and refuses to acknowledge the reason for their presence. After keeping them in polite conversation all the evening, she says,

> My sage sir…have you lived to this time without ever having been duped by a woman before? I wanted a day's reprieve, and I have gained it—gained a day, spent in most agreeable conversation, for which I thank you. To morrow…I must invent some new excuse for my cowardice; and though I give you notice of it beforehand…I shall succeed. Good night![22]

Lady Delacour's caprice is linked to a frightening vision which must be resolved so that she can finally reject her past life completely and fully reform.

Whereas Lady Delacour ultimately avoids the cut of the mastectomy, thereby ensuring that her womanhood will not be damaged, Harriet Freke gets maimed in a "man-trap." Forever looking for trouble, Harriet sneaks into Lady Delacour's garden on a number of consecutive nights in an attempt to discern the identity of Lady Delacour's lover, thereby creating Lady Delacour's "vision" of someone outside her room. The man that Harriet sees in Lady Delacour's rooms is the physician who is treating her, but Harriet's destructive personality assumes the worst of her former friend and she seeks to gather information to use against Lady Delacour. The gardener sets a trap which maims the trespasser, presumed to be a man, who is caught in it. Harriet's vindictive plan to harm the unreformed Lady Delacour backfires when she is permanently marked for her transgressions. With a disfigured leg, Harriet will no longer be able to transgress gendered boundaries: "she grew quite outrageous when it was hinted, that the beauty of her legs would be spoiled, and that she would never more be able to appear to advantage in man's apparel."[23] Harriet cannot be reformed and is, therefore, permanently outwardly disfigured. Lady Delacour, on the other hand, asserts that her reformation will be evidenced by her willingness to undergo the mastectomy. However, her reformation saves her from the fate of a mastectomy, therefore allowing her to escape permanent disfigurement. Belinda functions as the means of physical and mental reformation for Lady Delacour as she is the means by which order is restored to the latter's life. Lady Delacour amends her ways in that she ultimately submits to the doctor's authority, then to the priest's authority, and finally to her husband's authority. The literal cancer is properly diagnosed and treated for what it is, and the figurative cancer of Lady Delacour's impropriety is expunged. Patriarchal order is restored and reformation of Lady Delacour's personality is reflected in her physical recovery.

Although Edgeworth's fictionalization of cancer as a reflection of morality seems ludicrous to modern readers, we certainly recognize the fear of the afflicted woman in revealing her cancer to others. In the case of Frances Burney, the rhetoric of fear is evident in her first-person account of a mastectomy. Like Astell and Lady Delacour, Burney avoided treatment until her cancer proved significantly painful and impeded her ability to write. This long silence imposed by her illness is anomalous for this prolific writer whose journals and letters span twelve volumes.[24] In a letter to her beloved sister Esther, Burney focuses on the surgery itself in order to recount her brush with death and convince her family that she is recovering. This autopathography, or first-hand account of how one deals with one's illness, was written nine months after her surgery, and graphically details the mastectomy without anesthesia. Not only is it interesting in terms of her personal account, it is also interesting in that she underwent the mastectomy in a time when treatments for breast cancer were "regressing."

For example, in 1802, Doctor Cadgogan asserted that breast cancer was the result of lifestyle choices like poor diet, little exercise and excessive alcohol and coffee consumption. He writes: "If only women would devote their tremendous energies to rearing children instead of spending their time on other frippery, both the home and the nation would be the better for it."[25] In 1815 in England, Samuel Young attempted compression to cut off blood supply to the tumor. A certain Nooth, also in England, cauterized the breast by spraying it with carbolic acid. In France, where Burney had her surgery, Alfred Velpeau had reverted back to the humoral theory and was using hemlock, arsenic, and mercury to bring the humors back into balance as late as 1856. With regard to surgery, he wrote,

> To destroy a cancerous tumor by surgical means is usually an easy matter and but little dangerous in itself; but the question arises, whether such a procedure affords a chance of radically curing the patient. This proposition remains undecided...although it has been discussed since the time of Hippocrates.
>
> ...The disease always returns after removal, and operation only accelerates its growth and fatal termination.[26]

Burney's French surgeon, Baron Dominique-Jean Larrey, still believed in surgery as treatment. There is some irony here because modern physicians suspect that her fist-size tumor was probably benign, partly because she lived for twenty-nine more years after her surgery. Regardless of what modern physicians may suspect about her cancer, Burney's position in French society as Madame d'Arblay gained her access to the best medical treatment in France; she shared Larrey with Napoleon.

Burney's letter detailing the surgery to her sister, while ostensibly a private document, certainly suggests that she understood its public nature. She indicates on the letter the subject of the content: "Breast operation/ Respect this/ & beware not to injure it!!!"[27] She encourages her sister to distribute the letter to friends and acquaintances at "[her] own decision" (p. 615). Additionally, she exhorts her sister and female family members to seek medical attention more quickly than she did if they find themselves in a similar situation. Her exhortation works to assert the female voice as one of authority with regard to breast cancer as she gives her sisters medical advice.

Burney also knows, as Sangeeta Mediratta points out, that her letter will be subject to the rigorous state censorship that is a result of the political hostility between France and England.[28] The job of the censor is to cut away objectionable material. The superscript on the letter can then be interpreted as a metaphorical plea to censors not to dissect her document as her breast has been dissected. Instead, she exhorts them to "respect this and beware not to injure it" (p. 597). The document becomes more than a private document intended for a female audience. Instead, it is a very public letter that not only transcends national boundaries but gender boundaries as well, in that French and British male officials will read the letter and possibly censor it, and it will be circulated among Burney's family, male and female alike.

Burney's insistence on participating in the discourse about her illness is interestingly framed in the letter in that she includes the medical report about her surgery that was written by the student of Larrey the day after the surgery. The student, at Larrey's insistence, sat through the night with Burney. The letter describes "the removal of a cancerous tumor the size of a fist, which was attached to the large pectoral muscle and developed in the right breast."[29] The letter delineates the people involved and the optimism of all that the surgery was successful. Before outlining post-operative instructions about diet and medicines, the writer notes: "At ten, the patient was astonished at how well she felt—Larrey found her without fever, and the pain in the incision was negligible..." (p. 616). The medical text is certainly quite different from Burney's own narrative. Indeed, Mediratta juxtaposes the two, writing,

> the biomedical myopia and depersonalizing objectivity of the medical student's account acts as an ironic counterpoint to her tale of confinement, pain and horror and represents the dominant discourse of medicalisation at the time.[30]

Hemlow notes that the student's experience with Burney's mastectomy would likely seem textbook, as her symptoms aligned with those outlined in Diderot's *Encyclopedie* which included the two plates of surgical tools previously discussed.[31]

Burney's text does nod to some of the masculine discourses of the day. She uses military metaphors, appropriate for describing the actions of the First Surgeon to the Imperial Guard. She refers to Dubois, an attending physician, as "Commander in Chief" who issues commands "en militaire" (p. 610). She also inserts herself into the medical discourse that occurs concerning her surgery. Her doctors have left her unaware of when her surgery will be, arguably to protect her from anxiety over the impending ordeal. When they arrive, she forces them to bow to her own terms for the exact time of the surgery by insisting that they must wait a few hours to do the surgery because she has arrangements to make. Her assertion of will here is directly contrasted with her initial reaction; upon seeing the seven doctors descend upon her house she feels indignation, but her voice is stripped from her, she "could not utter a syllable" (p. 610).

As the surgery begins, Burney asserts her own courageous spirit by refusing to be held. When the doctor asks who will hold the infected breast so that the surgery can begin, the silence of the other doctors is subverted by Burney's outcry: "C'est moi, Monsieur!" She literally participates in her surgery by holding her own breast. Heidi Kaye notes that "although the surface meaning of Burney's outcry is 'I will,' it can also be read as

'It's me!'—an assertion of her own subjectivity, or the integrity of her physical and psychic sense of self: 'This breast, it's me.'"[32]

Before the surgery begins, Burney's face is covered with a handkerchief, ostensibly so that she will be unable to see what is happening. Ironically, the cloth is see-through and she keenly observes her doctors from behind "the veil," which functions, then, as beneficial only for the doctors. With her face removed, the doctors can attempt to engage her dismembered body as an object because they cannot see her subjective reactions—the pain and anguish—that their actions cause her. Their apparent selfish motivation for keeping Burney's face covered is reflected in the fact that even after she has made clear to them that she can see their actions through the cloth, they insist on re-covering her face.

Additionally, the doctors attempt to exclude her from the discourse when they use non-verbal communication during the surgery. Understanding that the doctors intend to remove her entire breast, Burney interrupts them to assert her own counter-conclusion about how much of her breast needs to be removed. She is "aroused" from her "passively submissive state" and argues with them, "explain[ing] the nature of [her] sufferings, which all sprang from one point, though they darted into every part." The doctors listen to her "in utter silence" (p. 610); for a moment, Burney is no longer the silenced one but the silencer. She has used the power of her own gaze to interpret the dominant discourse's meaning and inserts herself into that discourse, moving her from the position of object to subject. Ultimately, however, the doctors indicate (through hand signals) that her participation in the discourse has not changed their plan. Silenced again, Burney describes herself as "Hopeless, then, desperate, & self-given up… relinquishing all watching, all resistance, all interference, & sadly resolute to be wholly resigned." The next time Burney records her voice in the process is to record her scream which "lasted unintermittingly during the whole time of the incision" and is so blood-curdling that she "marvel[s] that it rings not in [her] Ears still! So excrutiating was the agony" (p. 612).

Yet again Burney asserts her voice during the surgery when she implores the doctors to warn her before they recommence scraping the cancerous tissue from her breast bones. Throughout the text, circumstances make Burney voiceless (for instance, she is certain she fainted twice because she has gaps in her recollection), but she continually reasserts her subjectivity by claiming her voice. The most obvious assertion is her very text through which she resists objectification by using her own "view" of (or gaze at) the physicians in her detailed description. In interpreting their silence, she enacts the power of the gaze with the doctors functioning as the object of her gaze; she represents herself, no longer objectified by the dominant discourse.

The text of the document itself exposes the physical and psychological effects of the surgery that Burney underwent. She notes that before her surgery she had been unable to dress herself independently for “many months.” Her inability to use her right arm had made writing impossible for her; indeed, her arm was “condemned to total inaction.” The graphic account of the surgery, the cutting of the flesh, the scraping of the breast bone, even the exposure of her wound to the air, terrifies the reader. Her own physical torment is juxtaposed to that of the surgeon who is so exhausted from “cutting against the grain” of her flesh that he must switch hands in order to retain the strength to finish the ordeal. After her surgery, she is “lifeless” and “utterly colourless” and has to be carried to bed (pp. 612-614).

While she certainly describes her physical pain in chilling terms, the psychological impact of the surgery and her recovery from it are recounted in equally graphic terms. She writes:

> My dearest Esther, not for days, not for Weeks, but for Months I could not speak of this terrible business without nearly again going through it! I could not think of it with impunity! I was sick, I was disordered by a single question—even now, 9 months after it is over, I have a headache from going on with the account! & this miserable account, which I began 3 months ago, at least, I dare not revise, nor read, the recollection is still so painful (p. 613).

Despite the anguish that recounting her ordeal causes Burney, she realizes that she must break the silence of women that is institutionalized in the medical discourse of the day. Burney’s plea to other women to seek medical attention is couched in terms of her own reticence at seeking professional help. She expresses “repugnance” at seeing a doctor about her condition because she did not want to consent to an examination.[33] As Kaye points out, a breast exam “threatens Burney’s sense of identity as a proper woman, who should be modest and private as the cornerstone of middle-class domestic values.”[34] Indeed, Burney expects to be able to keep her long robe on through the procedure, and when she is forced to disrobe she laments the absence of support from her feminine community:

> I was compelled, however, to submit to taking off my long robe de Chambre, which I had meant to retain—Ah, then, how did I think of my Sisters!—not one, at so dreadful an instant, at hand, to protect—adjust—guard me… (p. 610).

Burney's lament is immediately preceded in the narrative by another assertion of her need for female community. When her doctors attempt to dismiss her maid and two nurses, Burney recovers her voice that has been silenced by dread and embarks upon a "little dispute" with the doctor, resulting in one of the nurses remaining with Burney throughout her surgery (p. 610).

Kaye argues that another way that Burney attempts to retain her subject position is by invoking the literary language of the Gothic and the sentimental, thereby framing herself as a tragic, sentimental heroine who is juxtaposed to the rational men of medicine.[35] Kaye points to the seven men in black entering Burney's home unexpectedly and without Burney's permission as the first hint of Gothicism. Burney describes her own prognosis of her illness in weighted terms: "Yet I felt the evil to be deep, so deep, that I often thought if it could not be dissolved, it could only with life be extirpated" (p. 603). Her description of the doctor's "fatal finger" which "describe[s] the Cross--& the circle" to indicate the incision to be made on her breast is interestingly complex. While his finger is "fatal," thereby casting him as the villain, it is at the same time inscribing the shape of the cross over her breast. The man in black signing the cross certainly evokes religious imagery.

Burney asserts her power and authority within her household as she strives to protect her son and husband from the horror of her situation. Even though the sight of the bandages and other preparations make her feel sick, she arranges the surgery so that her family will be gone from home; she does not want them to hear her screaming. Additionally, she literally puts her house in order by making arrangements for the physical space in which her surgery will occur. Even though she has been unable to write for months, she "defie[s] [her] poor arm, no longer worth sparing, & [takes] [her] long banished pen to write a few words to M. d'A-- & a few more for Alex, in case of a fatal result."[36] Her efforts certainly distract her in the face of her surgery and delay the inevitable, but they also allow her to be the self-sacrificing wife and mother, perhaps highlighting the fact that her actions rather than her literal breast are what define her role in the house. Indeed, her husband acknowledges his weakness and adds to her account:

> No language could convey what I felt in the deadly course of these seven hour […]. Besides, I must own, to you, that these details which were, till just now, quite unknown to me, have almost killed me, & I am only able to thank God that this more than half Angel has had the sublime courage to deny herself the comfort I might have offered her, to spare me, not the sharing of her excruciating pains, that was impossible, but the witnessing

> so terrific a scene, & perhaps the remorse to have rendered it more tragic for I don't flatter my self I could have got through it—[37]

As she faces losing this symbol of motherhood, she acts courageously, thus reinscribing her maternal authority and establishing her strength.

This comparative strength transfers to the doctors as well. It is Burney, after all, who holds her breast for the surgeon rather than one of the seven doctors there to assist. Burney also makes careful observations during her surgery, noting how the surgeons, particularly Larrey, are responding emotionally to her plight. She notes that the battle-hardened physician is "pale nearly as myself, his face streaked with blood, & its expression depicting grief, apprehension, & almost horrour."[38] The depiction of the vulnerability of the men she loves and admires paints a complimentary picture not only of her, but of these men who are affected by her own tragedy.

Across genres and points of view, these narratives suggest shifting ideas about silence with regard to breast cancer. The suffering in silence we see in Astell is replaced with a model of dealing with breast cancer that argues for the need of a women's community in times of crisis. Even though Lady Delacour is reinscribed in the patriarchal order by way of her experience, she gains the kinship of close community via Belinda and her daughter. Burney goes a step further in asserting the primacy and authority of the women's community. Indeed, Burney's narrative challenges the notion of sterile medical discourse by humanizing Larrey, her physician and friend. The dominant medical discourse may attempt to silence women with regard to their bodies, but as long as women like Frances Burney and Audre Lorde counter that authority with their own voices, women's communities will play a significant role in healing.

Notes

[1] Nancy G. Brinker, *Promise Me: How a Sister's Love Launched the Global Movement to End Breast Cancer*. (New York: Crown Archetype, 2010). See also G. H. Sakorafas and M. Safioleas, "Breast Cancer Surgery: an Historical Narrative. Part II. 18th and 19th Centuries," *European Journal of Cancer Care* 19 (2010): 6-29; and James S. Olson, *Bathsheba's Breast: Women, Cancer, and History*, (Baltimore, MD: Johns Hopkins University Press, 2002).

[2] Quoted in Sakorafas and Safioleas, 7.

[3] See Plates XXVIII: Chirurgie and XXIX: Chirurgie, in "Surgery," *The Encyclopedia of Diderot & 4 Collaborative Translation Project.* Ann Arbor: MPublishing, University of Michigan Library, 2010. http://hdl. handle.net/ 2027/spo.did2222.0001.420, accessed 5 December 2012. Originally published as

"Chirurgie," *Encyclopédie ou dictionnaire raisonné des sciences, des arts et des métiers,* vol. 3 (plates) (Paris: David et al., 1763).

[4] Sakorafas and Safioleas, "Breast Cancer Surgery," 18.

[5] Audre Lorde, *The Cancer Journals* (Argyle, NY: Spinsters, 1980). See also Thatcher Carter, "Body Count: Aubiographies of Women Living with Breast Cancer," *Journal of Popular Culture* 36 (2003): 653.

[6] "Mary Astell," *Stanford Encyclopedia of Philosophy* (Stanford: Metaphysics Research Lab, 2012). http://plato.stanford.edu/entries/astell, accessed 5 December 2012.

[7] George Ballard, *Memoirs of Several Ladies of Great Britain* (Oxford, 1752), p. 459. Future references will be given in the text.

[8] Quoted in William Kolbrener and Michal Michelson, "'Dreading to Engage her': The Critical Reception of Mary Astell," *Mary Astell: Reason, Gender, Faith,* (Burlington, VT: Ashgate, 2007), p. 1.

[9] Kolbrener and Michelson, p. 1.

[10] Ballard, p. 460. Ballard's account of Astell's final days is recounted verbatim in *English Churchwomen of the Seventeenth Century*, (New York: J.A. Sparks, 1846), and summarized in many other sketches of Astell's life.

[11] Elisa New, "Feminist Invisibility: The Examples of Anne Bradstreet and Anne Hutchinson," *Common Knowledge* 2.1 (1993): 102.

[12] Heike Hartung, "'Doleful Ditties' and Stories of Survival—Narrative Approaches to Breast Cancer in Frances Burney, Maria Edgeworth and Susan Sontag," *Gender Forum* 19 (2007). http://www.genderforum.org/issues/-gender-ii, accessed 21 February 2011.

[13] Heather Macfadyen, "Lady Delacour's Library: Maria Edgeworth's *Belinda* and Fashionable Reading," *Nineteenth-Century Literature* 48.4 (1994): 423-439.

[14] Maria Edgeworth, *Belinda* (Oxford: Oxford World's Classic, 1994), p. 34. All further quotations from the novel will be taken from this edition.

[15] Susan C. Greenfield, "'Abroad and at Home': Sexual Ambiguity, Miscegenation, and Colonial Boundaries in Edgeworth's *Belinda,*" *PMLA* 12.2 (1997): 214-228.

[16] Edgeworth, p. 42.

[17] Edgeworth, p. 42.

[18] Sangeeta Mediratta, "Beauty and the Breast: The Poetics of Physical Absence and Narrative Presence in Frances Burney's *Mastectomy Letter* (1811)," *Women: A Cultural Review* 19 (2008): 191.

[19] Edgeworth, p. 43.

[20] See Greenfield, "Abroad and at Home."

[21] Edgeworth, p. 65.

[22] Edgeworth, pp. 305-306.

[23] Edgeworth, p. 312.

[24] Frances "Fanny" Burney was born 13 June 1752 into a highly educated family. Her father, the renowned musicologist Charles, travelled in circles of the literary and artistic elite of the day; Burney records in her diary, begun at age sixteen, regular social interaction with Sir Joshua Reynolds, David Garrick, James Boswell,

and Samuel Johnson. She began her literary career quite young, and her first novel, *Evelina, or, A Young Lady's Entrance in the World*, was published in 1778. She went on to publish numerous novels with her father's support; he drew the line, however, at supporting the plays she wrote. Among her novels are *Cecelia, or Memoirs of an Heiress* (1782), and *The Wanderer, or Female Difficulties* (1814), comedies of manners which changed the landscape of the novel.

[25] Quoted in Mediratta, "Beauty and the Breast," 193.

[26] Quoted in Sakorafas and Safioleas, 10. See pp. 9-11 for more discussion of the regression in the treatment of breast cancer in the nineteenth century.

[27] All quotes from the primary text are from Joyce Hemlow, ed., *The Journals and Letters of Fanny Burney* (Madame D'Arblay), 7 (Oxford: Clarendon Press, 1972), pp. 596-616. Future references will be given in the text.

[28] Mediratta, 188-189.

[29] Thanks to Chaudron Gille for her translation of the original, included in Hemlow, p. 616.

[30] Mediratta, 194.

[31] Hemlow, p. 616, n. 42.

[32] Heidi Kaye, "'This Breast—it's me': Fanny Burney's Mastectomy and the Defining Gaze," *Journal of Gender Studies* 6.1 (March 1997): 43.

[33] Quoted in Kaye, 46.

[34] Kaye, 46.

[35] Kaye, 51.

[36] Hemlow, p. 609.

[37] Hemlow, p. 614.

[38] Hemlow, p. 614.

CHAPTER NINE

MEDICAL IMAGERY OF VENEREAL DISEASE AND THE GENDERING OF CULPABILITY IN EIGHTEENTH-CENTURY FRANCE

MARIALANA WITTMAN

For most of the eighteenth century visual representation of venereal disease was extremely rare in medical contexts. In fact, accurate drawings of venereal disease symptoms on the body were not a common element in medical literature until the early nineteenth century. In most instances of early sixteenth- and seventeenth-century engravings, pock-covered bodies were illustrated simply through dots on the (male) body with the emphasis more on the symbols of the painful mercury treatments or the surgical procedure of cauterization. The purpose of such representations was closer to moral education—communicating to all audiences the consequences of moral transgressions—than the dissemination of medical knowledge. Surprisingly, the eighteenth-century medical literature lacked even these basic images of the diseased body and the new forms of treatment were described rather than illustrated. The exception is a handful of drawings depicting tools, but they were isolated from practical contexts. It was only toward the end of the century that detailed drawings of chancrous body parts, such as those that would educate the medical practitioners of the Revolutionary and Napoleonic periods, began to appear in medical literature. Instead, eighteenth-century medical entrepreneurs—whether part of the medical elite or the enterprising itinerant healer—chose to visually enhance their texts with scrolling line designs, plant fronds, and crests. The absence of strong pictorial representation raises the question of how venereal disease was visualized. Although a pronounced visual imagery of the diseased body in the eighteenth century did not exist, powerful representations of venereal disease were painted through words rather than brushes. Through a perusal of the pages of treatises, pamphlets, journals, police reports, and letters, this chapter will take a critical look at the ways discourse shaped what medical men "saw" in order to raise important points on the gendering of venereal disease in eighteenth-century France.

As we shall see, the most vivid and dynamic image in the medical literature was that of the diseased male body. In the period from 1736 to 1789, medical conceptualizations of vulnerability naturalized and gendered the likelihood of developing a case of *la maladie vénérienne*.[1] Medicine defined the female body as inherently resistent to and capable of expelling the disease-causing agent thanks to menstruation. The counterpart was the vision of the male body as particularly susceptible due to how the penis functioned during sexual congress. The result of these understandings of reproductive physiology was a vision of men as diseased but women as relatively un-diseased. Situating these features of medical theory next to the better studied subject of prostitution will help us gain a more complete account of the period's moral zeitgeist.[2] In actuality, the diseased prostitute played a minor role in the medical discourse on venereal disease. The more common female figure outlined in medical literature was the wife—present by virtue of her victimization by male sexual license. Even with the potent juxtaposition of the "innocent wife" to "the errant husband," the diseased female body appears sketchy in comparison to the more fully delineated diseased male body. While medical attention was drawn to men's experiences, it fostered a vision of the male body as the vector of disease. This increased visibility of the diseased male body placed men more fully at the centre of the moralizing that accompanied medical discussion on the spread of the disease. Analysis of eighteenth-century medical discourse on venereal disease shows clearly that culpability for the spread of venereal disease was almost exclusively assigned to men.[3]

Gender in the Formulation of Vulnerability Theories

Fundamental to the eighteenth-century notion of vulnerability was the belief that venereal disease was caused by an external entity. As early as the sixteenth century, shortly after the first reports told of a new disease spreading rapidly throughout Europe, physicians put forward the idea that the disease could pass through contagion.[4] The concept of contagion presented an alternative to the existing view of sickness and disease, which had been explained as physiological responses to a disruption of the internal balance of the body's humours.[5] In contagion theories, some inanimate matter entered the body and disturbed the humoral balance. It was this imbalance that was seen as causing the dysfunction of disease. For two centuries, these two different aetiologies more or less functioned alongside each other until gradually the contagion theory came to dominate the medical elite's doctrine. The ebbing debate was essentially settled for good after the publication of *De morbis venereis libri sex* by the prominent Montpellier-trained and later Paris-based physician, Jean Astruc (1684-1766).[6] One of his key objectives for the treatise was to clearly demonstrate that venereal disease was caused exclusively by an exopathic entity, called "*le virus vénérien*."[7] Although his argument was not novel, the treatise greatly contributed to establishing the contagion theory as the paramount standard.[8]

With the path to developing venereal disease thus defined from the point where the virus entered the body, the possibility of contagion depended on the strength or weakness of the barrier between the outside world and the internal body. The discussion of vulnerability became a matter of how easily the virus penetrated that barrier. This was a significant change from the older aetiology's framing of susceptibility: an individual's unique humoral temperament and lifestyle caused, and therefore predicted, the likelihood of disease. From the moment that medical theorists began to hold the presence of the virus as a necessary precondition to *la maladie vénérienne*, temperament and lifestyle only affected the prognosis.[9] Consequently, in order to establish susceptibility, the exterior of the body was explored for sites of entry. The pores in the skin were considered to be the permeable channel constituting that site of entry for the virus-laced bodily fluids, the only medium thought capable of carrying the virus in and out of bodies.[10]

The early symptoms that routinely appeared in concentrated areas on the body's surface pointed to particular weaknesses in the skin's barrier. It was theorized that the skin in specific regions became more penetrable when heated and stretched by its nature, its location, or stimulating movements. When paired with the types of physical touch involving some fluid of the body, certain acts came into focus. Breastfeeding joined the warm and moist tissues of the woman's breast with the "polluted" saliva of the infant, or vice versa, the tissues of an infant's mouth with the "poisoned" milk of the woman. Increased skin permeability and contaminated fluid were identified in other activities such as "lascivious" kissing, performing the service of midwife to a diseased woman, or examining ulcerated parts in the practice of surgery.[11] But by far the most mentioned and analyzed contact point between body and fluid was the genitalia with "the seminal humour impregnated with the venereal virus."[12] Even though all these instances of venereal communication were realized to be legitimate health threats and figured in the didactic elements of medical discourse, practitioners developed more complex theories of vulnerability only for sexual contagion.[13]

Essentially, the more elaborate and detailed concepts of vulnerability attempted to explain why more men than women appeared to develop venereal disease. The belief that vulnerability was rooted in gender dated back to the sixteenth century. In earlier treatises, however, the matter had been more nuanced because the emphasis had been on individual temperament rather than the broader categories. It was said that the hot and dry humours dominant in the male temperament predisposed men to venereal disease. Conversely, it had been argued that women were not prone to it because of the cold and moist quality of the humours in their temperament. But when the contagion theory had achieved hegemony, the impact of temperament no longer had the same explanatory power in the new exopathic context. The shift to the exterior of the body explained how the virus passed between bodies, as we saw above, but skin tissue alone did not explain the asymmetrical prevalence in men. After all, sexual acts were said to have the same heating effect on the pores in both sexes and there was no distinction made between the tissues of the penis and vulva.[14] In terms of skin permeability, the probability of the virus proceeding through the pores was more or less equal for a healthy man as it was for a healthy woman. In fact, the developments in the contagion theory made the higher incidence in men an even greater medical conundrum.

This paradox was resolved by an idea that two different levels of vulnerability stemmed from the distinct functioning of the reproductive parts. The sex organs were endowed with the power to influence the virus's penetration of the body and to regulate its development into *la maladie vénérienne*. The probability of the virus causing venereal disease in women was thought lower than that of men due to the monthly process of menstruation. The periodic flushing of impure fluids was said to stop the advance of the virus. This idea, what I will refer to as the theory of relative female immunity, saved women from venereal disease, or at least limited their cases to a less intense local inflammation.

According to leading authors on venereal disease, experience proved that even if "a considerable quantity of the virulent matter" entered the vagina, women did not develop "this disease/evil."[15] The healing power of menstruation was based on views stretching back to antiquity. Menses had been considered essentially like urine, sweat, excrement, saliva, nasal mucus, male and female sexual fluids, and vomit, which all contributed to humoral balance. The discharging, emitting, or ejaculating of any excess fluid had been thought essential to health and their natural occurrence was viewed as the body healing itself. Women's monthly discharge of blood, it was thought, expelled excess fluids that in the male body were usually consumed due to temperament and greater physical activity.[16] While this concept implied that the female body was inherently in a state of imbalance or disease, it defined the excremental nature of menstruation as potentially therapeutic. This vision of healing was the frame on which the eighteenth-century hypothesis on relative female immunity was built.

According to eighteenth-century treatises on venereal disease, menstrual blood carried out the virus before it could spread deeper into the body and this was the reason fewer women appeared to suffer from pox. It was still possible for the virus to produce some form of venereal disease in women. The term *la maladie vénérienne* encompassed a wide range of symptoms that were all believed to be caused by the venereal virus. Today, venereal disease, or more commonly, sexual disease, refers to separate diseases with different aetiologies, but in the early modern period venereal disease referred to one disease subcategorized as "local" (or "simple") and "universal" (or "confirmed"). A diagnosis of local as opposed to universal was primarily based on an assessment of the time since the virus first entered the body and the imagined quantity of the virulent matter. From this it was extrapolated that since menses shortened the virus's time span within the female body and reduced its quantity with each monthly evacuation, women's sufferings were at most localized venereal disease.

Although menstrual blood had been ascribed healing abilities in some contexts, there were equally well-established discourses in medicine (and religion) that characterized it as impure, polluting, and capable of causing sickness and disease. In many cultures and periods, menstrual blood was conceived to be insalubrious and associated with the transmission of diseases. Specific to sexual relations, Renaissance medical writers warned that congress with a menstruating woman could cause leprosy, epilepsy and monstrous births.[17] Shortly after *la maladie vénérienne* began to spread rapidly through Europe, the pathological nature of menses was associated with this disease as well; particularly, theories on its beginnings. While there were differing schools of thought on the pox's origin, both claimed sex with a menstruating woman was the kindling in the creation of the virus. The majority of eighteenth-century practitioners subscribed to an account that specified the menstrual blood of ancient Caribbean women as the source (their blood was thought to be virulent enough to generate the venereal virus).[18] In both cases, menstrual blood was closely entwined in the theories on the pathology of venereal disease.

It appears contradictory that medical practitioners specializing in venereal disease held menses to be therapeutic as well as pathological. The disagreement appears even greater when we consider that medical writers did not speak of menstrual blood as destructively interacting with the virus in any way.[19] During the eighteenth century, the coexistence of these two seemingly contrary interpretations of menstrual blood was possible due to the convergence of several factors. First, physicians and surgeons of the period were more likely to have the opinion that menses aided women because the contagion theory now stressed communication of the virus (through sex, heredity, and breast-feeding). Consequently, the pathological characterization that had been a common feature in the diagnostic process faded away, and reflections on the ill effects of menstrual blood became more or less isolated to the theoretical discussions on the virus's origin. Secondly, the foreign origin of the virus, as outlined by eighteenth-century contagion theory, shifted the pathological features of menses onto a new "other": native women.[20] Third, the historical pathologization of menstrual blood was tempered by the development of new ideas that cast the female body in a more positive light.

In the eighteenth century, the female body came to be seen as biologically designed for motherhood. The uterus, for example, was valorised rather than maligned as it had been previously.[21] A contributing factor to this appreciation of female reproductive abilities was a weakening of the bond between original sin and the female body that had shaped medical thought until the seventeenth century—at which point medicine decreasingly viewed the human body through the prism of theology.[22] Instead, nature's intentions became the foundation upon which medicine rested the conceptualizations of the female body as it related to motherhood. A result was a rise in eighteenth-century treatises that discussed menses as a sign of a woman's good health.[23] The monthly evacuation was no longer a sign of women's imperfection in comparison to the model of the male body, but a symbol of their distinct status as a female. Dissociated from the maledictive connotations, menstruation was more easily regarded as a natural form of healing.[24] While one surgeon's suggestion that women were happier than men because of their inherent resistance to venereal disease had a sardonic note, it points to the generally positive tone in which eighteenth-century authors discussed this idea that women were practically invulnerable to venereal disease.[25]

The notion of relative female immunity was grounded in ancient and modern conceptualizations of the female body and its physiology, yet it was supported by empirical evidence. It is important to underline that the theory was credible because, quite simply, fewer women with venereal disease appeared before practitioners' eyes. For example, physicians' consultation letters from the 1710s to 1740s advised twenty-five men and only nine women for symptoms of venereal disease.[26] The predominance of men is also visible in the paradigmatic cases employed in physicians' and surgeons' treatises that abounded with descriptions of diseased men.[27] In addition, male bodies were the common medium utilized to demonstrate therapeutic successes and (very rarely) failures in the medical community's letters, journal articles, and reviews of remedies.[28] This ratio of men to women in medical practices confirmed what practitioners held to be true and, as we will see below, the possible influence social factors had on this proportion did not subvert their conclusions.

When a woman with venereal disease did appear in medical accounts, it was cast as an abnormality. This is illustrated in Astruc's effort to substantiate the therapeutic power of menses. He cited the cases of older women who suffered from venereal disease more intensely because they had ceased menstruating.[29] Here, the diseased bodies of older women served as evidence of the norm: un-diseased, menstruating women. Similarly, although contrary to what one might expect, the conviction that a larger number of women suffered from local symptoms than consulted male practitioners furthered the invisibility of a diseased female body. Practitioners believed that many respectable women were ignorant of their exposure to the virus, failed to observe the signs of venereal disease, or misunderstood the nature of their vaginal discharges. Regarding women of "suspect character," it was claimed such women disregarded their symptoms, concealed the transmission of the virus, or pretended the gonorrhoeal discharges were instead the common vaginal discharge, *les fleurs blanches*.[30] By virtue of its smaller size, the group of women that did consult practitioners became the anomalies to the imagined group. Although, as we can see, this suggested a larger number of diseased women, the picture was opaque and ambiguous. What remained clear was that only a small number of women developed venereal disease. Certainly, this obscurity could have been construed to propose widespread venereal disease among women, and thus inspire anxieties over a diseased female body; however, that would have contradicted all the theoretical wisdom and practical observations that forecast greater incidence among men. The conjecture that more women were diseased than appeared was just not persuasive enough to overturn the visible crowd of diseased men that dominated medical practices, and visibility was a potent principle in an era striving to base knowledge in concrete terms rather than mystical speculation.

In addition to the diseased female being cast as abnormal, the theory of relative female immunity defined the common signs of venereal disease in women such that the female body would not bear clearly noticeable marks.

As we saw earlier, it was believed that menses limited the virus's power to produce a universal case, and so it was believed that women were more likely to have symptoms, such as *la gonorrhée*, the very common inflammation of the urethra and the surrounding tissue. As a vaginal discharge, this manifestation of venereal disease was not visible on the exposed parts of the body. Thus, the female body was less perceptibly diseased. There were more legible signs of local venereal disease, such as pustules, porri, condylomata (a sore resembling warts), buboes, and chancres. But the more conspicuous characteristics of the universal *la vérole* were thought to only infrequently stigmatize women.

Did fewer women suffer from venereal disease? It is probable that venereal disease was less common among women because of the sexual morals of the period. Focusing only on heterosexual sex, the occasions for exposure to the virus were significantly lower for the majority of women both prior to and during marriage.[31] Still, it cannot be overlooked that a woman's sexual health was greatly impacted by a husband's actions before and throughout the marital union. Unfortunately, the standards of recording medical information at the time mean the answer is conjecture. While some practitioners' registers do give a fair amount of information, it is at times hard to know if descriptions are of an individual patient or a synthesis of several.[32] In addition, sources usually record exemplary cases rather than document a physician's or surgeon's entire practice. Practitioners almost never reported ineffective and blundered cures (unless it was that of a competitor), which indicates selective documentation was rampant. Discovering the validity behind the theory may be unattainable, but the material does expose the recapitulation of their conviction that the female body was unsusceptible to the virus.

As I have argued, the aggregate was a picture of the female body as relatively un-diseased. Whether practitioners chose to retell exact or composite stories of venereal disease in women, the product was a representation of a lower percentage of women to men in their own practice and an assumption that the same would be true for the practices of their audience. The examples of female bodies with venereal disease, real and imagined, failed to leave an impression on medical knowledge because they defied expectations and paled in comparison to the other sex.

Several social factors can account for the dominance of the male body in medical literature. In early modern French society, men were permitted greater sexual licence. Wealthy men were the patrons of the physicians and surgeons who penned treatises. Government sponsored trials and studies on remedies were in part motivated by a need to check the number of men requiring treatment for the disease during their service in the armed forces.[33] Men from all social backgrounds were in a better financial position than women to pay for remedies in the marketplace, which were manifold.[34] Women may have treated themselves and/or consulted midwives rather than male practitioners. Treatments were considered equally applicable to both sexes with a simple adjustment in the quantity of the remedy for women, and thus the male body served as the template. Lastly, rather instinctively, male practitioners understood the male body better since it was familiar by virtue of it being of their own sex. The reason advanced by practitioners, however, was the idea that the male body was extremely vulnerable to the venereal virus, what I will call the theory of male susceptibility.

The complement to the female physiology that naturally purged the venereal virus was the male body that seemingly absorbed it. The explanation for the insufficient resilience in men was said to relate to the various stages through which the penis progressed in order to engage in sex. The permeable skin of the penis signified the first weak point, yet this was common to both sexes, as we saw above. A major caveat, however, was that the tension and thinning of the skin, which occurred when the penis swelled and hardened, caused the pores to expand, and this increased the likelihood of the virus infiltrating the body.[35] Another hypothesis on male susceptibility held that the softening in the stretched skin after ejaculation raised the risk of the virus-laden fluids being admitted. This flaccid state was strongly advised against in the preventative measure medical men proffered.[36] In the middle of the eighteenth century, surgeon [Jean?] Ballay (fl. 1762) claimed that the critical moment came immediately following ejaculation, when the male urethra's empty canal would consequently draw up the air nearest the orifice, which on some occasions was an "infected lake."[37]

In the opinion of physician Louis Alexandre de Cézan (fl. 1764-1778), the increased predisposition in the male body was that "the penis does not expel the virus once it has been introduced."[38] Recalling that the quantity of the virus and the time it had been inside the body predicted the progress of a local case into a universal one, the theory of male susceptibility conveyed the idea that once the virus breached the pores, the duration of its stay inside the male body became virtually dependent on medical intervention. Until signs of venereal disease began to appear, a man was conceivably unaware of the virus's existence in his body. Though symptoms could appear in as early as a few days, it was also believed it could be years before any sign might manifest itself. Without any natural process to continually expel the virulent matter, as the female body had, a man's case could quickly progress from local to universal if he waited too long before consulting a physician or surgeon. For example, the consequence of a man's delay of forty years for his *chaude pisse* (gonorrhoeal discharge) was its development into a "scab-like dry patch" that covered his whole body except his face and hands.[39] It could even cost a man his life, according to the physician Jacques de Horne (b. ca. 1740). He suggested that the death of Louis, a twenty–ear-old native of Languedoc, was inevitable because the young man "had not thought to appeal to the men of the art [of medicine]" when his gonorrhoeal discharge was suppressed—thought to be dangerous as it forced the virus to turn deeper into the body and spread further.[40] As the theory on male susceptibility foretold, a man's body succumbed to venereal disease if proper medical care was not promptly sought.

The distinctive element in the theory of male susceptibility was a focus on sexuality.[41] That this was unique to male susceptibility may come as a surprise because it seems logical that, in terms of a contagious sexual disease, sexuality would be central to concepts of vulnerability for both sexes. However, this was not the case. As we saw above, practitioners theorized that a man's vulnerability lies in one of the phases the male organ went through in order to engage in sex. Therefore, a consideration of male susceptibility commenced with questions on the state of the penis. The analysis carried on to looking at men's sexual behaviors, and practitioners detailed the finer points of the theory by mentioning or alluding to men engaging in various sexual activities. It was common for discussion of the male member's vulnerabilities to be followed with stipulations that a man wash and/or apply remedies immediately after sex. One treatment advised that a man submerge his penis in a glass filled with the prepared liquid while still erect.[42] In comparison, in the theory of relative female immunity, the female body's action on the virus was connected to processes independent of sex acts. Sex pervaded discourse on male susceptibility, whereas the medical commentary on relative female immunity gravitated toward a disembodied synopsis of the female reproductive parts and rarely mentioned women's sexual conduct.

The emphasis on men's sexual activity also appears in the ways practitioners recorded consulting and treating of the sick. With men, physicians and surgeons pinpointed the source of their venereal disease to discrete sex acts. For example, "at the age of eighteen Monsieur received a venereal bubo as a consequence of a relation with a diseased woman [*femme gâtée*]."[43] On the other hand, within the records on women, the transmission of the virus to the female body was distanced from any single act of sex and was instead set as a vague period and in broad terms. Practitioners commonly dated a woman's contagion as imprecisely as the "venereal disease, which had been communicated to her by her husband."[44] Determining the exact length of time the virus was in the body was fundamental to diagnosis and prognosis, so this incongruence is noteworthy. We might interpret this gendered periodization of contagion as the mere consequence of men's better knowledge of the sexual congress that posed risks and their greater awareness of their reproductive parts. This implies that women had little to no knowledge of the sexual contagion that could accompany their or their husbands' intercourse and were unaware of the changes in their own bodies. Yet, evidence shows that women did indeed know of the risks of sexual contagion and its relation to their personal health.[45] Thus, that practitioners underlined sex in the discourse on men is revealing of the gendered visions of venereal disease at work.

Entangled in the focus on sex in the theory of male susceptibility was an anxiety about French virility. The belief that men were more vulnerable to the venereal virus expressed a societal fear that men with venereal disease were unable to father healthy children. The site of sexual contagion and generation was one and the same, and, not missing the irony, several practitioners remarked that the source of life "becomes quite often a source of bitterness and death."[46] The tension between reproduction and degeneration perceptibly overlapping at the male member underpinned the stress that the theory on male susceptibility placed on sex. It was through sex that men were vulnerable to venereal disease and through sex that they communicated the virus to their offspring. Precisely how the contagion passed to unborn children was not fully understood. Intra-uterine heredity, although an accepted possibility, was not frequently mentioned as the source of an infant's disease.[47] Even when a mother was said to be the source of an infant's venereal disease symptoms, the origin was traced back to the father. The more common viewpoint was that men communicated the virus in their semen during copulation. While this followed from the opinion that men had the disease more frequently than their wives, the partiality to spermatic heredity was based on the current notions of conception and hereditary disease, which interpreted the male as the dominant and active partner in reproduction.[48] With men identified as *the* propagators of venereal disease in the family, their sexual activities in and outside marriage were very significant.

The theory of male susceptibility suggested a grave forecast for population growth. Claims that the population of France was dwindling in size and vitality had significant weight in discussions on venereal disease, and some variation on the idea that "venereal disease poisons the human species, diminishes the number of citizens, enervates individuals" appeared in all forms of medical literature.[49] The greater vulnerability in men was thus connected to broader discourses on fatherhood, which we will return to later, and elevated the issue to a social concern with national significance.[50] With associations such as these, the diseased male body became even more visible to medical practitioners.

As I have shown, medical theory constructed the male body as visibly diseased and the female body as relatively un-diseased. The idea that women innately possessed a degree of immunity to the venereal virus not only explained the near absence of women from medical men's practices, it also perpetuated the invisibility of the female body by setting boundaries to the symptoms of venereal disease experienced by women. The sparse illustrations of any female body, let alone a diseased one, magnified the depictions of a diseased male body. This was furthered by the greater and more detailed descriptions of men with the full range of venereal disease symptoms. Their theories illustrated men's susceptibility to the virus within scenes of sexual action, while women's relative immunity was held in the sterile space of medical contemplation. Those women and men who deviated from these norms were literally and figuratively invisible. Seeing was the cornerstone of enlightened medicine, and the gendered visions of venereal disease depicted in the theories on vulnerability gave a particular shape to the conceptualization of culpability in eighteenth-century France.[51] Decoding the distinct physiologies of the male and the female body provided a scientific foundation on which practitioners developed archetypical figures involved in the spread of venereal disease. As we are about to see, the more visibly diseased male was the main figure in the moralizing discourse.

Visualizing the Authors of Venereal Disease in the Family

These descriptions of venereal disease in male and female bodies were expanded upon within the medical literature through discussions on the prostitute, the wife, and the husband. Although these social categorizations referred to real men and women, they were equally constructs in the portrayal of venereal disease. The figures of the prostitute and the wife illustrate the vision of the female body as basically unscarred by venereal disease. Medical practitioners discussed women in ways that squared with the theory of relative female immunity. Young men, husbands, and fathers dominated the scenes and were invariably described as diseased. This is an important point because scholarship on venereal disease has predominantly argued that "the male body was consistently represented as the healthy body, while the female body represented as diseased."[52] Yet, eighteenth-century medical discourse reflects a different picture. This was partially, as I have argued, because the theories on relative female immunity and male susceptibility rendered a diseased male body more noticeable. This becomes even more apparent when the scope is broadened from how sexed bodies were viewed in theory to include the moralizing comments presented in most published and unpublished medical writings. The examination of the two figures of women revolving around the male body will show how their disease was dependent on and significant because of a man's bout with venereal disease.

The medical perspectives on venereal disease and the body staged, in effect, a battle between the sexes. In addition to a virtual immunity to the venereal virus, the female body was held to be capable of easily transmitting it to many men.[53] Join these medical ideas to the common claims that women were inclined to deceit and dissimulation, and the female body would appear the agent in the spread of venereal disease with men the victims.[54] More precisely, the woman of compromised virtue, who had turned to prostitution, seems to be the epitome of the diseased female. There is no debate that prostitution was intricately woven into the story of *la maladie vénérienne*. The compelling relationship between the disease and sexual contagion fundamentally pointed toward prostitution—with its historical reputation as sinful and illegal.[55] The medical community did repeat the social judgments of the times, but did so sparingly and in a nearly formulaic fashion. For the most part, the vilification of prostitutes in medical literature was brief and isolated. For practitioners, the encounters with the archetypical diseased prostitute worked more to emphasize the disease in men than in women.

Yet, the figure of the prostitute is very prominent within historical research and writing. Studies of the fictions and the realities of prostitution have frequently included mention of venereal disease.[56] The web of associations between venereal disease and prostitutes illustrates how vast the reach of the disease was; however, the extensive research on prostitutes overshadows the history of other women and men affected by the disease.[57] In fact, with a few exceptions, prostitutes have been the only group of women with venereal disease that have been researched in depth so far.[58]

This is not terribly surprising given that prostitutes were represented as propagators of venereal disease. By the eighteenth century, the prostitute had a long history as the villain in its spread. Sixteenth- and seventeenth-century authors had argued that the sexual disorder of promiscuous women was the origin of the disease. Yet, the link between the sexual behavior of prostitutes and the spread of venereal disease had loosened somewhat as new aetiologies developed. Contagion theory created some distance between the prostitute and the disease through the replacement of the virus's origin in foreign bodies. This did not absolve prostitution for its part in communicating the virus, but it did shift the prostitute's body to the margins of medical discourse to some extent.

Typically, the criticism of prostitutes worked to situate the controversial nature of treating venereal disease within altruistic and morally upright intents. In prior centuries, medical treatment for those other than the innocently affected had been thought to be teetering on the edge of intervening in God's punishment and had even been seen as inciting lechery. Eighteenth-century society accepted this attitude as practitioners clearly felt it necessary to state their motives were honourable. From single-page handbills to multi-volume treatises, medical men made certain it was known that their objectives were to ensure that the venereal virus did not penetrate the French family. Medical men swiftly legitimatized all their medical endeavors by expressing the idea that prostitutes "perpetuate the reign of the virus" that was otherwise on the decline.[59] Following that, the moral diatribes were few and far between. In the eighteenth century, medical men either skimmed over the topic of prostitution or treated it with significantly less condemnation than will happen during the Revolutionary and Napoleonic periods.

Practitioners discussed sexual contagion between prostitutes and men with scant interest in the prostitutes. Take, for example, Astruc's discussion on how the virus could be communicated when two men had congress with the same woman. In Astruc's words,

> a healthy man could take la Vérole from a healthy woman, if this woman after having had commerce shortly before with a diseased man, permits the approaches of another without washing herself.[60]

Astruc's choice to hold the man in the centre of the narrative situates the male as the active party in the exchange of the virus even though the woman was the source of the contagion. Despite the role of the debauched woman in passing the virus from one man to another, she remained a passive agent. Furthermore, she was "healthy" while the stigma of "diseased" (*gâté*) was cast upon the first man. Astruc was not the only one to keep the focus on the man. More often than not, if any mention was made of a prostitute, she was cast as a passive participant. It was said that men had symptoms of venereal disease "after having had commerce with a diseased prostitute," or "after visiting prostitutes," and not that a prostitute communicated the virus to a man.[61] The man remained the main figure and it was the man's diseased state that was presented as the most important.

Keeping the prostitute as a passive agent in the spread of venereal disease and relegating her diseased body to the margins, if only grammatically, contributed to the overall framing of the male as the diseased body of concern.

For the most part, the figure of the prostitute was minor because her diseased state stood outside the parameters of medicine. In general, it did not require mentioning that a prostitute was the source of a man's disease since it was assumed to be the case. In terms of consulting or treating a prostitute, in a sense, the information was immaterial. Overall, prostitutes did not demonstrate the effectiveness of cures and were not deemed good test subjects for experimental remedies.[62] In physicians' writings, the prostitute's appearance was fleeting because physicians catered to a wealthy and elite clientele and, therefore, were not likely to have been consulted by common prostitutes. And physicians, according to the traditional division of labor within medicine, tended not to actually treat those with venereal disease (although the lines were being redrawn in the period). Surgeons were the practitioners specializing in handling venereal disease and they published less than physicians.[63] When surgeons did write, they only sporadically noted the provision of healing services to women of suspect character. A rare example of a detailed account comes from a letter chirurgien-major Le Vacher addressed to the Académie Royale de Chirurgie in 1737. His few paragraphs on treating a prostitute well exceed the common cursory phrase or sentence that was the extent of the space typically dedicated to the prostitute. Incidentally, although Le Vacher remarked that her symptoms were the "fruits of her debauchery," he chronicled the event with pity and not vilification.[64]

In reality, like other women, prostitutes sought medical care from those who were not members of the medical elite. Although this limited the exposure medical men had to prostitutes with venereal disease, it does not detract from the fact that practitioners were considerably less interested in curing them. The virus inside the prostitute's body was mostly inconsequential so long as medicine could prevent it from entering the family when husbands procreated with their wives, to which we will turn shortly.

This is evident when we consider the early nineteenth-century approaches to the dilemma. Representative of the significant change in tactic is Alexandre-Jean Baptiste Parent-Duchâtelet's belief that venereal disease could be controlled through regulating prostitution. Parent-Duchâtelet was not the first to suggest the focus be on women.[65] However, his *De la prostitution dans la ville de Paris* (1836) was a study dedicated to prostitutes and it "marked the first occasion that prostitution had been treated as a serious social problem."[66] Stringent surveillance and regulation of prostitution was proposed in the eighteenth century, but it came from social critics.[67] Eighteenth-century medical practitioners would not have disagreed with these contemporaries. They simply had not reached the degree of concentration on public women that Parent-Duchâtelet would in the nineteenth century.

The prostitute remained admired for her beauty, untouched by the suggestion of disease. True, it was believed that beneath that beauty a risk of disease threatened those men who chose not to abstain. A common trope suggested that women deceived men through "signs of a brilliant health" that hid the virus under a fresh and rosy complexion.[68] The appearance of health, as we saw earlier in Astruc's comment, was no guarantee that a *femme* was not a *femme gâtée*. But, as Kathryn Norberg has correctly pointed out, a prostitute was "a *fille du monde* or just a *fille*, and she was lovely and alluring, not diseased."[69] The caricature of promiscuous women in eighteenth-century literature as attractive and available for visual or physical enjoyment was relatively untarnished by medical discourse. The near absence of prostitutes and the minimal description of their diseased state in the medical story of venereal disease allowed them to remain a fantasy.

The medical community's stance on prostitution was that of toleration. They professed disapproval of the practice, but their services allowed men to avoid the physical and social repercussions associated with visiting prostitutes. The prostitute herself was a tangential concern because her sexual health (diseased or barren, as was a common belief) did not factor into the regenerative agenda of medicine. Without a doubt, prostitutes were considered mechanisms in the spread of venereal disease, but medicine did not pin the greater part of moral responsibility on them. The key role of prostitutes in medical literature was to reflect the image of the male body.

The female figure that far surpassed the image of the prostitute in medical literature was the innocent wife. These two characters shared several common purposes in the rhetoric. Foremost, the wife's appearance within the discourse on venereal disease pivoted on a man's diseased state; her presence in the literature did not always include a portrayal of her body as diseased; and her body was a device to depict a husband's disease. The great difference between the prostitute and the respectable woman was that the wife's disease was never her fault. She stood absolved entirely by virtue of her marriage.

When a married woman appeared in the treatment records she was almost always accompanied by her husband. He may have physically brought her to the physician or surgeon. For example, upon completion of a month-long treatment for a tumor on his penis and spots on his legs and forehead, a young man returned to the surgeon with his new bride so that she could be cured.[70] Another man took his wife with him from Flanders to Paris to consult a physician for their diseases.[71] It was common for a husband and wife to be treated together, yet couples made up a small percentage of practitioners' records. In general, practitioners recorded consulting a man initially and then, if necessary, expanded their notations to include his spouse. In the documents on female patients, wives rarely show up without some mention of their husbands in the early remarks. In an exceptional example, a woman consulted a physician for a white discharge that was suspected to be a symptom of *la vérole*. At first, the consultation was focused entirely on the respectable woman. But, it was soon stalled until her husband could be seen as well. The consulting physician found it impossible to pin down her *perte blanche* until the husband was questioned in order to determine if he had communicated the virus to her.[72] In the instances that men did not physically accompany their wives to treatment, the husband was just as present. The majority of the records on women define the wives' symptoms by a standard phrase: "the venereal disease that had been communicated to her by her husband."[73] It could be argued that a woman did not even have possession of her body's expressions of ill health. For example, in the case of a merchant's wife her disease was not her own but expressed as "the pains of the same disease of her husband."[74]

Similar to how the construction of the female body as relatively immune precluded any real vision of venereal disease in women, the assumption that wives were the innocent victims of their husbands prevented practitioners from considering respectable women involved in the spread of venereal disease. Astruc stated that "the custom was established that husbands were the presumed authors of all the venereal diseases that happened to their wives, just as they were the alleged fathers of all the babies that they had."[75] He advised that it was useless and indecent to suggest a wife's malady stemmed from her own conduct. The ironic tone belies a doubt as to the reality of the statement. Nonetheless, Astruc, his colleagues, and his successors held fast to this framework. Exemplary of this is the case of a woman with ulcers on her labia that a physician first suspected as *la vérole*. However, the husband's denial of ever having any venereal disease made the presence of the virus uncertain. Another suggestion that perhaps the husband was not the author of her disease came in the fact that she had lived with her husband for two months without any sign of illness, and it was only four months after he departed that her ulcers appeared. While this potentially placed her fidelity in question, the physician maintained that she was above suspicion. To support his conclusion he drew from medical theory, which explained that it was possible for the virus to be in the body some time before symptoms manifested themselves.[76] The husband continued to profess he never had venereal disease, even when he was informed that his wife was with child, a fact the physician believed would change the husband's story. In the end, the husband's persistent claim of innocence remained unconvincing to the physician, who steadily blamed the husband for the wife's disease. As this story demonstrates, the honest woman was simply not seen as the wellspring of disease.

In reality, of course, conjugal sex presented the possibility of either party communicating the contagion, and this was sometimes reflected in observations of the time. The semi-autobiographical novel of Madame d'Épinay (*Histoire de Madame de Montbrillant*) recounts her fear that venereal disease would expose her affair (although, as it turns out, her husband was the source of her virus that she then communicated to her lover).[77] We can also find men mentioning a wife's diseased state, among other grievances, in order to support a petition to have their wives imprisoned through *lettres de cachet*.[78] A surgeon's boast about his treatment method is also revealing. He noted that wives, as well as husbands, used his treatment because of their wish to keep their contagion secret from a spouse.[79] Despite indications such as these, that women could be liable for the communication of the venereal virus into the family, the medical community did not waver from their conviction that a wife's contagion stemmed from a husband's disease.

Although the sexual double standard that led to the communication of the virus to (often) unsuspecting wives was a legitimate problem, the "innocent wife" tends to show up in vignettes as a tool to remark on the behaviors of men. As they did with the cameos of prostitutes, practitioners usually placed the sketches of innocent wives at the front of their publications and within the rhetoric that justified their remedies and defined their motives as moral and honourable. The dilemma of venereal disease among married women went largely unaddressed. Though charitable gestures, such as the offerings of free treatment for "unfortunate victims of libertinage," have the veneer of tackling the problem, the image of the female victim was exploited to promote the product or service.[80] More important for our discussion here, the literature that claimed women as the beneficiaries of medical attention maintained the relationship of the woman to the man such that the picture of the diseased male body was still within sight. Furthermore, the "innocent wife" model was discursively drawn as threatened by male sexuality but not necessarily riddled with venereal disease. This caricature worked to make women less visible in the picture of venereal disease in France.

The visibility of the diseased male body brought with it moral responsibility. Practitioners did not always link a man's venereal disease to the victimhood of another. Young men were not usually the object of moralizing commentary, but even when they were their missteps were closer to guilt-free; for example, "a young man that error had seduced."[81] The imagined distance between a young man and his procreative years permitted leniency provided a man "submit to a painful and annoying treatment, perhaps even unnecessarily," so that he not "give la Vérole to his wife and engender [diseased] infants."[82]

For those men who did not make certain the virus had been extirpated from their bodies through medical treatment, the characterization increased appreciably from wrongdoer to offender. Practitioners described men who exposed a chaste woman to the virus as "negligent" and even "cruel."[83] An implication of violence was equally expressed in the very common framing of women as the "misfortunate victims of their husbands' debauchery."[84] The practitioners' permissive attitudes toward sexual exploration, which accompanied remarks on young men, quickly transformed into accusations of overindulgence and immorality every time a man's diseased state was juxtaposed to the family.[85]

The criticism became fiercer when practitioners linked the diseased male body to alarming portrayals of malformed young. Sexual immorality and "voluptuous" lifestyles branded men as bad fathers. The representation of children as the "unfortunate victims of the lechery of their father" was copious.[86] A man need not even bear visible signs of venereal disease himself for an infant's ulcers were sufficient evidence to hold a father accountable.[87] Simply engaging in debauchery was enough to characterize a man as neglectful of his paternal duties. Sexual pleasure was measured against sexual purpose when "the substance that serves in the reproduction of man" was thought responsible for transmitting the virus to "the foetus from the very moment of its formation."[88]

The extent to which men were responsible is succinctly illustrated in a treatise, *Instruction sommaire sur le traitement des maladies vénériennes dans les campagnes* (1786), published in order to standardize venereal disease treatment throughout the nation. Intended for a wide audience of medical practitioners, physicians Joseph-Marie-François de Lassone's (1717-1788) and Jacques de Horne's description of the movement of venereal disease into the countryside powerfully underscored male culpability. Migrant workers, they said, extended the problem of venereal disease beyond the (deserving) urban libertines to the heretofore disease-free (innocent) rural populace. The men who came to Paris for temporary work

> return home infected by the disease to which they exposed themselves; disease that they communicate to their wives, when they are back, either because they are categorically ignorant of their state, or because of hasty treatment, and often by Charlatans, gives them a security as dangerous as the disease. This fatal communication is not limited to the wife, who is as it were subjected to it by her condition [as a wife]; the infants commonly share in it, & very soon all a canton finds itself infected by a unrecognized or little known virus, who destroys, degrades the species, imperceptibly devastates the future races on which the expectations of agriculture and the strength of the State are founded.[89]

The full range of repercussions blamed on men's actions in medical literature is summarized in these opening lines of the treatise. This detailed chronicle bluntly blamed men for destabilizing French society as a whole.

While practitioners could be quite stern toward the errant husband, they always offered redemption. Clemency accompanied the scenarios in which medicine was permitted to restore to men the honour and health that was in jeopardy. More than simply erasing the traces of sexual promiscuity, medicine had the potential to improve man. The "misfortune" of venereal disease could remind a husband of his duty and "render [him] more wise and more attentive."[90] Or so that "peace and harmony remain in the household," medical innovations enabled a husband to "take his [medicinal] chocolate in front of his wife, without her suspecting the secret."[91] Although the medical community offered men the opportunity to hide their diseased state from family and community, practitioners represented their knowledge of the diseased male body as transparent to their investigation.

Conclusion

The act of seeing venereal disease was a complex undertaking in the eighteenth century. The venereal virus was believed to be imperceptible. The medical community openly admitted that some aspects of contagion were still unknown, especially since venereal disease did not always follow exposure to the virus. The exact actions of treatment remained unclear. Still, medical men worked to arrest the spread of venereal disease, and their theories on vulnerability were attempts to conceptualize the problem. In the effort to master the covert actions of the body, practitioners categorized bodies and divided physiology into governing concepts to explain the observations of difference between men and women. In the process, guided by the shared assumption that the male body was more susceptible, practitioners gendered vulnerability. They visualized a greater quantity of the virus passing through the pores of a penis, while portions of the virulent matter were conveyed outside a woman's body during menstruation. This process of rendering the unobserved virus visible created tracks that could be followed. In pursuing the insidious movement, from whorehouse to bourgeois *maison*, from urban habits to country lifestyles, medical men relied upon these images of venereal disease to signpost their curing endeavors.

Further delineating the theories on relative female immunity and on male susceptibility through the images of the innocent wife, the errant husband, and the inconspicuously diseased prostitute created limits to the invisible spread of the venereal virus. The characterizations depicted who was endangered, who bore responsibility, and who was the source, in a language of reason and nature. In the scene of venereal disease each archetype had an important part in the grand narrative. The female body vacillated from healthy to diseased while the male body was consistently represented as diseased. The repetition of the image of the diseased male body throughout the discussions on women as well as men worked to regularize the information into convincing observational facts.

Why did the eighteenth century lack visual representations of venereal disease? Perhaps the image of the disease was so commonplace that it did not require illustration. Maybe the marks on diseased bodies were thought to be too distasteful to appear within Enlightenment works that aimed at depicting human improvement rather than disgrace. Also in step with the spirit of the times, medical practitioners might have chosen words for their power to enlighten. Although we may not know why the eighteenth century eschewed visual representations of venereal disease, by incorporating the gendering of vulnerability and the focus on healing the male body into the history of eighteenth-century France, we can come closer to seeing the complex vision of venereal disease that was influential in the period.

Notes

[1] The direct translation of *la maladie vénérienne* (venereal disease) is essentially synonymous with sexually transmitted disease today. However, the eighteenth-century French term carried significantly different socio-cultural and medical meanings. The historically contingent connotations of venereal and sexual become more complicated when attempting to discuss and translate a disease that was

comprehended from different ideologies on illness and the body. In the eighteenth century, *la maladie vénérienne* technically referred to any malady with symptoms appearing in the genital region or following sex acts, but in nearly all instances practitioners used the term to speak of symptoms caused by what they called *le virus vénérien* (see below, note 7). For these reasons, I have chosen to use the contemporary terminology and its translation in order to avoid any anachronism.

[2] For a list of the scholarship on prostitution and venereal disease see below, notes 56 and 57.

[3] For a more detailed treatment of the subject, see my forthcoming doctoral thesis on venereal disease in eighteenth-century France, "*La maladie honteuse, la maladie vénérienne*: Venereal Disease in France, 1736-1789" (PhD thesis, Queen Mary, University of London).

[4] For an overview of the early modern debate on the origin of pox, see Marie E. McAllister, "Stories of the Origin of Syphilis in Eighteenth-Century England: Science, Myth, and Prejudice," *Eighteenth-Century Life* 24.1 (2000): 22-44; Claude Quétel, *The History of Syphilis*, trans. Judith Braddock and Brian Pike (Baltimore, MD: Johns Hopkins University Press, 1992), pp. 33-49.

[5] On the early ideas of contagion, see Jon Arrizabalaga, John Henderson, and Roger French, *The Great Pox: The French Disease in Renaissance Europe* (New Haven, CT: Yale University Press, 1997), chap. 9; Vivian Nutton, "The Seeds of Disease: An Explanation of Contagion and Infection from the Greeks to the Renaissance," in *From Democedes to Harvey: Studies in the History of Medicine* (London: Variorum Reprints, 1988), 11, pp. 1-34; and her "The Reception of Fracastoro's Theory of Contagion: The Seed That Fell among Thorns?" *Osiris*, 2nd ser., 6 (1990): 196-234. For more on eighteenth-century pathology, especially as it pertains to environment, see James C. Riley, *The Eighteenth-Century Campaign to Avoid Disease* (London: MacMillan Press, 1987).

[6] Jean Astruc, *Traité des maladies vénériennes,* trans. Auguste-François Jault, 4th ed., 4 vols. (Paris: Cavelier, 1777). The first French translation from the original Latin appeared in 1740 and a second edition followed in 1743. The 1777 edition contains editorial changes but no changes by the author since the 1743 revision. The editor united and preserved the author's additions over the three previous editions and suppressed some controversial material that had pertained to particular individuals. This has no significant impact on the theoretical aspects of Astruc's work and the 1777 edition has been used due to reader access.

[7] The term virus was common in the eighteenth-century medical literature, but it referred to an inanimate entity rather than a microorganism as the word has come to mean following nineteenth-century medical developments.

[8] Henceforth, the contagious nature of venereal disease was axiomatic and many medical authors simply referenced Astruc instead of devoting any textual space to the debate.

[9] For example, see Astruc, vol. 4, pp. 166-167; Pierre Lalouette, *Nouvelle méthode de traiter les maladies vénériennes, par la fumigation* (Paris: Merigot, 1776), pp. 26-27.

[10] By the eighteenth century, the contagion theory stipulated that the virus was too heavy to be communicated through the air and that it did not endure on common objects. These were distinctions from earlier ideas on contagion as well as older aetiological views on venereal disease. For an outline of the eighteenth-century contagion theory, see Astruc, vol. 2, pp. 14-15. For the discussion of the previous conceptualizations of contagion, see above note 5.

[11] Astruc, vol. 2, pp. 15-19; see also Julien Offray de La Mettrie, *Nouveau traité des maladies vénériennes* (Paris: Huart, 1739), pp. 142-143; Guillaume-René Le Fébure Saint-Ildephont, *Le médecin de soi-même, ou méthode simple et aisée pour guérir les maladies vénériennes*, new ed., 2 vols. (Paris: Michel Lambert, 1775), vol. 1, p. 1. For an example of concerns about the communication during midwifery, see "De Nancy, le 10 février," *Gazette de Santé*, 23 February 1775; and Claude-Esprit Thion de La Chaume, *Tableau des maladies vénériennes, suivi de l'exposition des principales méthodes employées jusqu'ici pour les combattre* (Paris: Louis Jorry, 1773), p. 9.

[12] Astruc, vol. 2, p. 16. All translations are my own except as noted otherwise.

[13] In addition to transmission during sex acts, the medical community was very concerned with communication from parents to offspring and between wet-nurses and nurslings. Although these two modes of transmission were frequently examined along with sexual contagion, they did not factor in the theories on vulnerability that underpinned the moralizing that occurred in the medical literature. The passing of venereal disease from parent to offspring was well known but not well understood. For a good discussion of the complex science of hereditary disease, see Sean Quinlan, "Inheriting Vice, Acquiring Virtue: Hereditary Disease and Moral Hygiene in Eighteenth-Century France," *Bulletin of the History of Medicine* 80 (2006): 649-675. The spread of venereal disease to infants also caused considerable disquiet in connection with the practice of wet-nursing. For a discussion of medical thoughts on this form of contagion and the rhetoric that accompanied it, see Joan Sherwood, *Infection of the Innocents: Wet Nurses, Infants, and Syphilis in France, 1780-1900* (Montreal: McGill-Queen's University Press, 2010). The communication of venereal disease when medical services were being provided was not frequently mentioned. While it was undoubtedly a way by which the virus spread, the issue was generally raised as a tool to re-establish hierarchy among medical practitioners. For discussions on the instability of the boundary lines in eighteenth-century medicine, see Laurence Brockliss and Colin Jones, *The Medical World of Early Modern France* (Oxford: Clarendon Press, 1997), pp. 445-459, 565-578; Toby Gelfand, *Professionalizing Modern Medicine: Paris Surgeons and Medical Science and Institutions in the Eighteenth Century* (London: Greenwood Press, 1980); Matthew Ramsey, *Professional and Popular Medicine in France, 1770-1830: The Social World of Medical Practice* (Cambridge, UK: Cambridge University Press, 1988); George Weisz, *Divide and Conquer: A Comparative History of Medical Specialization* (Oxford: Oxford University Press, 2006).

[14] See Astruc, vol. 2, p. 50.

[15] Jacques Daran, *Traité complet de la gonorrhée virulente des hommes et des femmes* (Paris: Delaguette, 1756), p. 81.
[16] Within the Galenic tradition hemorrhoid bleeding in men was also seen as restoring internal fluid balance and was often linked to menstrual bleeding. See Gianna Pomata, "Menstruating Men: Similarity and Differences of the Sexes in Early Modern Medicine," *Generation and Degeneration: Tropes of Reproduction in Literature and History from Antiquity through Early Modern Europe*, ed. Valeria Finucci and Kevin Brownlee (Durham, NC: Duke University Press, 2001), pp. 109-152.
[17] For Biblical references, see Leviticus 15:24, 18:19, and 20:18. For a good discussion on the associations between menstrual blood and sickness, see Ottavia Niccoli, "'Menstruum Quasi Monstruum:' Monstrous Birth and Menstrual Taboo in the Sixteenth Century," in *Sex and Gender in Historical Perspective*, ed. Edward Muir and Guido Ruggiero, trans. Mary M. Gallucci (Baltimore, MD: Johns Hopkins University Press, 1990), pp. 1-25.
[18] An alternative proposal was that the mixture of multiple men's semen in the womb of a single woman was the initial cause of venereal disease. Notions on improper sex underpinned both ideas. See Astruc, vol. 1, pp. 315-322.
[19] Ian Maclean notes that some Renaissance authors who spoke of menses as capable of healing attributed the power to "the sympathy between the disease and the menses, which far from being beneficial are in this system as noxious as the disease on which they act homeopathically." See Ian Maclean, *The Renaissance Notion of Woman: A Study in the Fortunes of Scholasticism and Medical Science in European Intellectual Life* (Cambridge, UK: Cambridge University Press, 1980), pp. 39-40.
[20] On the role of the "other" in discourse on venereal disease, see Anna Foa, "The New and the Old: The Spread of Syphilis (1494-1530)," in *Sex and Gender in Historical Perspective,* pp. 26-54; and Kevin P. Siena, "Pollution, Promiscuity, and the Pox: English Venereology and the Early Modern Medical Discourse on Social and Sexual Danger," *Journal of the History of Sexuality* 8.4 (1998): 569-571. For a related discussion on the role of race and gender in the eighteenth-century science that sought to correlate corporeal difference with social and the political matters, see Londa Schiebinger, *Nature's Body: Gender in the Making of Modern Science* (Boston: Beacon Press, 1993), pp. 115-183.
[21] Londa Schiebinger, "Skeletons in the Closet: The First Illustrations of the Female Skeleton in Eighteenth-Century Anatomy" in *The Making of the Modern Body: Sexuality and Society in the Nineteenth Century,* ed. Catherine Gallagher and Thomas Laqueur (Berkeley: University of California Press, 1987), pp. 42-82 (esp. pp. 42-53). See also Elisabeth Badinter, *Mother Love: Myth and Reality: Motherhood in Modern History* (New York: Macmillan Publishing, 1981); Catherine Fouquet and Yvonne Knibiehler, *La femme et les médecins* ([Paris?]: Hachette, 1983), pp. 70-74. The gender roles outlined in Jean-Jacques Rousseau's *Émile* and *Julie ou La Nouvelle Héloïse* are a salient example of cultural discourse on social roles for women. For discussions on the influences of Rousseau's works

see Liselotte Steinbrügge, *The Moral Sex: Woman's Nature in the French Enlightenment*, trans. Pamela F. Selwyn (Oxford: University Press, 1992).

[22] Fouquet and Knibiehler, pp. 81-96. For an overview of medical change in the eighteenth century, see Brockliss and Jones, pp. 411-479.

[23] Pierre Roussel, *Système physique et moral de la femme: ou tableau philosophique de la constitution, de l'état organique, du tempérament, des mœurs, & des fonctions propres au sexe* (Paris: Vincent, 1775). On women in medical thought, see Fouquet and Knibiehler, *La femme et les médecins*; Lindsay Wilson, *Women and Medicine in the French Enlightenment: The Debate over Maladies des Femmes* (Baltimore, MD: Johns Hopkins University Press, 1993).

[24] In general, purges, phlebotomy, enemas, frictions, fumigation, tisanes, and pills were prescribed in venereal disease treatments to induce the flow of fluids so that the venereal virus would be conveyed out of the body within the sweat, saliva, urine, and blood. The most common form of treatment, *les grands remèdes*, and the less orthodox treatments, the remedies sold by entrepreneurial practitioners of all sorts, functioned on the same premise that inciting bodily fluxions chased out the venereal virus. Menses naturally followed this universal principle.

[25] Daran, pp. 9-10. For an additional example, see [Jean?] Ballay, *Traité sommaire des maladies vénériennes* (Paris: Debure, 1762), p. 49.

[26] *Consultations choisies de plusieurs médecins célèbres de l'université de Montpellier sur des maladies aigues et chroniques*, 10 vols. (Paris: Durand, 1748-1757), vol. 1, Consultation XXXIV; vol. 7, Consultation VI; vol. 10, Consultation XXI, XXIV. For consults in which the patient is a woman or in which a reference is made to a diseased woman: vol. 1, Consultation LXVI, LXVII; vol. 2, Consultation LXVII; vol. 3, Consultation II; vol. 5, Consultation LX; vol. 8, Consultation XL, XLIV; vol. 9, Consultation ["Consultation traduction de la précédente"] (pp. 400-403); vol. 10, Consultation XI.

[27] For examples, see Daran, *Traité complet de la gonorrhée virulente*; P.-Violette Dubois, *Nouveau traité des maladies vénériennes, dans lequel on explique les meilleures méthodes pour les guérir, & sur-tout la grosse vérole* (Paris: C.-M. d'Houry, 1725); Achille-Guillaume Le Bègue de Presle, *Mémoire pour servir à l'histoire de l'usage interne du mercure sublimé corrosif* (Paris: P. Fr. Didot, 1764).

[28] Académie royale de chirurgie (ARC), carton 12, dossier 46, pièce 1-3; c. 12, d. 59, pièce 2; c. 12B, d. 52, pièce 1; c. 12B, d. 53, pièce 1-2; c. 38, d. 30; c. 38, d. 43, Bibliothèque de l'Académie de Médecine, Paris. Société Royale de Médecine (SRM), c. 134, d. 18; c. 136, d. 13, pièce 11(b), Bibliothèque de l'Académie de Médecine, Paris. "De Paris, le 25 avril," *Gazette de Santé*, 28 April 1774; "De Paris," *Gazette de Santé*, 5 September 1776.

[29] Astruc, vol. 4, pp. 166-167. See also Daran, p. 82.

[30] For example, see Daran, p. 75. Most treatises on venereal disease attempt to distinguish between gonorrhoeal discharge and vaginal discharge by the moral character of the women and the relationship of the discharge to the menstrual cycle. The viscous discharge of *les fleurs blanches* (naturally white in colour but could be green, yellow or black even) was thought to generally precede menses,

but then cease during menstruation. See Thion de la Chaume, p. 16. On *fleurs blanches* in general, see Jean Goulin, *Le médecin des dames, ou l'art de les conserver en santé* (Paris: Vincent, 1771), pp. 111-112.

[31] To the best of my knowledge, there has yet to be any detailed study on venereal disease and sexual activities other than heterosexual in early modern Europe.

[32] At the point an individual with symptoms of venereal disease entered a physician's or surgeon's sphere, most likely, he or she had already formed some belief on the ailment and perhaps had already attempted a cure through other avenues. The term "patient" carries a passive connotation that was uncommon in medicine during the eighteenth century. Most sources used the terms "le malade" (the sick man) and "la malade" (the sick woman). Philip Rieder uses the rarity of the term patient as a point of departure for his study on eighteenth-century medicine. See Philip Rieder, *La figure du patient au XVIIIe siècle* (Geneva: Droz, 2010).

[33] In the second part of the period, a fair number of the venereal disease specialists had backgrounds in military medicine. Treating soldiers for venereal disease was undoubtedly influential in the tendency toward the male body as a template. But the presence of soldiers, and other young men, was not pronounced in the general medical discourse, and they played especially minor roles within the moral commentary. See Wittman, "La maladie honteuse, la maladie vénérienne," chap. 3.

[34] The research of Morag Martin and Lindsay Wilson has shown that in fact women were counted as prospective customers for medical products. See Morag Martin, "Doctoring Beauty: The Medical Control of Women's *Toilettes* in France, 1750-1820," *Medical History* 49 (2005): 354; Wilson, *Women and Medicine in the French Enlightenment*, pp. 5-6.

[35] Astruc, vol. 2, pp. 15-16. See also La Mettrie, p. 200. On the spongy tissue of the penis see also SRM c. 96, d. 9, pièce 3.

[36] Astruc, vol. 2, p. 51. On the importance of a hard member see La Mettrie, p. 202; François Ranchin, *Opuscules ou traits divers et curieux en médicine* (Lyon: Pierre Ravaud, 1640), p. 645.

[37] Ballay, pp. 33-34.

[38] Louis Alexandre de Cézan, *Le secret des médecins, ou manuel anti-syphillitique* [*sic*], (Paris: Costard, 1775), p. 9.

[39] ARC c. 12, d. 46, pièce 3.

[40] Jacques de Horne, *Observations faites et publiées par ordre du gouvernement, sur les différentes méthodes d'administrer le mercure dans les maladies vénériennes,* 2 vols. (Paris: Monory, 1779), vol. 2, pp. 463-466. For similar cases, see vol. 2, pp. 466-469, 502.

[41] In using the term sexuality I only wish to refer to sexual behaviors and capacity for sexual desires, not sexual identity.

[42] SRM c. 96, d. 9, pièce 3, p. 15.

[43] *Consultations choisies*, vol. 6, Consultation IV, p. 25. See also ARC, c. 12, d. 46, pièce 1, and c. 12, d. 54.

[44] De Horne, *Observations faites*, vol. 1, pp. 37-38.

---

[45] Y series 10764, 10993a, 11381, 11695, 12987a, 13122, 13398, 13513, 13781, 14076, 14333, 14555, 14819, 15054a, and 15179, Archives Nationales, Paris. It is important to recall that such sources are not the unmediated voice of women, but are the notations of male figures of authority. Still, the documents indicate that women knew of their husbands' extramarital affairs and were aware of how the venereal virus had or could have been communicated in the marital bed.

[46] Astruc, vol. 1, p. xxviii. See also M. Andrieu, *Agenda anti-syphillitique* [*sic*] (Paris: chez l'Auteur, 1787), p. 3.

[47] For a mention of the virus passed from a mother because of her gonorrhoea symptoms, see Daran, pp. 125-126. For a discussion of the question of maternal transmission in the nineteenth century, see Alain Corbin, "L'hérédosyphilis ou l'impossible rédemption. Contribution à l'histoire de l'hérédité morbide," *Romantisme* 31 (1981): 135-136. Sherwood discusses the medical opinions that highlighted female responsibility, pp. 21-23.

[48] On hereditary traits and diseases, see Joseph Raulin, *Traité de la conservation des enfants*, 2nd ed., 2 vols. (Paris: Saugrain & Lamy, 1779), vol. 1, pp. 184-185; on venereal disease specifically, vol. 2, pp. 457-461. On the ideas on man's role in conception, see Angus McLaren, "The Pleasures of Procreation: Traditional and Biomedical Theories of Conception," in *William Hunter and the Eighteenth-Century Medical World,* ed. W. F. Bynum and Roy Porter (Cambridge: Cambridge University Press, 1985), pp. 323-341; Quinlan, "Inheriting Vice, Acquiring Virtue."

[49] Andrieu, *Agenda anti-syphillitique*, p. 15. For analysis on degeneration, see Sean Quinlan, *The Great Nation in Decline: Sex, Modernity and Health Crises in Revolutionary France c. 1750-1850* (Aldershot, UK: Ashgate, 2007).

[50] On fatherhood, see Jean Delumeau and Daniel Roche, *Histoire des pères et de la paternité* (Paris: Larousse, 1990), chap. 9 and 10; Lynn Hunt, *The Family Romance of the French Revolution* (Berkeley: University of California Press, 1992); Jeffery Merrick, "The Family Politics of the Marquis de Bombelles," in *Order and Disorder under the Ancien Régime* (Newcastle: Cambridge Scholars Publishing, 2007), pp. 164-181; Robert Nye, *Masculinity and Male Codes of Honor in Modern France* (Oxford: Oxford University Press, 1993); Leslie Tuttle, "Celebrating the Père de Famille: Pronatalism and Fatherhood in Eighteenth-Century France," *Journal of Family History* (2004): 366-381.

[51] See Margaret Healy, "'Seeing' Contagious Bodies in Early Modern London," in *The Body in Late Medieval and Early Modern Culture*, ed. Darryll Grantley and Nina Taunton (Aldershot, UK: Ashgate, 2000), pp. 157-167; Ludmilla Jordanova, *Sexual Visions: Images of Gender in Science and Medicine between the Eighteenth and Twentieth Centuries* (Madison: University of Wisconsin Press, 1989), (esp. p. 91); Barbara Maria Stafford, *Body Criticism: Imaging the Unseen in Enlightenment Art and Medicine* (Cambridge, MA: MIT Press, 1991).

[52] Mary Spongberg, *Feminizing Venereal Disease: The Body of the Prostitute in Nineteenth-Century Medical Discourse* (New York: New York University Press, 1997), p. 2. See also Sander Gilman, *Disease and Representation: Images of Illness from Madness to AIDS* (Ithaca, NY: Cornell University Press, 1988), pp.

248-254; Laura McGough, *Gender, Sexuality, and Syphilis in Early Modern Venice: The Disease that Came to Stay* (Basingstoke: Palgrave Macmillan, 2011), p. 8; Siena, "Pollution, Promiscuity, and the Pox," pp. 557-571.

[53] On the ability for women to easily transmit the virus, see Ballay, p. 49; Daran, p. 74.

[54] On women and dissimulation, see Hunt, pp. 97-98.

[55] Over the course of the eighteenth century, legislation on prostitution was passed several times, but the government acted with ambivalence toward the practice and generally tolerated prostitution.

[56] Erica Benabou's famous study on eighteenth-century prostitution, for example, contains a section on venereal disease. See Erica Benabou, *La prostitution et la police des mœurs au XVIIIe siècle* (Paris: Perrin, 1987), pp. 407-430; Cissie Fairchilds, *Domestic Enemies: Servants & Their Masters in Old Regime France* (Baltimore: Johns Hopkins University Press, 1984), pp. 76, 185; Colin Jones, "Prostitution and the Ruling Class in Eighteenth-Century Montpellier," *History Workshop* 6 (1978): 7-28; Alistaire Tallent, "Listening to the Prostitute's Body: Subjectivity and Subversion in the Erotic Memoir Novels of Eighteenth-Century France," *Proceedings of the Western Society for French History* 33 (2005): 211-223. In the nineteenth century, see Alain Corbin, *Women for Hire: Prostitution and Sexuality in France after 1850*, trans. Alan Sheridan (Cambridge, MA: Harvard University Press, 1990); Jill Harsin, *Policing Prostitution in Nineteenth-Century Paris* (Princeton, NJ: Princeton University Press, 1985); Annet Mooij, *Out of Otherness: Characters and Narrators in the Dutch Venereal Disease Debates 1850-1900*, trans. Beverley Jackson (Amsterdam: Rodopi, 1998); Judith Surkis, *Sexing the Citizen: Morality & Masculinity in France, 1870-1920* (Ithaca, NY: Cornell University Press, 2006). Anna Lundberg's study spans the end of the eighteenth- through the twentieth-centuries in Sweden, *Care and Coercion: Medical Knowledge, Social Policy and Patients with Venereal Disease in Sweden 1785-1903* (Umeå, Sweden: Demographic Data Base, Umeå University, 1999).

[57] Laura McGough has made a similar observation, p. 9. For examples of the focus on diseased prostitutes, see Susan P. Conner, "Politics, Prostitution, and the Pox in Revolutionary Paris, 1789-1799," *Journal of Social History* 22.4 (1989): 713-734; Johannes Fabricius's *Syphilis in Shakespeare's England* (London: Jessica Kingsley Publishers, 1994); Jennifer Foster, "Medical Regulation and Social Discipline at the Hôpital Royal et Militaire and the Bon Pasteur de Montpellier, 1731-1789," (PhD diss., University of Southern California, 2000); Quétel, *History of Syphilis*; Spongberg, *Feminizing Venereal Disease*.

[58] For two studies on diseased women not engaging in prostitution, see Jill Harsin, "Syphilis, Wives, and Physicians: Medical Ethics and the Family in Late Nineteenth-Century France," *French Historical Studies* 16.1 (1989): 72-95; Sherwood, *Infection of the Innocents*.

[59] Daran, p. xxii.

[60] Astruc, vol. 2, p. 16.

[61] ARC, c. 12, d. 59, pièce 1. SRM c. 118B, d. 96. See also *Consultations choisies*, vol. 1, Consultation XXXIII, p. 231, Consultation LXVI, p. 472; vol. 2,

Consultation XVI, p. 121-122; vol. 3, Consultation LXXVI, p. 423; vol. 6, Consultation IV, p. 25; Dubois, p. 18; Hugues Maret, *Mémoire dans lequel on cherche à déterminer quelle influence les mœurs des François ont sur leur santé* (Amiens: Godard, 1772), pp. 37-39; SRM c. 97, d. 76, pièce 2.

62 Treatments in which debauched women appear, SRM c. 134, d. 18. A relatively small number of remedy trials state specifically that prostitutes were the test subjects, see MM. Bacher, de Horne, Roussel de Vauzesme, and Saint-Léger, *Effets de la tisane caraïbe proposée pour la guérison des maladies vénériennes* (Paris: [n. pub.], 1779); Jean Keyser, *La préservatif ou avis au public sur les dragées anti-vénériennes du Sr Keyser* ([Paris?], [n. pub.], 1756). De Horne felt the propensity for licentious sex made re-contagion probable among prostitutes, which caused the durability of a cure to be difficult to determine (*Observations faites*, vol. 1, pp. 16-20).

63 See Brockliss and Jones, pp. 411-479; Gelfand, *Professionalizing Modern Medicine*; Jean-Pierre Goubert, "L'art de guérir. Médecine savante et populaire dans la France de 1790," *Annales. Histoire, Sciences Sociales* 32 (1977): 908-926; Caroline Hannaway, "Medicine, Public Welfare and the State in Eighteenth-Century France: The Société Royale de Médecine of Paris (1776-1793)," (PhD diss., Johns Hopkins University, 1974); Christelle Rabier, "Les chirurgiens de Paris et de Londres 1740-1815: économie, identités, savoirs," 2 vols. (PhD diss., Université de Paris-1 Panthéon-Sorbonne, 2008); Ramsey, *Professional and Popular Medicine in France, 1770-1830.*

64 ARC, c. 12, d. 53, pièce 1.

65 For example, Marie-Nicolas Devergie, *Recherches historiques et médicales sur l'origine, la nature et le traitement de la syphilis* (Paris: Baillière, 1834), pp. 16-17.

66 Harsin, *Policing Prostitution*, p. 97. See also pp. 96-130. Alexandre-Jean Baptiste Parent-Duchâtelet, *De la prostitution dans la ville de Paris*, 3rd ed., 2 vols. (Paris: J.-B. Baillière, 1857).

67 For examples, Anonymous, *Les causes du désordre public, par un vrai citoyen* (Paris: Guillot, 1784); see Louis-Sébastien Mercier, *Tableau de Paris*, new ed., 4 vols. (Amsterdam: [n. pub.], 1783), vol. 3, chap. CCXXXVIII, p. 107. Nicolas Edmé Rétif de la Bretonne, *Le pornographe, ou idées d'un honnête homme sur un projet de règlement pour les prostituées* (Paris: Éditions d'aujourd'hui, 1983).

68 Daran, p. 74.

69 Kathryn Norberg, "From Courtesan to Prostitute: Mercenary Sex and Venereal Disease, 1730-1802," in *The Secret Malady: Venereal Disease in Eighteenth-Century Britain and France*, ed. Linda Merians (Lexington: University of Kentucky Press, 1996), p. 34.

70 Dubois, p. 154.

71 Paul Delaunay, *Le monde médical parisien au dix-huitième siècle*, 2nd ed. (Paris: Librairie médicale et scientifique, 1906), pp. 238-239.

72 *Consultations choisies,* vol. 2, Consultation LXVII, p. 420.

73 For example, see De Horne, *Observations faites*, vol. 1, pp. 38, 83, 282; vol. 2, pp. 25, 490; La Mettrie, p. 203.

[74] Roger Dibon, *Dissertation sur les maladies vénérienne* (Paris: Noël Pissot, 1725), p. 94.
[75] Astruc, vol. 4, p. 162.
[76] *Consultations choisies*, vol. 8, pp. 280-281. The concept that the virus could remain hidden in the blood for long periods was a tenet in Astruc's compendium; see Astruc, vol. 1, p. xxix. See also Daran, p. 121.
[77] Louise Florence Tardieu d'Esclavelles, Marquise d'Épinay, *Memoirs and Correspondence of Madame d'Épinay,* trans. E.G. Allingham (New York: The Dial Press, 1930), pp. 52-54. See also Francis Steegmuller, *A Woman, a Man, and Two Kingdoms: The Story of Madame d'Épinay and the Abbé Galiani* (New York: Alfred A. Knopf, 1991), p. 13.
[78] Arlette Farge & Michel Foucault, eds., *Le désordre des familles: lettres de cachet des archives de la Bastille* (Paris: Éditions Gallimard, 1982), pp. 63-64, 74-75, 130.
[79] Dubois, p. 178.
[80] Le Fébure de Saint-Ildephont, "Traitement gratuit pour le mal vénérien, administré aux adultes de l'un et de l'autre sexe et aux enfans dans Versailles" (Paris: G. Desprez, 1775).
[81] De Horne, *Exposition raisonnée des différentes méthodes d'administrer le mercure dans les maladies vénériennes* (Paris: Monory, 1774), p. 115.
[82] Dibon, *Lettre de M***, médecin de Reims, à Darnouval, médecin à Clermont, où l'on essaie de démontrer les écarts de M. Astruc* (Reims: [n. pub.], 1742), p. 18. See also *Consultations choisies*, vol. 2, Consultation XVI, p. 126; Charles-Augustin Vandermonde, *Essai sur la manière de perfectionner l'espèce humaine* (Paris: Vincent, 1756), vol. 1, pp. 83-84.
[83] Daran, p. xxv.
[84] De Horne, *Observations faites*, vol. 1, p. 17.
[85] Thion de la Chaume, p. 10.
[86] Daran, p. xxv.
[87] J. J. Gardane, *Détail de la nouvelle direction du bureau des nourrices de Paris* (Paris: Ruault, 1775), pp. 18-20.
[88] Andrieu, *Compte rendu au public sur des nouveaux moyens de guérir les maladies vénériennes* (Paris: Belin, 1782), p. 15.
[89] Jacques de Horne and Joseph-Marie-François de Lassone, *Instruction sommaire sur le traitement des maladies vénériennes dans les campagnes* (Paris: Ph.-D. Pierres, 1786), pp. 3-4.
[90] De Horne, *Exposition raisonnée*, p. 115.
[91] Le Fébure de Saint-Ildephont, *Médecin de soi-même*, vol. 1, pp. ix-x.

CHAPTER TEN

YOU'VE GOT THE VAPORS?: HISTORICAL, MEDICAL AND LITERARY PERSPECTIVES

IVY DYCKMAN

On the surface, it would appear that the Enlightenment era—especially in France, the country most popularly associated with its intellectual and philosophical aspects—had finally opened doors in socio-cultural arenas for, at the very least, noble and upper-class women. That, finally, lettered men had been somewhat enlightened as to women's potential to contribute their talents in the arts and sciences to society would have seemed a natural consequence of rational thought. This was a false assumption, though not entirely. As James F. McMillan observes, "France did not produce a female *philosophe*, and in that sense it is possible to claim that for French women the Enlightenment—like the Renaissance—was a non-event."[1] Yet, in the mid-to-late seventeenth century and throughout the eighteenth, certain intellectual women hailing from the elite echelons of society did provide a venue, the *salon*, thereby establishing a setting which would allow for the exchange and debate of great and small ideas. Hostesses or *salonnières* such as Claudine-Alexandrine Guérin, marquise de Tencin (1682-1749); Marie-Thérèse Geoffrin (1699-1777); Marie du Deffand (1697-1780); Julie de Lespinasse (1732-1776); and Suzanne Necker (1737-1794) functioned as catalysts for the dissemination of Enlightenment ideals.[2]

With regard to women as legitimate figures in the world of eighteenth-century medicine, they remained in the background. Notwithstanding their nearly non-existent status as what we would classify nowadays as professional, their contributions to healing the sick were substantial. On a daily basis, they assisted those entering the world, those on their way out, and those who required treatment of their ailing physical bodies. In short, women were "central to health and healing before 1800."[3] They were folk healers, midwives, members of religious orders and female charitable confraternities, Ladies Bountiful (noblewomen of the upper classes), compilers of medicinal recipes, and at times, though not as common, surgeons, apothecaries, and even *charlatanes*.[4] Despite their considerable activity in healing and health, there is a lack of information and research on women who engaged in and wrote about self-help and preventative care. Susan Broomhall makes the general observation that

> histories of medicine have tended to focus on the interventionist practices of medicine and rarely analysed primary and preventative care: even though contemporaries did see these as medical.[5]

Because eighteenth-century French and English women were conspicuously silent about expressing themselves on the healthy and unhealthy states of their bodies, this paper will examine how certain physicians spoke about medical conditions peculiar to women and what they subsequently prescribed as treatments. As usual, women's voices were appropriated by men, albeit learned men. McMillan corroborates this when he states, "Glaringly absent from the eighteenth-century philosophical (and medical) discourse on women's nature was any significant contribution by women themselves."[6] Coming from a male authorial voice, this statement is worthy of note.

We will focus on two French and three English treatises that concern women's diseases and disorders with suggestions for cures and remedies, one of which appears to have borrowed extensively from another. These publications, dated from 1762 to 1792, were selected because they included self-help references after each disease description.[7] All of them are organized in much the same way. They are divided into chapters or sections that describe medical conditions attributed mainly to women, which, to a great extent, revolve around the reproductive system. Specific remedies and recipes (also known as receipts) for cures are included. As space does not permit detailed discussion of all the female disorders described in these five manuals, only the condition of the vapors will be closely examined.[8] The emotional aspects of an ailment attributed to physical causes will be of particular interest in our analysis. Because eighteenth-century European medicine was so unlike that of today, it will be helpful to begin with an overview of the philosophies that physicians of that era brought to their profession and of the training they received and the practices they applied. This introduction will also serve to explain how these learned gentlemen regarded women and why they treated their female patients as they did. A discussion of the vapors will follow, before we proceed with an examination of the sections on that condition as they appear in the publications of Jean Astruc, Samuel Auguste André David (S.A.D.) Tissot, John Ball, A. Hume, and John Leake.

Humoral medicine was still in vogue in the eighteenth-century European medical arena. It was "the predominant type of medicine [...] practised in England by orthodox practitioners from the 13th century until the 19th century [...]."[9] University-trained physicians were schooled in Hippocratic and Galenic principles based on the presence of four humors or fluids in the body.[10] The relative proportion of each—blood, phlegm, yellow bile, black bile—determined the health, temperament, and physical constitution of an individual. Daily management or regimen of the six non-naturals—"air, food and drink, exercise (including sexual activity) and rest, sleep and wakefulness, bodily evacuations, and the passions of the soul"[11]—were necessary for humoral balance and hence for assurance of good health over illness.[12] Towards the end of the seventeenth century until the final decades of the eighteenth, materialist and vitalist beliefs challenged this Galenic tradition. Although they were both optimists and "emphasized the need to build medical knowledge afresh,"[13] mechanists and vitalists clashed theoretically. Mechanist doctrine, based on Cartesian or Newtonian principles, held that

> all movements within the body, whether salutary or pathological [...] [were] the result of some original impulsive force and of subsequent, finely regulated mechanical operations that differed in no important way from those governing the movements of 'brute matter.'[14]

To avoid confrontation with the Church, the creation of matter was attributed to the divine. Towards mid-century, vitalism began making inroads in medical and intellectual circles. Unlike mechanism, this doctrine held that the presence of a vital force, not physical and chemical laws, determined the functions of living organisms. Furthermore, theological implications were skirted, making the theory a target for religious attack.[15]

Galenic, mechanist, or vitalist medical models hardly contributed to the betterment of women's health, welfare, or socio-cultural status. From a current perspective, descriptions of female anatomy and physiology were at times primitive if not ludicrous. This is not surprising since these theories were conceived by men in male-dominated societies. Galenists believed that the adult male was "the most perfect form of the species," women being "regarded as merely imperfect versions of men."[16] Even female genitalia were seen as "reversed and deficient forms of the male organs."[17] With regard to the humors, women were "colder and moister than males," reflecting a phlegmatic temperament associated with the brain.[18] Mechanism, despite making advances in anatomy and physiology, also had its weaknesses.[19] Reproduction, for instance, could not be explained as a mechanical process, but rather as an enlargement of a minuscule living creature that had existed in the form of a male or female seed since the beginning of time.[20] In spite of such limitations in his knowledge, the mechanist physician Astruc produced well-known works on venereal disease, diseases occurring in women, and obstetrics.[21] He may have viewed men and women as machines, but his works evidenced recognition of the uniqueness of each gender. Vitalists, too, contrasted with the Galenists with regard to distinct differences between the sexes. But vitalists challenged adherents of both schools of thought with their emphasis on observation, and their concern for a healthy body and lifestyle, as well as their desire for "simplicity and naturalness," an "abiding theme of the Encyclopedists."[22] On the surface, these beliefs appeared progressive for women. To the contrary, in reality they contributed to their social, political, and cultural setbacks. The recognition of gender distinction by vitalists presented men as the stronger sex. Women, having weaker constitutions, were deemed passive members restricted to the bearing and rearing of children and to the management of the household.[23]

Medical practitioners in eighteenth-century Europe consisted of licensed and mostly unlicensed healers. At the top of the licensed ladder was the small, elite group of university-trained physicians whose primary task was to diagnose and wax philosophical about the diseases of their patients. Next and more numerous were the surgeons, who dealt with the exterior body, performing hands-on procedures such as cutting, operating, and bloodletting. Apothecaries represented the third official group of the medical community. Most of the quotidian healing was done by unlicensed practitioners. With the establishment of such institutions as the Collège de Pharmacie in Paris (1777) and the Royal College of Surgeons in London (1800), surgeons and apothecaries were finally able to enjoy the social and scientific status of physicians. Throughout the eighteenth century, women were denied formal training as physicians, surgeons, and apothecaries. In France, at least, women who had acquired knowledge of surgery or pharmacy did so because of unofficial apprenticeship supervised by fathers or husbands. Although most midwives lacked formal training, there did exist under the statutes of 1730 a requirement for authorized apprenticeship and examination. Midwives also had access to instruction at the *Office des Accouchées* at the Hôtel-Dieu in Paris and through the itinerant work of Madame du Coudray (c. 1712-1794) who offered courses and training in midwifery to a great many women and even a substantial number of men all over France. Apart from these few entries into the orthodox medical community, women were primarily responsible only for overseeing healing within and outside of the home.[24]

With respect to the overall world of medicine during the Enlightenment, there was notable progress. Mechanists, vitalists, and empiricists were all challenging traditional Galenic views as they introduced and debated new theories in the faculties and salons. The public at large had greater access to printed matter that at once exposed readers to innovations in health and science and gave them knowledge on how to care for their own bodies. The feeling of optimism that resulted from enlightened beliefs extended into the medical community. The ensuing sense of hope and egalitarianism led to significant reforms in hospital organization, clinical medicine, and medical training and outreach. The humanitarian and optimistic dimensions of the Enlightenment yielded encouraging developments in private and public health and hygiene sectors as well as greater interest in the physical welfare of children and animals.[25]

Even so, the concepts of nature and sensibility in Enlightenment thought supported the subservient position of women throughout the eighteenth century and beyond. Mary Lynn Stewart explains the secondary gender role of women in terms of biopolitics. Since the *philosophes* claimed that natural laws governed the universe, they were ambivalent about how to justify "female subordination" given the egalitarian notion embedded in natural rights theory.[26] In order to maintain masculine superiority in the socio-political hierarchy, the *philosophes* asserted the existence of "corporeal inequality and social complementarity."[27] Women, then, were charged with generative and domestic responsibilities for which nature intended them, constrained from entry into the political and economic domain of men. The notion of sensibility only reinforced the rationality of natural rights theory. It dealt with the human capacity of emotional, physical, intellectual, and esthetic perception and/or responsiveness. The *philosophe* Jean-Jacques Rousseau (1712-1778) contributed to a moral dimension of sensibility through his writings, in *La nouvelle Héloïse* (1761), for example. Julie, the heroine, was the quintessential model of the virtuous daughter, wife, and mother who knew her place in the natural order of the world. Though capable of committing the dramatic act of martyrdom, Julie, like all other women, was deemed innately more emotionally and intellectually fragile than her masculine superiors.[28]

E.C. Spary speaks of the eighteenth century as "a time of increasing medicalization of Western societies."[29] That is, ordinary people enjoyed greater accessibility to medical practitioners, remedies, paraphernalia, and literature. In other words, the increase and spread of medical and scientific knowledge in the second half of the century allowed lay individuals some degree of management over the health and hygiene of their own bodies. She cites as examples of this "highly successful literary genre" of "domestic health manuals" the Scottish physician William Buchan's *Domestic Medicine* (1769), the English theologian John Wesley's *Primitive Physick* (1747), and the Swiss physician S.A.D. Tissot's *Avis au peuple sur sa santé* (1761).[30] About that same time, there appeared texts on medical conditions specific to women. Two of these better-known treatises were written by Montpellier-schooled doctors, the mechanist Astruc and the vitalist Pierre Roussel (1742-1802).[31] There are examples, though not numerous, of women writing about medically-related topics. These papers, whether circulated or not, concerned collections of recipes of home-produced remedies, which were not meant solely for women. The most famous and enduring of these compilations was that of Madame Fouquet (1590-1681).[32] Mary E. Fissell notes that remedy books printed from manuscripts became best-sellers in England during the 1650s. She cites the popular and profitable *A Choice Manual, of Rare and Select Secrets in Physick and Chyrurgery* (1653) published after the death of its author Elizabeth Grey, Countess of Kent (1582-1651).[33] A final example of an early-modern compiler of recipes is Elizabeth Freke (1641-1714) who, like the above two, hailed from the upper classes. She was an unhappily married memoirist who also drew up inventories of her homemade medicines between December 1710 and May 1712. Although they were not meant for public readership, they are of historical interest. The papers reveal her familiar knowledge of pharmacology and medical theory, the types of medicines she produced and stored as well as the ingredients, equipment, and methods used in the making of the remedies.[34]

Just as there exists an abundance of material on eighteenth-century medicine, so it seems likewise on the subject of the vapors.[35] From the seventeenth through the nineteenth centuries, this condition was of such interest that descriptions and references can be found throughout the literature of the period. It might be useful if not amusing to learn about this ubiquitous condition through a few references culled chronologically from French and British literature.

The first example comes from the correspondence of Madame de Sévigné (1626-1696). In a letter addressed to a Monsieur de Pomponne, dated 20 November 1664, she references Madame Fouquet. The latter was attempting to secure the queen's help on behalf of Madame Fouquet's son Nicolas, who was on trial, by giving her majesty a plaster "qui l'a guérie de ses convulsions, qui étoient, à proprement parler, des vapeurs." Unfortunately, the effort did not advance her son's case, but the *emplâtre* was such a success that Madame Fouquet was hailed a saint, a performer of miracles.[36]

The next references concern the spleen, a type of nervous disorder affecting both sexes in eighteenth-century England. It was so prevalent that Dr. George Cheyne, "a well-known physician, who had himself fallen a victim to the disease," wrote a treatise on it entitled *The English Malady* (1733).[37] This condition, also known as "vapours" and "hystericks," found its way into the novels of such influential writers as Daniel Defoe (c. 1660-1731) and Henry Fielding (1707-1754). Defoe's Robinson Crusoe suffers "ecstasies of vapours" when discovering Friday's footprint, and Fielding's Captain Booth describes his wife Amelia's "vapours" as "one of the worst disorders that can possibly attend a woman"; "a sort of complication of all diseases together, with almost madness added to them."[38]

The final two illustrations demonstrate how women themselves are capable of coming to terms with this disorder. They rely on their own instincts and abilities to seek relief rather than on the counsel of a physician. In her poem entitled "Song: 'Why will Delia thus retire,'" (1730) Lady Mary Wortley Montagu (1689-1762) offers unconventional advice to counter the grief of her widowed friend, indicated poetically as Delia. She remarks:

> I, like you, was born a woman,
> Well I know what vapours mean!
> The disease, alas! is common,
> Single we have all the spleen (13-16).

As an iconoclastic aristocrat known for her caustic writings as well as the introduction of the smallpox inoculation to England—and hence Western Europe, resulting from her time in Turkey as the wife of the English ambassador there—Lady Montagu was not reticent about telling Delia that a young lover is the cure for her vaporous, depressive state:

> All the morals they teach us
> Never cur'd our sorrows yet:
> Choose among the pretty fellows
> One of humour, youth, and wit.
> Prithee hear him ev'ry morning,
> At least an hour or two;
> Once again at night returning,
> I believe the dose will do (17-24).

The sensual receipt that she suggests for the widow's vapors was surely rarely prescribed by a male doctor of the time, at least, not until the widow had remarried.[39]

It might strike readers as almost inconceivable that Nicolas Edme Rétif de la Bretonne (1734-1806), prolific and pornographic writer of the second half of the eighteenth century, would have had anything positive to say about the notion of a woman healing herself of the vapors. As in the case of Lady Montagu's remedy, Rétif's cure would possibly have been considered unacceptable to many eighteenth-century physicians. In his *Les Nuits de Paris,* published between 1788 and 1793, Rétif fashions a tale reminiscent of *Thousand and One Nights*, in which a vaporous marquise gradually rids herself of the lethargic, depressive effects of the disorder thanks to the narratives delivered to her by the first-person narrator, who visits her after his nocturnal wanderings on the île Saint-Louis. Like King Shahryar, the marquise experiences great delight at the expectation of receiving each successive account. As a result of these nightly stories and her subsequent desire to give assistance to the young female victims who are the subjects of many of these tales, the marquise gains "energy and life."[40] She eventually sheds her passive gender role as a dissolute noblewoman, evolving into an activist of her time.

From the four literary references just described, it is not difficult to deduce that the vapors were characterized by a depressive state, at times accompanied by convulsions and even feelings of madness. The symptoms of the disease evoke contemporary diagnoses of bipolar disorder, severe depression, post-traumatic stress disorder, or simply the blues. In the eighteenth century, it was considered one of many illnesses—hypochondria, hysteria, the spleen, dyspepsia—categorized as "nervous disorders."[41] The etymology of the term originates with the late fourteenth-century Anglo-French *vapour*, derived from the Latin *vaporem*, meaning "exhalation, steam, heat." The plural form vapors dates from the 1660s, recalling the "medieval notion of 'exhalations' from the stomach or other organs affecting the brain."[42] This history helps to clarify what bodily gaseous emanations supposedly had to do with a nervous disorder or how a physiological occurrence could alter a mental state. An insightful explanation was written not by a physician or medical historian but by the late columnist William Safire in one of his weekly essays on popular etymology in the *New York Times Magazine*. He said that the term was chosen

> because the mental state of low spirits was thought to originate in the stomach or spleen (in men), or the uterus (in women), for which the Greek word is hystera, bubbling up to the brain and causing morbidity.[43]

Since according to the eighteenth-century notion of sensibility, women were considered the weaker sex, they were more susceptible to this condition. To avoid developing the vapors, women were advised to lead a sober lifestyle, which meant not only eating healthy foods and breathing clean air but also rejecting the degenerate ways of upper-class ladies who were more prone to the vapors. Debauched nobles were also disposed to this effeminate disease due to unhealthful habits that reflected the boredom and idleness they seemed to perfect on a daily basis. Scholars, too, suffered from this condition. They prioritized intellectual over physical pursuits, which had deleterious effects on the body's sensibility.

Jean Astruc (1684-1766), mechanist physician, medical professor, and biblical scholar, touted the creation of the generalist practitioner who would welcome among his patients ailing women and children but not the elderly. While there were unauthorized English translations of his courses on the diseases of children and women in circulation, Astruc wrote works directly on female diseases during the years preceding his death.[44] The source used here is an English translation of his *Traité des maladies des femmes*, which was published in London in 1762.[45] Given the prevalence of venereal disease, he also authored an earlier, well-known, needed treatise on that delicate subject.[46]

The second volume of Astruc's treatise on women's disorders deals with diseases affecting the uterus. Interestingly, after the table of contents, this volume includes a chronological listing of authors, all male, who had written about women's diseases, and concludes with a narrative version of this same catalog. By incorporating these catalogs, he seems to be justifying his own work through precedent. This text in translation contains an index as well. The thirteenth and final chapter specifically concerns the vapors or hysteria and is entitled: "Of the hysteric passion, or uterine suffocation." In the first section, Astruc describes the disease, in the second the causes, and in the third the symptoms which he subdivides into those that affect the abdomen, the thorax, the head, and the entire body. The fourth and fifth parts consider the topics of diagnosis and prognosis. The latter speaks to the cure and degree of danger of the disorder; in general, the "hysteric passion" is difficult to cure but not "commonly dangerous."[47] The sixth and final section of the chapter deals with the "Method of cure."[48] The recommended treatment depends on whether the subject is in or out of a fit or paroxysm and experiencing convulsions, that is, severe, involuntary muscle contractions.[49] If the patient is in the throes of paroxysm three kinds of remedies are recommended: those that relax the body; those that induce the circulation of blood; and those that generate "strong sensations in the exterior organs."[50] The purpose of these remedies is to "produce rapid *refluxes* towards the brain, capable of counteracting, and overcoming the sympathetic *refluxes*, made in the uterus, and which cause the accidents of the vapours."[51] This sounds like a war involving gaseous emanations in which the noxious fumes of the uterus are vanquished with the aid of the proposed treatments, some of which appear quaint, ridiculous, or even barbaric by contemporary standards. For example, it is recommended that the patient in paroxysm have her thighs rubbed from top to bottom, be induced to sneeze by introducing tobacco fumes up her nose, be stimulated by having her hair pulled or be "shaken briskly," or be administered purgatives in the form of glysters (enemas). Astruc describes how women "in low life" in the rural Languedoc region use garlic on the navel to alleviate the paroxysm. Vaginal massage using musk or civet is advised, but with a caveat. Astruc warns that it is against religious belief to induce secretions in such a fashion. It is better that a woman, not a physician, undertake this procedure. The most effective remedies are either "antihysteric potions" or "bolusses" (boluses) for which he offers recipes composed of ingredients gotten locally from, for example, the apothecary, herbalist, healer, or garden. In the event of severe hysteric fits or paroxysms, opiates, bleeding, or induced vomiting may be remedies of preference. When the paroxysm ends, Astruc recommends treating the bodily root cause to prevent any future occurrence. In the final section, he also suggests remedies for the cure of the "hysteric vapours" recommended on the authority of reputable physicians. This includes one that requires administering a measured amount of afterbirth, dried in the oven and ground into a powder.[52]

Of the two French-speaking physicians that we shall now examine, Samuel Auguste André David Tissot (1728-1797) had a more profound effect on public health reform and a greater readership than his fellow Montpellier-trained colleague Astruc. Like Rousseau, he was francophone Swiss and did not hesitate to disseminate his controversial, no-nonsense thoughts and advice on the health and welfare of all individuals of every social class. He wrote what was probably considered the most important self-help manual of the century, *Avis au peuple sur sa santé*, published in 1761 and reprinted forty-two times in French and seventeen times in translation.[53] In that publication, he includes a chapter on women's health, "Chapter XXVI. Avis pour les femmes," but limits its contents to female reproduction: *les règles* (menstruation), *la grossesse* (pregnancy), and *suites de couches* (post-partum period). His various references to the vapors have more to do with their nefarious effects originating in the environment as well as in the body. With regard to those disposed to a nervous disorder—the vapors or hypochondria—he advises against the treatment of bleeding since it tends to cause further weakness.[54] Tissot's other popular works deal with masturbation, the health of intellectuals and those of the upper classes, and nervous disorders.[55] In these books, he addresses health problems resulting from sedentary and degenerate lifestyles.

Although a treatise on women's disorders purportedly by Tissot exists in English translation, it does not seem to appear on lists of works attributed to him. *The Lady's Physician* (1766), a thin translated volume whose complete title is out of proportion to its length, could have indeed been written by him as a separate work or as a synthesis of previous writings on women's disorders selected from his other publications. It could also have been a pirated English edition of the latter. Whatever the case, *The Lady's Physician* is a concise self-help manual containing eighteen sections that deliver clear, practical advice about all of the usual female issues.[56] Tissot covers the topic of the vapors in just four pages of the sixth section.[57] The first paragraph describes in a picturesque fashion the causes of the malady, which is due to "an Accumulating of the Blood in the Bowels" that hinders menstrual flow resulting in "much Mischief to the fair Sex, on account of their tender Structure" (p. 19). It is understood that virgins and widows are especially susceptible to this "Complaint" due to lack of sexual intimacy (p. 19). As we saw, Lady Mary Wortley Montagu draws attention to this issue in her "Song." The second paragraph describes the physical manifestations of this disorder, some of which sound dreadful. Tissot states:

> The Speech is interrupted, the Heart is in a violent Palpitation, the Pulse is irregular and hard [...] racking Pains are felt in the Bladder and Kidney, as if the Patient was afflicted with the Stone; [...] Fits of Weeping and Laughing succeed to each other, without any apparent Cause for either, and are accompanied with Convulsions (p. 20).

Like Astruc, Tissot distinguishes between the cures used during what he calls the "Fit" rather than the paroxysm and those used "out of the Fit" (pp. 20-21). Some of his suggestions to patients in the "Fit" include rubbing the body and limbs with "warm Flannels"; tickling the soles of the feet; having the hair pulled "in the most sensible parts, to awaken the Faculty of Feeling"; sending tobacco smoke up the nose by means of a pipe; and introducing "a few Grains of Musk, or Civet" into the vagina (pp. 20-21). As we have indicated, some manner of these is found among Astruc's recommendations as well. Once the "Fit" is over, to prevent its return or to diminish its intensity, Tissot prescribes:

> A bleeding in the Foot, to be followed in a Day or two by a Vomit of Hypecacoana [...]; twenty-four Ounces of simple Pepper-mint-water, of Valerian in Powder two Ounces, and of Lavender-drops one Ounce [...] perfectly well mixed together [...] [as well as] waters impregnated with Iron [...] (pp. 21-22).

Unlike Astruc, Tissot allots minimal space to recipes and recommends exercise to those disposed to this affliction. The latter is in keeping with his ideas on the necessity of a healthy lifestyle. He tells women to walk and go horseback riding. He considers mood a factor as well. Patients are to "seek all Occasions of Mirth, avoid dull Company, too serious Conversation, melancholy Stories" (p. 22). Most importantly, he advises patients to take advantage of the "powerful Remedy," the "Matrimonial State" (p. 22). Once again, sexual intimacy figures mightily in the cure of the disorder. Pharmacopeia and partnerships aside, his advice on exercise and positive emotional states is much in keeping with contemporary thought on optimum maintenance of physical and mental health.

British physicians claim authorship of the three remaining self-help manuals. Apparently, they did not enjoy the same celebrity or reputation as did their French-speaking colleagues Astruc and Tissot. One of them may have even been a pseudonymous copyist. Nonetheless, it is worth examining the advice that they gave to women about disorders particular to their gender. Their recommendations may have evidenced similarity to those found in the French manuals, which seemed to have had a considerable European audience. The British manuals appeared a little later, over the closing decades of the century.

The first of these works, *The Female Physician: or, Every Woman her Own Doctress* (1770), is by the physician John Ball (1704?-1779). Apart from this self-help work on women's disorders, Ball wrote on fevers as well as on various other diseases and their treatments and prepared compilations of medicines.[58] He was obviously a physician of varied interests and specialties. The titles of his publications, like that of Tissot's *The Lady's Physician*, were detailed descriptions of the contents. *The Female Physician* is no exception. In the preface of this practical, short work, he makes it plain that in most instances "every woman of common abilities" would be able to heal herself with the assistance of this book alone.[59] Despite its brevity, the work contains an index of medicines. The vapors must be of some import, because it is the subject of the first chapter entitled: "Of the Nervous, or Hysteric Disease." A predictable discussion of the disorder ensues. Ball states that the "hysteric disease" is "common to maids, wives, and widows," and although not dangerous, can be terrifying (p. 1). He continues with a long paragraph of the symptoms, which are both emotional and physical. For example, the patient may experience "a lowness of spirits," "a pain in the back," "the utmost disturbance and dejection of mind," "violent laughter and profuse weeping [that] succeed each other by turns, without any apparent or real cause for either," and "distensions of the belly" (pp. 1-2). Again, advice for healing is offered when the patient is in the fit and out of it. Most of these suggestions ring familiar. When in the fit, a strong substance, like "common snuff," "should be held to the nostrils in order to rouze her"; bleeding will be necessary, but only if the patient has a strong constitution; and the "thighs and legs ought to be well rubbed" (pp. 2-3). When the patient is recovered from the fit and to prevent its return, Ball prescribes "a gentle vomit" followed by "a gentle stomach purge" induced by specific concoctions (pp. 3-4). After these procedures, recipes are given for remedies to "not only strengthen the stomach and bowels but likewise the whole body" (pp. 4-8). Deviating from purely medicinal cures, Ball suggests "cold bathing" to strengthen "the nervous system or state of nerves in general." Since a cold bath "tends to make people thinner," he proposes that "those who are too plump may use it daily" (p. 9). Additional recipes are noted for "nervous complaints" (pp. 9-12). Before closing the chapter, Ball, like Tissot, offers recommendations for a healthy lifestyle, which are intended to complement the remedies he has previously specified. This would include "good air, proper aliment, moderate exercise, and agreeable amusements." He expands briefly upon each, noting, for instance, that the best time to drink a bit of wine is on an empty stomach, that horseback riding is the best exercise, that "early rising, like gentle exercise, or cool air, will brace and invigorate the body," and that "the mind ought to be [...] kept as easy and chearful [*sic*] as possible, since nothing hurts more the nervous system [...] than fear, grief, or anxiety" (pp. 12-15). This last recommendation is a significant reference to the effect of negative emotions on physical health. In the final paragraph, he observes that in addition to all of the above suggestions for the cure of "nervous or hysteric diseases," opiates, particularly taken at bedtime, can be more effective than "the whole class of nervous medicines" for "composing the mind and procuring sleep." He and Tissot conclude with the same patriarchal advice of the age, "that a *woman's best remedy is to marry, and bear children*" (p. 15).

The next physician under discussion, A. Hume, presents a problem. His self-help manual entitled *Every Woman her Own Physician; or,The Lady's Medical Assistant* (1776) appears to have been largely plagiarized from Ball's *The Female Physician* (1770).[60] Unlike the other authors, there seems to be no information available about him, not even a date of birth or death. He qualifies himself as an M.D., whether or not the title is valid. Close comparison of both manuals reveals numerous similarities in the form of paraphrasing, which borders on and sometimes crosses over into plagiarism. Extensive passages are reproduced without attribution. For example, there is an identical passage that warns against a cold bath under certain conditions:

> When the stomach, liver, or other bowels are much obstructed, or otherwise very unsound, the cold bath is improper, since by turning the blood with more force than usual upon these arts, it may increase, instead of lessening the patient's complaints. (Ball, p. 9; Hume, p. 55)

Hume removed Ball's index on medicines but added an extensive section on the diseases of children, which may have been plagiarized as well. Ball's self-help manual must have enjoyed such public success that it was reconfigured and redistributed under another name and publisher even before the demise of the original author.

The final work in this discussion is by British physician John Leake (1729-1792). In the introduction of the first volume of his *Practical Observations Towards the Prevention and Cure of Chronic Diseases Peculiar to Women* (1792), Leake states the intent of the work, which is simply to "afford women more competent ideas of their own disorders, as well as the most gentle and effectual methods of treating them." He feels, though, that it is "ludicrous" to assume that every woman should be her own physician all of the time.[61] Leake also reveals something of his professional experience and his particular interest in the "nature and treatment of *Female Diseases*." He notes that he practiced midwifery for eighteen years but prefers assisting a greater number of sick women as "Physician to the Westminster Lying-In Hospital."[62] He published course lectures on the practice of midwifery in 1775.[63] From the lengthy explanatory titles alone, Leake could almost be described as an eighteenth-century precursor of the modern-day obstetrician-gynecologist. This self-help manual is distinct from the previous four. It is more verbose in that Leake explains in greater detail the nature of each disease and its physiological basis, interspersing literary quotations that correspond to the respective commentary. For a work intended for women of that age, it had an unusual intellectual approach. It is more than a manual of receipts and remedies with limited, dry remarks. Since it appeared at the end of the Enlightenment, *Practical Observations* serves as a compendium of the thoughts and ideas expressed over the entire century. Leake writes whole chapters on subjects that merit only some or no mention in the other books. In Section IV, he treats the "influence of the passions on the body and mind" as well as the "effects of climates on delicate constitutions." Leake devotes the last chapter to the "salutary power of *air*, *diet*, *exercise*, and *simple medicines*."[64] In the introduction, he does not hesitate to criticize the earlier works of the well-respected physicians Tissot and Buchan, who did not treat women's diseases as thoroughly as he does in *Practical Observations*. He says:

> Little having been said of *Female Diseases* in a practical and intelligible manner, I thought the present undertaking more necessary; for although *Tissot* in his Advice to the People, and *Buchan* in his Domestic Medicine, have written excellently and judiciously on diseases in general; they have, in a great measure, omitted those peculiar to women, except such as arise from obstructed menses, pregnancy, and child-birth (pp. 15-16).

Leake approaches the subject of nervous disorders differently as well. His discussion is found in Section X, entitled "Of Nervous Disorders, Hysteric Affections, Low Spirits, and Melancholy; their Treatment and Cure" (pp. 224-282). Given his academic penchant for explanation, allusion, example, and digression, this chapter, like all of the others in the work, resembles a course lecture. As a physician of the Enlightenment he speaks of "Sensibility," which is necessary in order to understand the "true nature of *Nervous Disorders*, also to shew, what the nerves are, from whence they proceed, and what is their particular office in the animal system" (p. 234). He determines that women are more susceptible to nervous disorders than men due to their delicate constitutions and their more cloistered lifestyles, "which deprives them of the benefits of exercise and fresh air" (p. 247). For Leake, the principal remedies of nervous disorders include "moderate exercise, in dry, pure air [...] and also, the *cold bath*" because they strengthen the body, unlike "*bleeding*, *vomits*, *strong purgatives*, the immoderate use of tea, or a sedentary life in warm, moist air," which are all "highly pernicious" (pp. 247-248). Since mid-century, the cures for nervous disorders had become markedly less aggressive and more salutary. However, humoral medicine had not entirely disappeared. Leake notes that apart from "simple weakness," there are other, more violent causes of nervous disorders that are caused by "*diseased humours* in the blood" (p. 250). Leake does refute the traditional belief that hysteric passion originates in the womb and from there travels by "nervous sympathy" to cause morbidity in other parts of the body. In his experience, he has observed that "various impressions will occasion *hysterics*, independent of any affection of the womb itself" (p. 252). For instance, "anger or extreme jealousy" may have the same effect (p. 253). Although their symptoms are different, men and women suffer from the same nervous disease, which is known as "*hysteric passion*" in women and "*hypochondriac melancholy*" in men (p. 253). He agrees with the preceding physicians that the disease can be dangerous but rarely fatal. One of his most prescient observations deals with the reclassification of the vapors. He considers it, along with "*Low Spirits*" and "*Lunacy,*" as a form of "*Melancholy,*" an emotional and physical state that apparently attracted greater attention from the literati than the medical community (pp. 254, 260). This view of the vapors approximates the modern understanding of the condition as a form of depression, not hysteria. This insight alone sets Leake apart from the others.

A first-hand examination of eighteenth-century self-help manuals about women's disorders can be revelatory but not in an exclusively negative sense. Written primarily in the latter half of the eighteenth century, they reflect the good and bad about Enlightenment thought with regard to women and their place in society. They can be seen as a means of promoting women's place as dutiful wives and mothers whose sensitive temperaments supposedly denied them active participation in the masculine-controlled outside world, which was the design of nature, not man. Or, the manuals can be interpreted as a step forward, a written confirmation of women as individuals who were capable of taking care of their own bodies, even if men were telling them how to do it. The physicians writing this advice recognized that the women of their times had the intellectual ability to comprehend the nature of the feminine disorder and to execute its cure. Of course, many of their descriptions and remedies of the conditions seem unconscionable by modern standards. Looking at one particular disorder, the vapors—a mostly feminine nervous disorder that has been used interchangeably with such designations as hysteria and hysteric passion—the reader can see a progression in its etiology, pathology, and treatment. Tissot makes a breakthrough when he recommends the necessity of incorporating nature in practicing a healthy lifestyle. Drugs, medicines, bleeding, and purgatives alone are not the answer to curing nervous disorders. In the final decade, Leake identifies the vapors with melancholy and low spirits, thus anticipating modern psychology. In the last pages of his chapter on "Nervous Disorders, Hysteric Affections, Low Spirits, and Melancholy; their Treatment and Cure," he addresses the healing power of music and harmony with regard to the emotional and physical pain brought on by depressive states. He says that "no remedy can be more rationally applied to counteract their malignant power than that of *Music* which excites a *contrary sensation* of the pleasurable kind, and acts immediately upon the *same Organs*" (pp.

279-280). As a lover of poetry, he turns to some lines from Alexander Pope (1688-1744) to ensure his female readers of its curative powers:

> Music the fiercest grief can charm,
> And fate's severest rage disarm;
> Music can soften pain to ease,
> And make despair and madness please;
> Our joys below it can improve,
> And antedate the bliss above (p. 278).

This is another seminal moment, which broaches the modern notion of mental health affecting the overall well-being of women. Indeed, music therapy is now a recognized and respected healing science. In a very large sense, Doctor Astruc, and more especially Doctors Tissot, Ball, and Leake, began to anticipate modern treatments for a debilitating female disorder.

Notes

[1] James F. McMillan, *France and Women 1789-1914: Gender, Society and Politics* (London: Routledge, 2000), p. 8.
[2] McMillan, *France and Women,* pp. 8-9.
[3] Mary E. Fissell, "Introduction: Women, Health, and Healing in Early Modern Europe," *Bulletin of the History of Medicine*, 82.1 (2008): 1.
[4] See Laurence Brockliss and Colin Jones, *The Medical World of Early Modern France* (Oxford: Clarendon Press, 1997), p. 261; Matthew Ramsey, *Professional and Popular Medicine in France, 1770-1830* (Cambridge: Cambridge University Press, 1988), p. 132.
[5] Susan Broomhall, *Women's Medical Work in Early Modern France* (Manchester: Manchester University Press, 2004), p. 9.
[6] McMillan, *France and Women*, p. 8.
[7] All five texts are Gale Eighteenth Century Collections Online (ECCO) Print Editions of the same works that have been digitized and are part of the online archive.
[8] The American variation of "vapors" will be used except when quoting British authors and/or translators.
[9] William A. Jackson, "A Short Guide to Humoral Medicine," *TRENDS in Pharamacological Sciences*, 22.9 (2001): 487.
[10] The American variation of "humors" will be used.
[11] Brockliss and Jones, *Medical World*, pp. 112-113.
[12] See E.C. Spary, "Health and Medicine in the Enlightenment," *The Oxford Handbook of the History of Medicine*, Mark Jackson, ed. (Oxford: Oxford University Press, 2011), pp. 86-87.
[13] Brockliss and Jones, *Medical World*, p. 441.

[14] Elizabeth A. Williams, "Physicians, Vitalism, and Gender in the Salon," *Studies in Eighteenth-Century Culture* 29 (2000): 3.
[15] Williams, "Physicians," p. 3.
[16] Brockliss and Jones, *Medical World*, p. 110.
[17] Brockliss and Jones, *Medical World*, p. 110.
[18] Brockliss and Jones, *Medical World*, p. 110; Jackson, "Humoral Medicine," p. 487.
[19] See Harold J. Cook, "Medicine in Western Europe," *The Oxford Handbook of the History of Medicine*, Mark Jackson, ed. (Oxford: Oxford University Press, 2011), p. 198.
[20] Brockliss and Jones, *Medical World*, pp. 430-431.
[21] Williams, "Physicians," p. 6. The titles of these works are: *De morbis venereis libri sex* (Paris, 1736); *Traité des maladies des femmes*, 6 vols. (Paris, 1761-1765); and *L'art d'accoucher réduit à ses principes où l'on expose les pratiques les plus sûres & les plus usitées dans les différentes espèces d'accouchemens* (Paris, 1766). These primary sources are listed in the bibliography of Brockliss and Jones, *Medical World*, p. 837.
[22] Williams, "Physicians," p. 8.
[23] Spary, "Health and Medicine," pp. 87-88.
[24] See Christabel P. Braunrot and Kathleen Hardesty Doig, "The *Encyclopédie méthodique*: an introduction," *Studies on Voltaire and the Eighteenth Century* 327 (1995): 29-30; Brockliss and Jones, *Medical Word*, pp. 262-263; Olivier Lafont, *Des médicaments pour les pauvres: ouvrages charitables et santé publique aux XVIIe et XVIIIe siècles,* introd. (Paris: Pharmathèmes, 2010), pp.7-8; Ramsey, *Professional and Popular Medicine*, pp. 49, 50, 53; Spary, "Health and Medicine," pp. 83-86; and Elizabeth A. Williams, *The Physical and the Moral: Anthropology, Physiology, and Philosophical Medicine in France, 1750-1850* (Cambridge: Cambridge University Press, 1994), pp. 23-25.
[25] See Brockliss and Jones, *Medical World*, pp. 409-479; Spary, "Health and Medicine," pp. 92-93.
[26] Mary Lynn Stewart, *For Health and Beauty: Physical Culture for Frenchwomen, 1880s-1930s,* introd. (Baltimore, MD: Johns Hopkins University Press, 2001), p. 5.
[27] Stewart, *Health and Beauty*, p. 5.
[28] See McMillan, *France and Women*, p. 10; Catherine Bodard Silver, "Salon, Foyer, Bureau: Women and the Professions in France," *American Journal of Sociology* 78.4 (1973): 843-845; and Williams, *Physical and Moral*, pp. 54-55.
[29] Spary, "Health and Medicine," p. 86.
[30] Spary, "Health and Medicine," p. 86. William Buchan (1729-1805) and John Wesley (1703-1791).
[31] See n.21; François Lebrun, *Se soigner autrefois: médecins, saints et sorciers aux 17e et 18e siècles* (Paris: Temps Actuels, 1983), p. 138; Williams, *Physical and Moral*, pp. 54-55. Astruc's six volumes of *Traité des maladies des femmes* were published in 1761. Roussel's *Système physique et moral de la femme* came out in 1775.

---

[32] See Brockliss and Jones, *Medical World*, p. 268; Lafont, *Médicaments*, pp. 163-178. More than fifty editions of Fouquet were published between 1675 and 1765 under three titles: *Recueil des receptes*, *Remèdes charitables de Madame Fouquet*, and *Remèdes faciles et domestiques.*

[33] Fissell, "Women, Health, and Healing," pp. 6, 14.

[34] Elaine Leong, "Making Medicines in the Early Modern Household," *Bulletin of the History of Medicine* 82.1 (2008): 145-168.

[35] The sources used to research this section include: Sabine Arnaud, "Ruse and Reappropriation in the French Eighteenth Century: la philosophie des vapeurs by C.-J. de B. de Paumerelle," *French Studies: A Quarterly Review* 65.2 (2011): 174-187; Oswald Doughty, "The English Malady of the Eighteenth Century," *The Review of English Studies* 2.7 (1926): 257-269; Heather Meek, "Of Wandering Wombs and Wrongs of Women: Evolving Conceptions of Hysteria in the Age of Reason," *English Studies in Canada* 35.2-3 (2009): 105-128; Edward Hare, "The History of 'Nervous Disorders' from 1600 to 1840, and a Comparison with Modern Views," *British Journal of Psychiatry* 159 (1991): 37-35; Sean M. Quinlan, "Vaporous Women and the Moral Cure," *The Great Nation in Decline: Sex, Modernity and Health Crises in Revolutionary France c. 1750-1850* (Aldershot, UK: Ashgate, 2007), pp. 42-51; Anne. C. Vila, "Beyond Sympathy: Vapors, Melancholia, and the Pathologies of Sensibility in Tissot and Rousseau," *Yale French Studies* 92 (1997): 88-101; Elizabeth A. Williams, "Hysteria and the Court Physician in Enlightenment France," *Eighteenth-Century Studies* 35.2 (2002): 247-255.

[36] Lafont, *Médicaments*, p. 167.

[37] Doughty, "English Malady," pp. 257, 259.

[38] Doughty, "English Malady," p. 262.

[39] This poem can also be found with the title "A Receipt to Cure the Vapors." This particular copy was accessed with the title "Song.": Montagu, Lady Mary Wortley. *Prose and Poetry of Lady Mary Worley Montagu*, Electronic Text Center, Universtiy of Virginia, http://etext.lib.virginia.edu/toc/modeng/public/MonWork.html, p. 495. See Brockliss and Jones, *Medical World*, p. 470; Lady Mary Wortley Montagu, Poetry Foundation, http://www.poetryfoundation.org, accessed 24 May 2013; Lady Mary Wortley Montagu, *Essays and Poems and Simplicity, a Comedy,* Robert Halsband and Isobel Grundy, eds. (New York: Oxford University Press, 1993), p. 257.

[40] See Nicolas-Edme Restif de la Bretonne, *Les Nuits de Paris or The Nocturnal Spectator: A Selection,* Linda Asher and Ellen Fertig, trans. Jacques Barzun, introd. (New York: Random, 1964), p. 358. Restif also appears as Rétif.

[41] Hare, "History," p. 41.

[42] *Online Etymology Dictionary*, http://www.etymonline.com, accessed 25 May 2013.

[43] William Safire, "The Way We Live Now: On Language; The Vapors," *New York Times Magazine*, 24 March 2002. http://www.nytimes.com/2002/03/24/magazine/the-way-we-live-now-3-24-02-on-language-the-vapors.html, accessed 6 October 2013.

[44] See n.21 above and Brockliss and Jones, *Medical World*, pp. 446-448.

[45] See n.7 above. John Astruc, *A Treatise on the Diseases of Women; in which it is Attempted to Join a Just Theory to the Most Safe and Approved Practice. With a Chronological Catalogue of the Physicians, Who Have Written on these Diseases. Translated from the French Original; Written by Dr. J. Astruc Royal Professor of Physic at Paris, and Consulting Physician to the King of France,* vol. 2, chap. 13 (London: printed for J. Nourse, Bookseller in Ordinary to his Majesty, 1762), pp. 245-285.

[46] See n.21 above.

[47] Astruc, *Diseases of women*, pp. 270-271.

[48] Astruc, *Diseases of women*, p. 271.

[49] Craig Thornber, *Glossary of Medical Terms Used in the 18th and 19th Centuries. History of Medicine*, http://www.thornber.net/medicine/html/medgloss.html, accessed 30 March 2013.

[50] Astruc, *Diseases of women*, p. 272.

[51] Astruc, *Diseases of women*, p. 272.

[52] Astruc, *Diseases of women*, pp. 272-285.

[53] Brockliss and Jones, *Medical World*, p. 452.

[54] See Samuel Auguste André David Tissot, *Avis au peuple sur sa santé* (Lausanne: F. Grasset, 1761), pp. 364-384, 492.

[55] See Quinlan, *Nation in Decline*, p. 35. See also the entire section, "Self-Help for Sick Elites: the Example of Samuel Tissot," pp. 33-42. The French titles of these works are: *L'Onanisme* (1760); *De la santé des gens de lettres* (1768); *Essai sur les maladies des gens du monde* (1770); *Traité des nerfs et de leurs maladies* (1778).

[56] See n.7 above. The complete title is *The Lady's Physician. A Practical Treatise on the Various Disorders Incident to the Fair Sex. With Proper Directions for the Cure Thereof. The Whole Laid Down in so Plain a Manner, as to Enable every Reader not only to be a Competent Judge for Herself, but also to Direct Others with Propriety and Success. Written Originally in French, by M. Tissot, M.D. First Physician to the Queen of France, and Fellow of the Royal Society of London; Member of the Medico-Physical Society of Basil, and of the Œconomical Society of Berne, and Author of Advice to the People Concerning their Health. Translated by an Eminent Physician* (London: printed for J. Pridden, 1766).

[57] *The Lady's Physician*, "Sect. VI. Of the Vapours, or Hysteric Passion," pp. 19-22. Future references will be given in the text.

[58] See n.7 above. John Ball. *The Female Physician; or every Woman her Own Doctress. Wherein is Summarily Comprised, all that is Necessary to Be Known in the Cure of the Several Disorders to which the Fair Sex are Liable; Together with Prescriptions in English of the Respective Medicines Proper to Be Given in Each Case. Delivered in a Manner so Concise, Familiar, and Intelligible, that Every Woman of Common Capacity May Be Able, upon Most Occasions, to Relieve Herself, by the Method and Remedies Herein Contained.* [...]. *By John Ball, M.D.* [...] (London: printed for L. Davis, near Gray's-Inn-Gate, Holborn, 1770). Additional works by John Ball: *A Treatise of Fevers* [...]. *Together with the*

Method of Cure According to Modern Practice. By John Ball, Apothecary (London: printed by H. Cock, for J. Scott, at the Black Swan in Pater-Noster Row, 1758)*; Pharmacopoeia domestica nova* [...]. *Auctore Joanne Ball, M.D.* (Londini: venalis prostat apud A. Millar, 1760); *The modern practice of physic* [...]. *In two volumes.* [...]. *The Second Edition, with Large Additions, and Amendments. By John Ball, M.D.* (London: printed for A. Millar, in the Strand, 1762); *A New Compendious Dispensatory; or, a Select Dispensatory: or, a Select Body of the Most Useful, Accurate, and Elegant Medicines, Both Officinal and Extemporaneous, for the Several Disorders Incident to the Human Body* [...]. *A Work of general Utility, Designed and Properly Calculated as well for the Benefit of Private Families, as of Young Physicians, Surgeons, and Apothecaries. By John Ball, M.D.* [London: printed for T. Cadell (successor to Mr. Millar) in the Strand, 1769].

[59] Ball, *Female Physician*, pp. iii-iv. Future references will be given in the text.

[60] A. Hume, *Every Woman Her Own Physician; or the Lady's Medical Assistant. Containing the History and Cure of the Various Diseases Incident to Women and Children. The Whole Rendered Intelligible by Prescriptions in English of the Respective Medicines Proper to Be Given in Every Disease; and Delivered in Such a Plain and Familiar Manner, that Every Woman of Common Capacity May Safely Prescribe for Herself, Her Acquaintance, and Her Poor Neighbours. By A. Hume, M.D.* (London: Printed for Richardson and Urquhart, 1776).

[61] John Leake, *Practical Observations Towards the Prevention and Cure of Chronic Diseases Peculiar to Women: In which their Nature is Explained,and their Treatment Clearly Laid Down, Divested of the Terms of Art, for the Use of Those Affected with Such Diseases, as well as the Medical Reader to which are Added, Prescriptions, or Efficatious Forms of Medicine, in English, Adapted to the Several Diseases* ,vol. 1 of 2, 7th ed. (London: printed for Baldwin, Murray, and Egerton, 1792), pp. 9-10.

[62] Leake, *Practical Observations*, pp. 12-13.

[63] John Leake, *A Course of Lectures on the Theory and Practice of Midwifery: in which Every Thing Essential to the True Knowledge of that Art Will Be Fully Explained and Clearly Demonstrated.* [...]. *By John Leake, M.D. Member of the Royal College of Physicians, London, and Physician to the Westminster Lying-in Hospital, at His House in Craven Street, in the Strand* (London, 1775).

[64] Leake, *Practical Observations*, p. 12. Future references will be given in the text.

CONTRIBUTORS

Kathleen Hardesty Doig is Professor of French in the Department of Modern and Classical Languages at Georgia State University. She has published mainly on encyclopedism, including *The Encyclopédie méthodique: Expansion and Revision* (*SVEC* 2013). With the late Dorothy M. Medlin, she edited André Morellet's *Mémoires sur le XVIIIe siècle et sur la Révolution*. She is on the editorial board of *New Perspectives on the Eighteenth Century*.

Ivy Dyckman is an independent scholar. She has done research on the Marquis de Sade and plans to explore fairy-tale qualities and indications of mental illness in his writings. She contributes book reviews to *The French Review* and *New Perspectives on the Eighteenth Century*.

Patsy S. Fowler is Associate Professor of English and Chair of Women's and Gender Studies at Gonzaga University. Her research focuses primarily on women writers and representations of sexuality in eighteenth-century British literature. She has published and presented on the works of Eliza Haywood and early women playwrights, and she is the co-editor of *Launching Fanny Hill: Essays on the Novel and Its Influences* (AMS 2002). She is currently co-editing a special issue of the *Journal for Early Modern Cultural Studies* that focuses on the future of Haywood studies.

Elizabeth Kuipers is Associate Professor of English at Georgia Southwestern State University. Her areas of interest include American literature, Women's Studies, and novel studies. She serves on the Executive Board of the Southeastern American Society for Eighteenth-Century Studies as the organization's archivist and historian.

Valérie Lastinger is Professor of French at West Virginia University. After many years of teaching French language, culture, and literature, she is currently Associate Dean of Undergraduate Studies in the Eberly College of Arts and Sciences. Her research interests encompass multiple issues centered on women's lives in the eighteenth and nineteenth centuries: motherhood, breastfeeding, and, more recently, the role of women in the sciences and in agriculture.

Morag Martin is Associate Professor and Director of graduate studies in history at the College at Brockport, SUNY. She is the author of *Selling Beauty: Cosmetics, Commerce and French Society, 1750-1830* (Johns Hopkins University Press, 2009). Though she originally discovered the case of Augustine Debaralle in 1994, she has just recently been able to return to the topic of women's medical education and practices in the Napoleonic period. Her current research focuses on the institutional history of regional midwifery training in France. She is specifically interested in the relationships between obstetrical education for women and men and female religious orders who frequently ran the hospitals within which this education took place.

Mary McAlpin is Professor of French at the University of Tennessee, Knoxville. Her research interests include the history of medicine and gender studies, and she has published on Rousseau, Marie-Jeanne Roland, Choderlos de Laclos, and Diderot, among others. She is the author most recently of *Female Sexuality and Cultural Degradation in Enlightenment France: Medicine and Literature* (Burlington, VT: Ashgate Press, 2012).

Sean M. Quinlan is Associate Professor of History at the University of Idaho. His scholarly work has appeared in *History Workshop Journal, Social History, Textual Practice, Eighteenth-Century Fiction, Early Science & Medicine,* amongst others. His *The Great Nation in Decline: Sex, Modernity, and Health Crises in Revolutionary France, c. 1750–1850* was published in 2007, and he is completing a second book entitled *Morbid Undercurrents: Medicine, Culture, and Radicalism in Post-Revolutionary France, 1794–1848.*

Felicia Berger Sturzer was Professor of French and Head of the Department of Modern and Classical Languages and Literatures at the University of Tennessee at Chattanooga until her retirement in 2013. Her research focuses on women's literature, the epistolary novel, Enlightenment sociability, and cultural studies. She has published mainly on Marie Jeanne Riccoboni, Julie de Lespinasse, and Pierre Carlet de Marivaux. She is on the editorial boards of *New Perspectives on the Eighteenth Century* and *Women in French Studies.*

Marialana Wittman is a PhD candidate in the School of History at Queen Mary, University of London. Her doctoral research is an in-depth examination of the medical conceptualization of venereal disease in eighteenth-century France. With attention to gender and sexuality, her study highlights important elements in medical theory and practice that significantly shaped the vision of the disease as a sexual one.

INDEX

The index includes the major topics, authors and writings discussed in the essays. Titles of works are given under the author's name where it is known.